MEDICAL & DENTAL ASSOCIATES, P.C.

3rd Edition

Shirley Chapman

Delmar Publishers' Online Services
To access Delmar on the World Wide Web, point your browser to:
www.cengage.com/delmar
To access through Gopher: gopher://gopher.delmar.com
(Delmar Online is part of "cengage.com", an Internet site with information on
more than 30 publishers of the International Cengage Learning Publishing organization.)
For information on our products and services:
email: delmar.help@cengage.com
or call 800-347-7707

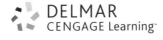

DELMAR
CENGAGE Learning™

Australia • Brazil • Japan • Korea • Mexico • Singapore • Spain • United Kingdom • United States

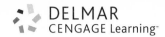

**MEDICAL & DENTAL ASSOCIATES, P.C.,
Third Edition**
Shirley Chapman

Publisher: Susan Simpfenderfer

Acquisitions Editor: Marlene McHugh Pratt

Developmental Editor: Marge Bruce

Project Editor: William Trudell

Art and Design Coordinator: Richard Killar

Production Coordinator: Cathleen Berry

Marketing Manager: Darry L. Caron

Editorial Assistant: Sarah Holle

Cover Design: Charles Cumming
    Advertising/Art, Inc.

For product information and technology assistance, contact us at
Cengage Learning Customer & Sales Support, 1-800-354-9706

For permission to use material from this text or product,
submit all requests online at **www.cengage.com/permissions**
Further permissions questions can be emailed to
permissionrequest@cengage.com

ISBN-13: 978-0-8273-7560-4

ISBN-10: 0-8273-7560-3

Delmar
Executive Woods
5 Maxwell Drive
Clifton Park, NY 12065
USA

Cengage Learning is a leading provider of customized learning solutions with office locations around the globe, including Singapore, the United Kingdom, Australia, Mexico, Brazil, and Japan. Locate your local office at **international.cengage.com/region**

Cengage Learning products are represented in Canada by Nelson Education, Ltd.

For your lifelong learning solutions, visit **delmar.cengage.com**

Visit our corporate website at **www.cengage.com**

Notice to the Reader

Publisher does not warrant or guarantee any of the products described herein or perform any independent analysis in connection with any of the product information contained herein. Publisher does not assume, and expressly disclaims, any obligation to obtain and include information other than that provided to it by the manufacturer. The reader is expressly warned to consider and adopt all safety precautions that might be indicated by the activities described herein and to avoid all potential hazards. By following the instructions contained herein, the reader willingly assumes all risks in connection with such instructions. The publisher makes no representations or warranties of any kind, including but not limited to, the warranties of fitness for particular purpose or merchantability, nor are any such representations implied with respect to the material set forth herein, and the publisher takes no responsibility with respect to such material. The publisher shall not be liable for any special, consequential, or exemplary damages resulting, in whole or part, from the readers' use of, or reliance upon, this material.

Printed in the United States of America
14 15 16 17 18 12 11 10 09

CONTENTS

How to Use This Book v

To the Instructor v

To the Student vii

**PART ONE
GATHERING PATIENT
INFORMATION** 1

Job Description 1

**Chapter One
Your Orientation Manual** 3

Welcome to Medical & Dental
    Associates, P.C. 6

Gathering New Patient Information 6

Gathering Patient Information from
    Other Sources................................. 20

Review Questions for Discussion 31

**Chapter Two
Introduction to Diagnostic Coding** 33

What Are ICD-9-CM Codes? 34

What Is the Diagnosis? 34

How to Use the ICD-9-CM Manual 35

Coding Neoplasms—Part I....................... 46

Coding Neoplasms—Part II 50

Review Questions for Discussion 52

**Chapter Three
E-Codes, V-Codes, Late Effect Codes,
and Hypertension Table**........................ 53

What Are E-Codes and How Are
    They Used? 54

How to Use the Table of Drugs and
    Chemicals..................................... 56

Late Effect Codes................................. 58

What Are V-Codes and How Are
    They Used? 60

Hypertension Coding 62

Review Questions for Discussion 64

**Chapter Four
CPT Codes**.. 65

What Are CPT Codes?............................ 66

How Are CPT Codes Used?...................... 66

How to Locate the Correct CPT Code 66

Review Questions for Discussion 78

**Chapter Five
HCPCS Codes** 79

HCPCS Code Levels.............................. 80

Applying HCPCS Codes 80

HCPCS Manual Format.......................... 81

Begin to Use HCPCS Manual 81

Case Study Abstracts 86

Review Questions for Discussion 87

**Chapter Six
CDT-2 Dental Codes** 89

American Dental Association Coding—
    CDT-2, Second Edition, 1995–2000 90

Dental Patient Information...................... 95

Review Questions for Discussion 98

**PART TWO
COMPLETING INSURANCE FORMS** 99

Job Description..................................... 99

**Chapter Seven
Completing the HCFA-1500**................... 101

Fee-for-Service or Indemnity Companies 102

Patient Not the Insured 109

Review Questions for Discussion 110

**Chapter Eight
Completing the HCFA-1500**................... 111

Spousal Coverage 112

The Birthday Rule 118

Coordination of Benefits 118

Divorced Parents 120

Review Questions for Discussion 121

PART THREE
COMPLETING INSURANCE FORMS 123

Job Description 123

Chapter Nine
Medicare Coverage 125

Introduction to Medicare Coverage 126

Medicare As the Only Coverage 126

Medicare As Secondary Coverage 129

Medicare Fee Calculations 130

Medicare-Medicaid 132

Review Questions for Discussion 132

Chapter Ten
Medicaid—Workers' Compensation 133

Medicaid 134

Workers' Compensation Insurance
    Coverage 136

Review Questions for Discussion 138

Chapter Eleven
CHAMPUS and CHAMPVA 139

CHAMPUS and CHAMPVA 140

Completing the HCFA-1500 for
    CHAMPUS or CHAMPVA 141

Review Questions for Discussion 142

Chapter Twelve
Other Insurance Coverage 143

Disability Insurance 144

Social Security Disability Insurance 144

Supplemental Security Income 144

Auto Liability Forms 144

Other Insurance 145

Review Questions for Discussion 146

Chapter Thirteen
Completing the ADA Form 147

Completing the ADA Form 148

Medicare Coverage 152

Review Questions for Discussion 154

Chapter Fourteen
Managed Care 155

Health Care Reform 156

Managed Care Examined 156

Impact on Insurance Billing Specialist 156

Computerization 157

Final Thoughts 158

PART FOUR
REFERENCES AND RESOURCES 159

Job Description 159

Chapter Fifteen
Resources 161

Information About Our Practice and
    Our Doctors 161

Master Fee Schedule 162

Place of Service Codes 162

Type of Service Codes—CHAMPUS 163

Glossary 165

Chapter Sixteen
Completed Patient Information Forms 175

PART FIVE
NUMBERED FORMS AND
WORKSHEETS 249

Job Description 249

Index 293

HOW TO USE THIS BOOK

TO THE INSTRUCTOR

This text/workbook is written for the newcomer to the field of Health Information Management. It is geared toward the student seeking to become an **insurance billing specialist.** This umbrella term is used to mean those support personnel responsible for completing and tracking health insurance claims, from the gathering of patient information needed to develop the form to the point of receiving payment and interpreting Explanations of Benefits (EOBs) from primary and secondary insurance carriers, as applicable. The text material is presented as an orientation manual and presupposes that the student is a new employee of the medical/dental organization. The orientation manual format is used throughout the text/workbook to explain concepts and reinforce the connection between the student and the work to be done. Every attempt is made to create the feel of an office environment including an informality not usually associated with a textbook. This enables students to take learning risks that may seem daunting without constant encouragement and reward for a good attempt.

After completing this course, the insurance billing specialist will be ready to find entry-level employment opportunities in many varied and interesting sites: physician and dental offices, medical clinics, immediate-care centers, outpatient hospital departments, and nursing homes are common examples.

In using the text/workbook to prepare for this new profession, no previous job experience in the medical field is required of the student. However, you will need other manuals including current issues of ICD-9-CM, CPT, HCPCS National Level II and CDT-2 references. A good medical dictionary is extremely important. Instruction in medical terminology and anatomy/physiology would be very useful and allow you to grasp the material more quickly.

ORGANIZATION OF TEXT/WORKBOOK

This text/workbook is divided into five parts.

Part I features a general introduction to the new workplace and describes the process of gathering patient information. It explains the four major coding systems used to complete medical and dental insurance forms, and lays the foundation of establishing simulated patient situations.

Part II describes how to complete these forms according to the general requirements of most private companies, federal insurers, and Workers' Compensation boards, using fictitious patient scenarios to lend reality to the assignments.

Part III includes a variety of patient cases that the student must complete and these are presented with gradually increasing levels of difficulty. As you begin to understand the challenge of completing the insurance form correctly for each patient case, subsequent cases will present new problems.

Part IV is a collection of resources for student use. Here, information about the doctors, the fee schedule, and other key data is presented, as well as the Glossary of terms used within the text.

Part V contains specific numbered forms and other materials needed to complete the assignments given in each chapter.

COURSE GOALS/OBJECTIVES

The goal of this text/workbook is to teach the student without previous exposure to the health care field to complete medical and dental insurance forms on an entry-level basis. Those who have been away from the field for a while or who have minimal experience will also benefit from the basics explored. The author also anticipates varied learning environments in which to use this text/workbook, ranging from minimal classroom instruction time to advanced courses of study.

Since the focus of this text is to learn how to complete medical and dental insurance forms for reimbursement, minimal textbook space is devoted to exploring in detail the four coding systems required to complete these tasks. No mention is made of DSM-IV codes (Diagnostic and Statistical Manual, Fourth Revision) since psychiatry/psychology billing is so specialized. I do believe the student who might choose to work in the field of mental health would have few problems in learning DSM-IV after finishing this text/workbook. If classroom time allows some attention to DSM-IV codes, of course this would be useful and I leave that to the good judgment of the instructor. In this text/workbook, basic instructions are included that are sufficient to allow the student to complete all the assignments.

The solutions to all exercises and completed forms for student comparison to their own work may be found in the *Teacher's Guide.* Also, additional tests and their answers are provided.

As one who has taught medical coding for years in the classroom and in seminars, I understand full well the complexity of teaching ICD-9-CM and other coding systems to students. This text is intended as the first formal classroom introduction to medical coding because you must address medical coding if you are to learn insurance form completion. However, the author does not assume that this text/workbook is sufficient all by itself as a manual for those seeking a career as a Medical Coding Specialist or beyond. In my own teaching experience, additional classes and many hours of study and practice are required with an extensive internship prior to graduation into the field. I have used exactly the format presented in this text/workbook to teach beginning students in Medical Assistant, Medical Coding Specialist, and Medical Records Technology programs leading to an associate's degree. Many Medical Assistant graduates have reported to me how frequently they have used the skills learned in this one basic insurance class to complete the forms required, upon occasion, at their jobs. Of course, the instructor may wish to supplement this text/workbook with other, more complex materials as the student population demands, or may select to bypass sections deemed unnecessary within that classroom.

Note that the instructional viewpoint applies to the medical office not yet computerized. This author deliberately chose to present a manual office system for four main reasons:

- A significant number of health care environments within the heartland are still using a manual system even as we near the next millennium.

- After the student understands the manual system, the student will better understand the theories and assumptions present within a computerized system.

- Not all teaching facilities can provide computer exposure within this context.

- The student must understand the basics before advancing to the computer just as the elementary student must know how to use pencil and paper to add and subtract before moving to a calculator.

Chapter 14 presents a brief discussion of some of the adaptations that must be made to the computerized office and by that point in study, the student will be prepared to make the adjustment. In this way, the student will be ready to work in either environment.

Each chapter begins with the learning objectives stated and a list of "Power Words" defined and presented in alphabetical order. These terms are introduced for the first time within the chapter and are reprinted in the Glossary with a numerical reference to the chapter in which they first appeared. These are not medical terms per se, but are terms used within the Health Information Management industry. Building your vocabulary and understanding the jargon of this specialty certainly will empower you in entering your new profession. Each word, each term, each specific piece of information is as much a building tool for your new career as nails and hammers are tools for the carpenter! Students should be encouraged to seek out definitions of all medical terms presented and the instructor may wish to use the test instrument available in the *Teacher's Guide* to match those terms with their common definitions.

TO THE STUDENT

To begin using this text/workbook, the student is asked to pretend to be a new employee at the offices of Medical & Dental Associates, P.C. You have been hired to complete insurance forms for reimbursement. This text/workbook serves as your orientation manual to your new position as **insurance billing specialist**. Different offices have a variety of job titles for those doing this work, and the job title is not as important as the work to be learned. By following each step and each assignment in the text/workbook, you will come to understand the scope and demands of your new career and the techniques to master it.

This text/workbook assumes that the office where you are working is not computerized but is moving in that direction. This is called a "manual" system because the work of gathering data is done by hand rather than produced by a computer. This viewpoint is presented to you for three important reasons:

- You must understand the work involved in getting all the information together and completing forms for reimbursement in those "real-life" offices actually working with a manual system.

- Once you understand the process of gathering data, it is fairly simple to adapt this information to the computerized environment and we address these adaptations in Chapter 14.

- You will have the advantage of understanding the basics of manual systems while preparing to adapt this knowledge to a computerized office.

In learning to become an entry-level **insurance billing specialist**, the most important quality to have is patience with yourself while you are taking the time to learn. You will not be expected to become a master of *any* of the material you will be spending classroom hours to learn. You *are* expected to learn the steps presented to you in this text/workbook and follow through to the finish. Remember, this is only your first introduction to this world of Health Information Management. You will be learning how to manage the wealth of patient information that comes to you in the doctor's office. It takes much time and practice to become an expert in this field, but *no one* was born knowing how to code and complete insurance forms! All of us went through some type of training and learning process just as you are preparing to do. If you stay with the steps, attend class and *try,* you will be on your way to an exciting new career!

Good luck to you—let's get started.

Reviewers for
Chapman: Medical & Dental Associates, P.C., 3E

Marion Gresko
Niles, OH
E.T.I. Technical College

Joanne McNamara
Tyngsboro, MA
Lare Training Center

Brenda Potter
Fargo, ND
Moorehead State Technical College

Ramona Riley
Penryn, CA
Western Business College

Mary Beth Robbins
Homewood, AL
Herzing College

Diane Stewart
Statesboro, GA
Ogeechee Technical Institute

David Wiggins
Oklahoma City, OK
Wright Business School

To the Student

Part One

GATHERING PATIENT INFORMATION

JOB DESCRIPTION

TITLE: Insurance Billing Specialist

IMMEDIATE SUPERVISOR: Office Manager

JOB DUTIES: **Part I. To gather sufficient patient information to complete and file health insurance claims for reimbursement for services rendered by the physicians and dentists of this office. Actual patient records will be examined.**

Part II. To complete the insurance forms correctly in accordance with the general requirements of most fee-for-service third-party payers. Patient records of this office will be accessed for clarification.

Part III. To adapt the insurance form completion process, as determined by specific patient records, to the general requirements of the major insurers, such as Medicare, Medicaid, Workers' Compensation, CHAMPUS, and certain other managed care insurance plans.

Part IV. To provide the references and resources necessary to complete the insurance billing process.

Part V. To furnish the forms and worksheets needed to complete all required tasks.

Chapter One

YOUR ORIENTATION MANUAL

OBJECTIVES   After completing your study of this chapter, you will be able to

- explain how to gather patient information to complete insurance forms for reimbursement after office visits have been made or other services rendered
- understand the importance of patient confidentiality
- identify other job titles and define their roles
- explain the steps necessary to gather information about new patients seen at the hospital by our physicians

POWER WORDS

admitting privileges   Rights extended to licensed physicians by hospital administrators so that patients may be assigned to beds within specific areas of the hospital. Hospitals are reimbursed for housing patients and physicians are responsible to oversee patient care and treatment while staying in the hospital.

appeal letter   Formal request to insurers to reconsider their decision to deny a specific claim submitted by our office for payment.

benefits   The dollar amounts paid by the insurer for health care.

chart   Refers to the folder kept in the medical office or the separate one kept in the hospital medical records department containing all medical information about the patient and treatments rendered.

consultation   1) A physician's request that one of his or her patients be seen by one of our associates. A written report is sent to the referring doctor after an examination has been completed; 2) A request from a patient for an examination and second opinion in a situation where another doctor has rendered an opinion about the patient's condition; a "confirmatory" consultation.

co-payment   The part of the fee the patient is responsible to pay, not covered by payment of insurance benefits. Often, a dollar amount or percentage due is stated on the insurance identification card as the co-payment figure.

established patient	One who has been treated within the past three years by an associate in our office.
endodontics	The subspecialty within dentistry concerned with treatment of diseases of the tooth root and surrounding tissues including root canal therapy.
Explanation of Benefits (EOB)	Information accompanying an insurance payment explaining payment (or lack of payment); any deduction or adjustment for services rendered on a specific claim form.
family practice/ practitioner	Medical specialty that includes several branches of medicine; is usually a primary care physician (PCP) in managed care contracts; trained to provide total health care to patients of all ages.
gatekeeper	Under managed care contracts, the primary care physician (PCP) overseeing the general health care and treatment plan of the enrolled patient and covered family members; the PCP determines if or when specialists should be consulted or if the patient should be hospitalized.
general surgeon	Physician trained to provide treatment of disease by manipulation and operative methods.
gynecology	The branch of medicine concerned with female health care, including diseases connected with sexual function and the reproductive organs. This specialty is often practiced with obstetrics.
health insurance	A plan or policy outlining benefits and limitations of coverage for issuing payments to health care providers in exchange for appropriate services rendered to policyholders.
insurer	The insurance company or other third party providing health insurance coverage for the patient.
internal medicine	The branch of medicine concerned with the study of the internal organs, and with the medical diagnosis and treatment of disorders of these organs.
ledger card	A record of the fees, payments, and adjustments for each patient.
managed care	A system of providing health care insurance coverage that stresses cost control and disease prevention. Patients are assigned to case managers employed by the insured who are responsible for review of the doctors' treatment plans and patient discharge plans.
Medicaid	A state-administered, state and federally funded health insurance program for very poor and welfare recipients; based on income levels and family size.
Medical Records Department	The part of the hospital containing the charts and other information about current or recently discharged patients. In some hospitals, transcribers, medical coders, and others work here.
multispecialty	The term for an office of several doctors with more than one branch of medicine represented. In our office, we have two dentists, one internist/general surgeon, one obstetrician/gynecologist, one pediatrician, and one family practitioner.

new patient	One who has never been treated by an associate in our practice, or who has not been seen in three years or more.
obstetrics	The branch of medicine concerned with pregnancy and childbirth, including care both before and after the birth of the child.
office fee schedule	A list of fees charged to all patients based on the type of service rendered.
office manager	The staff member hired to supervise the daily work produced by all office personnel. This position may include hiring and firing employees along with other responsibilities.
Operative Report	A part of the patient chart that describes a surgical procedure provided by one of our physicians, including the preoperative and postoperative diagnoses.
oral surgeon	A specialist in surgical procedures within the oral cavity including removal of teeth.
pediatrician	Physician specializing in the treatment of children ranging from birth to adolescence.
post	In bookkeeping, this term means to record data to the patient financial record or account.
postpartum	The period of time from giving birth until about six weeks later.
primary insurance	The insurer to which a medical or dental claim is first sent for payment.
primary care physician (PCP)	In managed care contracts, the PCP is the physician who evaluates and manages the patient and establishes a treatment plan; the PCP also determines when the patient is referred to another physician and/or admitted to the hospital and is often called the "gatekeeper."
professional corporation (P.C.)	A legal term describing an organization of professionals who have chosen to work together in the same office space and share overhead expenses and, possibly, income.
receptionist	Staff person responsible for greeting the patients, gathering current patient information, booking appointments, preparing routing forms, collecting payments, and more, depending upon the size of the office.
reimbursement	In the medical office, this term most often means receiving payment from the insurance company or other third-party payer.
secondary insurance	Coverage of another insurance policy effective only after payment has been received from the primary insured and only if benefits are available to cover the services rendered.
subscriber	The insurance industry term for the person in whose name an insurance policy has been issued.
third-party payer	The insurance company, government, or others providing insurance coverage.
Workers' Compensation	Insurance coverage provided by an employer in case of employee injury on the job.

WELCOME TO MEDICAL & DENTAL ASSOCIATES, P.C.

YOUR ORIENTATION MANUAL

Welcome to the offices and staff of Medical & Dental Associates, P.C. We are pleased to have you with us in the capacity of **insurance billing specialist**. As you know, this position is extremely important to our office and to the community we serve here in Indianapolis, Indiana. We are providing you with this training manual to ensure that all tasks related to this position are performed correctly.

To begin, let us explain who we are. The four physicians and two dentists of our professional corporation (thus the "P.C." in our title) joined together to form a multispecialty group over ten years ago. Figure 1-1 is a recent photograph of our doctors.

Our suite of offices is located in the medical facility attached to Good Samaritan Hospital where our doctors have admitting privileges. All six associates are licensed to practice medicine in the state of Indiana.

Our doctors provide health care to patients from all parts of the city and surrounding counties. Some of the patients coming into our offices do not have health insurance coverage of any kind, some have exhausted their benefits, and some choose to pay for services themselves without using their health insurance coverage. Another staff member monitors these patient accounts and sets affordable payment schedules for them.

Your primary responsibilities as **insurance billing specialist** are to:

1. file health insurance claims for those patients with insurance coverage

2. file claims with any secondary or additional insurance companies with periodic tracking of any slow claims

3. monitor the Explanation of Benefits or EOBs that accompany the insurance checks received in our office to ensure the claims we submitted were correctly processed by the insurers receiving our claims

4. be responsible for submitting appeal letters to the insurers for claims denied payment

5. provide additional information as requested by the insurance companies

Before you can perform these tasks, you must first learn how to gather billing information for the patient with medical or dental insurance coverage.

GATHERING NEW PATIENT INFORMATION

When a new patient comes to the office, specific information must be obtained by asking the patient to complete a two-page Confidential Patient Information Record (CPIR) as in Figure 1-2A and 1-2B.

Some of the questions asked relate to the patient's medical history and the reasons for the visit to our facility, and some are needed specifically by the **insurance billing specialist**. Normally, the receptionist is responsible for assisting the new patient in completing the CPIR as in the case of patient Rose Altobelli. Look for her legal name and address, date of birth, sex, marital status, and social security number on Figures 1-3A and 1-3B. You must know if she is employed and the name and address of her employer. This patient is a single female who is self-employed. The name of her insurance company is General Insurance Company and the address and insurance identification (ID) number are all listed on the Confidential Patient Information Record. Ms. Altobelli is the subscriber.

When the insurance policy is issued, the subscriber's name will be clearly shown on the ID card. Another name for the subscriber is the "insured" but both terms mean the same thing—the policyholder in whose name the insurance policy was issued and the person identified on the ID card. Ms. Altobelli has no additional health insurance coverage from any other source, according to the confidential information she provided.

Medical & Dental Associates, P.C.

James P. Cartman, M.D.
Family Practitioner

Jane R. Portia, M.D.
Obstetrician/Gynecologist

Harold S. Beckermann, M.D.
Pediatrician

Linda R. Gregory, M.D.
Internist/General Surgeon

Michael P. Lane, D.D.S.
Dentist/Oral Surgeon

Patrick M. Zunkel, D.D.S.
Dentist/Endodontist

FIGURE 1–1 The physicians of Medical & Dental Associates, P.C.

Medical & Dental Associates, P.C.

3733 Professional Drive #300   317/123-4567
Indianapolis, IN 46260   Tax ID# 99-9999999

CONFIDENTIAL PATIENT INFORMATION RECORD

(please print)

Patient Name

Address

Telephone

Birthdate

Sex   Marital Status

Social Security No.

Responsible Party (if other than patient)

Relationship to patient

Address

Patient Employer

Address

Telephone

Occupation

Primary insured date of birth

Secondary insured date of birth

Third insured date of birth

Fourth insured date of birth

(Please use the back of the form to write information about the

third and fourth insured parties, if applicable.)

INSURANCE INFORMATION

Primary insured

Subscriber

Address

Telephone

Employer

Address

Job/Union No.

Subscriber's SS#

Relationship to patient

Insurance

Address

Policy No.

Subscriber ID No.

Group Name/No.

Effective date

Expiration date

Secondary insured

Subscriber

Address

Telephone

Employer

Address

Job/Union No.

Subscriber's SS#

Relationship to patient

Insurance

Address

Policy No.

Subscriber ID No.

Group Name/No.

Effective date

Expiration date

FIGURE 1–2A Page 1, Confidential Patient Information Record (CPIR)

Gathering New Patient Information

Medical & Dental Associates, P.C.

3733 Professional Drive #300
Indianapolis, IN 46260

317/123-4567
Tax ID# 99-9999999

MEDICAL HISTORY

Patient Name	Today's Date

Are you currently in good health?

Are you under a physician's regular care at this time?	If so, state reason(s) for regular treatment:

Are you currently taking prescribed medication?	If so, state brand name and dosage schedule:

Circle the names of the following diseases for which you have been treated:

Alcoholism	Allergies	Amenorrhea	Anemia	Arthritis
Asthma	Cancer	Colitis	Depression	Diabetes
Gingivitis	Heart Disease	Hemorrhoids	Hepatitis	Hernia
Hypertension	Hypoglycemia	Kidney Disease	Lumbago	Migraine
Mononucleosis	Periodontal Dis.	Rheumatic fever	Rubella	Other _____

Have you ever had prolonged bleeding? If yes, explain:

Have you ever had an unusual reaction to a drug, antibiotic or anesthetic, such as novocaine or penicillin?

If yes, explain:

Is there any other information we should know about you or your health?

Is there any other information we should know about previous treatments you have had?

Have you ever been exposed to the HIV/AIDS virus?

Purpose of the first visit

Family physician	Who referred you to this practice?

Authorization for Release of Medical Information to the Insurance Carrier and Assignment of Benefits to Medical & Dental Associates, P.C.

Commercial Insurance

I hereby authorize release of medical information necessary to file a claim with my insurance company and assign benefits otherwise payable to me to Medical & Dental Associates, P.C. I understand I am financially responsible for any balance due not covered by my insurance carrier or denied by my insurance carrier for lack of coverage. A copy of this signature is as valid as the original.

Signature of Patient or Legal Guardian _____

Medicare Insurance

Beneficiary _____ Medicare Number _____

I request that payment of authorized Medicare benefits be made either to me or on my behalf to Medical & Dental Associates, P.C. for any services furnished to me by that association. I authorize any holder of medical information about me to release to the Health Care Financing Administration and its agents any information needed to determine these benefits payable for related services.

Beneficiary Signature _____

Medicare Supplemental Insurance

Beneficiary _____ Medicare Number _____

Medigap ID Number _____

I request that payment of authorized Medigap benefits be made either to me or on my behalf to Medical & Dental Associates, P.C. for any services furnished to me by that physician. I authorize any holder of Medicare information about me to release to Medical & Dental Associates, P.C. any information needed to determine these benefits payable for related services.

Beneficiary Signature _____

FIGURE 1–2B Page 2, Confidential Patient Information Record (CPIR)

Medical & Dental Associates, P.C.

3733 Professional Drive #300　　317/123-4567
Indianapolis, IN 46260　　Tax ID# 99-9999999

CONFIDENTIAL PATIENT INFORMATION RECORD

(please print)

Patient Name　Rose Ann Altobelli

Address　4551 Hillside Dr.
　　　　Indpls, IN 46238

Telephone　(317) 555-3331

Birthdate　9/13/-- Age 32

Sex　F　　Marital Status　S

Social Security No.　613-07-1876

Responsible Party (if other than patient)

Relationship to patient

Address

Patient Employer　Altobelli Assoc.

Address　1200 Great Falls Rd.
　　　　Indpls, IN 46212

Telephone　(317) 555-3400

Occupation　Financial Consultant

Primary insured date of birth

Secondary insured date of birth

Third insured date of birth

Fourth insured date of birth

(Please use the back of the form to write information about the

third and fourth insured parties, if applicable.)

INSURANCE INFORMATION

Primary insured　Patient

Subscriber　Patient

Address　Same

Telephone

Employer

Address

Job/Union No.

Subscriber's SS#　613-07-1876

Relationship to patient

Insurance　General Insurance Co.

Address　1010 Southway Blvd.
　　　　Gary, IN 48431

Policy No.　—

Subscriber ID No.　613-07-1876

Group Name/No.　—

Effective date　4-14-95

Expiration date　—

Secondary insured

Subscriber

Address

Telephone

Employer

Address

Job/Union No.

Subscriber's SS#

Relationship to patient

Insurance

Address

Policy No.

Subscriber ID No.

Group Name/No.

Effective date

Expiration date

FIGURE 1–3A Page 1, Confidential Patient Information Record for Altobelli

Medical & Dental Associates, P.C.

3733 Professional Drive #300
Indianapolis, IN 46260

317/123-4567
Tax ID# 99-9999999

MEDICAL HISTORY

Patient Name *Rose Ann Altobelli*   Today's Date *9/1/--*

Are you currently in good health? *Relatively good health*

Are you under a physician's regular care at this time? *No*   If so, state reason(s) for regular treatment:

Are you currently taking prescribed medication?   If so, state brand name and dosage schedule:
No

Circle the names of the following diseases for which you have been treated:

Alcoholism	Allergies	Amenorrhea	Anemia	Arthritis
Asthma	Cancer	Colitis	Depression	Diabetes
Gingivitis	Heart Disease	Hemorrhoids	Hepatitis	Hernia
Hypertension	Hypoglycemia	Kidney Disease	Lumbago	(Migraine)
(Mononucleosis)	Periodontal Dis.	Rheumatic fever	(Rubella)	Other _____

Have you ever had prolonged bleeding? If yes, explain:
No

Have you ever had an unusual reaction to a drug, antibiotic or anesthetic, such as novocaine or penicillin?

If yes, explain: *No*

Is there any other information we should know about you or your health? *No, I'm new to the area and need a doctor*

Is there any other information we should know about previous treatments you have had?
No

Have you ever been exposed to the HIV/AIDS virus? *No*

Purpose of the first visit *Bothered by hemorrhoids and bowel problems*

Family physician —   Who referred you to this practice? —

Authorization for Release of Medical Information to the Insurance Carrier and Assignment of Benefits to Medical & Dental Associates, P.C.

Commercial Insurance

I hereby authorize release of medical information necessary to file a claim with my insurance company and assign benefits otherwise payable to me to Medical & Dental Associates, P.C. I understand I am financially responsible for any balance due not covered by my insurance carrier or denied by my insurance carrier for lack of coverage. A copy of this signature is as valid as the original.

Signature of Patient or Legal Guardian *Rose A. Altobelli*

Medicare Insurance

Beneficiary _____ Medicare Number _____

I request that payment of authorized Medicare benefits be made either to me or on my behalf to Medical & Dental Associates, P.C. for any services furnished to me by that association. I authorize any holder of medical information about me to release to the Health Care Financing Administration and its agents any information needed to determine these benefits payable for related services.

Beneficiary Signature _____

Medicare Supplemental Insurance

Beneficiary _____ Medicare Number _____

Medigap ID Number _____

I request that payment of authorized Medigap benefits be made either to me or on my behalf to Medical & Dental Associates, P.C. for any services furnished to me by that physician. I authorize any holder of Medicare information about me to release to Medical & Dental Associates, P.C. any information needed to determine these benefits payable for related services.

Beneficiary Signature _____

FIGURE 1–3B Page 2, Confidential Patient Information Record for Altobelli

PATIENT CONFIDENTIALITY

It is vitally important that you understand the significance of maintaining patient confidentiality at all times and in all aspects of your work. The information given in confidence by the patient is to remain in our office and not to be discussed with anyone outside the office unless the patient has given *written* permission to Medical & Dental Associates, P.C., to release information to another source. Breaking patient confidentiality by discussing any patient in this practice with any unauthorized party outside this office will be cause for *immediate dismissal*. If you have any doubts about any inquiry for information about one of our patients, check with the office manager for clarification.

Many inquiries about patients come over the telephone. **Insurance billing specialists** must be sure they are giving information to properly authorized callers. This means the chart must be pulled and written authorization to release information to the caller must be on file. Sometimes, unauthorized callers will try to gather information about a patient for fraudulent purposes or because of some legal contention or potential court appearance. If you are not sure you are talking to the person who has represented himself or herself as an authorized caller, get the telephone number of that caller and call him or her back. If the caller refuses to give you the number or hangs up, you will know the wrong party was calling. Another step is to ask the caller for a written request for specific information if the chart is not clear whether the person calling truly is authorized to receive the information. It is impossible to avoid giving information over the telephone, but it is crucial that only an authorized caller receive the information requested.

FAX MACHINES

Another potentially dangerous area concerns faxing patient information to an outside source. Faxing data to another office is a wonderful time-saver and often truly serves the needs of the patient or of the doctor. However, this is an area of potential abuse or error. Material can be faxed to the wrong location or passers by on the receiving end might see medical information never intended for them. We use a cover sheet that specifically states who is to receive the documents following, and we request the calling party stand at the fax machine to receive the information at the time we agree it will be sent. If the information is not received as expected, the recipient will then call us and we can track down the wrong number dialed and call to request that the erroneous information received be torn apart and the pieces returned to us, or we have sometimes gone to the site and personally picked up the wayward fax.

OTHER RELEASE OF INFORMATION

Certain highly sensitive personal or medical information about a patient should never be faxed without specific permission, or perhaps not faxed at all. This includes any AIDS testing or HIV results, references to abortion, a statement about pregnancy in an unmarried female, one's sexual orientation, or any discussion about the presence of a sexually transmitted disease. This is one issue that can never be taken lightly in any medical setting and our office remains unwavering in protecting the confidentiality of our patients at all times. Do not hesitate to err on the side of extreme caution regarding this issue.

Ms. Altobelli also was asked by the receptionist to complete and sign the Release of Information portion of Figure 1-3B. This signature must be on file for every patient in the practice and charts are routinely monitored and updated by the receptionist. By signing this section, Ms. Altobelli has authorized our office to release medical information to her insurance company relevant to her visit to the doctor today and in the future. She also signed the authorization for the insurance company to send any insurance payment directly to our office and promised to pay any portion of the bill not covered by insurance or denied by insurance. It is part of our routine gathering of patient information to have all our patients sign these documents, although in some cases (as with Medicaid and Workers' Compensation) such permission is not needed (see Chapter 10.) Therefore, you may safely file insurance claims without fear of releasing confidential information in error.

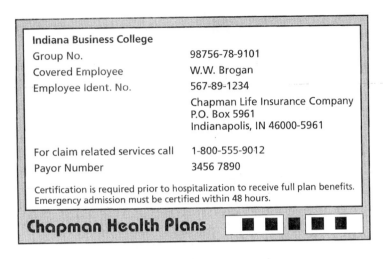

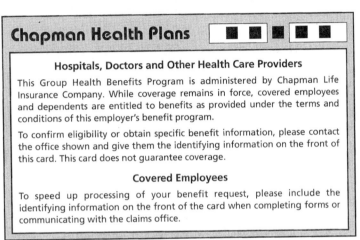

FIGURE 1–4 Front and back of a typical Insurance Identification Card

INSURANCE INFORMATION

The receptionist also makes a photocopy of the front and back of all health insurance identification cards to keep on file inside the chart, and may call the insurance company to verify coverage. This is shown on Figure 1-4.

The ID card usually shows the address where all claims should be sent for processing and other important information such as co-payment responsibilities. If authorization is required before treatment, surgeries, or hospitalization, a telephone number to call will be listed on the card. In our office, the receptionist makes any necessary preauthorization calls before the patient is seen by an associate and records that information in the patient's chart.

ROUTING SLIP

After answering any patient questions about the two completed forms, the receptionist will closely examine the forms and prepare a routing slip as shown in Figure 1-5.

The "routing slip" is a form used within our office to record each patient visit including the date, treating doctor, fees, diagnosis of the problem, any payments received, and the balance due. Other offices may use other terms such as "superbill" or "transmittal form" or "fee bill" to describe this form, but the purpose is the same: the document records the details of each patient visit. Our office is preparing to become fully computerized, but at this point, all our billing and record-keeping are done manually. This means all patient information is gathered and record-

Medical & Dental Associates, P.C.

3733 Professional Drive #300
Indianapolis, IN 46260

317/123-4567
Tax ID# 99-9999999

Patient name

CPT-4 CODES

OFFICE SERVICES

	CODE	FEE
New patient, problem focused	99201	_____
New patient, expanded problem focused	99202	_____
New patient, detailed	99203	_____
New patient, comprehensive, mod.	99204	_____
New patient, comprehensive, high	99205	_____
Established patient, RN	99211	_____
Established patient, problem focused	99212	_____
Established patient, expanded problem	99213	_____
Established patient, detailed	99214	_____
Established patient, comprehensive	99215	_____
Consultation		

LABORATORY

	CODE	FEE
X-ray, chest/ribs; single view, frontal	71010	_____
X-ray, chest/ribs; stereo, frontal	71015	_____
Therapeutic injections ( )	907__	_____
Drugs, trays, supplies	99070	_____
Educational supplies, books, tapes	99071	_____
Urinalysis, routine, dip stick	81000	_____
Urine pregnancy test, visual color	81025	_____
Blood count, hemoglobin	85018	_____
Pap smear	88150	_____

ICD-9-CM

DIAGNOSES

Anxiety reaction	300.00
Bleeding rectal	569.3
Benign prostatic hypertrophy	600
Bronchitis, acute	466.0
Bronchitis, chronic	491.9
Cardiac arrhythmia	427.9
Chest pain	786.50
Cirrhosis of liver	571.5
Conjunctivitis, acute	372.00
Depression	300.4
Flu	487.0
Fracture–nasal, closed	802.0
Fractured tibia	891.2
Headache, vascular	794.0
Herpes zoster	053.9
Irritable bowel syndrome	564.1
Menopause	627.2
Myocardial infarction, unspecified	410.90
Otitis, acute	381.01
Pharyngitis, acute	462
Pneumonia	486
Sinusitis, acute	461.9
Tendonitis	726.90
Tennis elbow	726.32
Pregnancy	V22.2
Sprained ankle	842.5
Tonsillitis	474.0
Vertigo	386.0
Well child	V20.2

CDT-2 CODES

DENTAL SERVICE

DIAGNOSTIC

	CODE	FEE
Periodic exam	00120	_____
Limited exam	00140	_____
Comprehensive exam	00150	_____
Extensive exam	00160	_____

PREVENTIVE

	CODE	FEE
Intraoral–FMX	00210	_____
Intraoral–PA	00220	_____
BW	0027_	_____
Single posteroanterior	00290	_____
Panoramic X-ray	00330	_____
Prophylaxis adult	01110	_____
Prophylaxis child	01120	_____
Topical fluoride	012__	_____

DENTAL SERVICE

RESTORATIVE

	CODE	FEE
Amalgams (decid) Tooth #_____	021__	_____
Amalgams (perm) Tooth #_____	021__	_____

CROWNS AND BRIDGES

	CODE	FEE
PFG crown	02750	_____
FG cast crown	02790	_____
3/4 gold cast crown	02810	_____
FC bridge pontic	06210	_____
Porcelain bridge ( )	062__	_____

OTHER PROCEDURES

DOCTOR'S STATEMENT: I certify that I personally provided the above services and that fees shown represent my usual fees

Signature _____ Date _____

TOTAL	$ _____
AMOUNT PAID	$ _____
BALANCE DUE	$ _____

FIGURE 1–5 Routing slip

ed by hand and no computers are used to store patient information.

Figure 1-6 summarizes the path taken by the routing slip from the time it is prepared by the receptionist until the patient returns it to the front office. In this office, the patients carry the completed routing slip from the treatment room to the billing receptionist who receives the form, totals the fees for the day, and marks the form for any payments collected. The receptionist will schedule another appointment if the doctor has instructed patients to return at a later date, and will give patients a copy of the routing slip for their records.

If Ms. Altobelli had needed special tests or needed to be scheduled for surgery or any other procedures undertaken outside this office, she would have been instructed by the doctor or the nurse in the treatment room and these instructions would have been noted on the routing slip.

Figure 1-7 shows the completed routing slip for Ms. Altobelli. The **insurance billing specialist** receives one copy of this form from each patient with health insurance coverage. This is your signal that an insurance claim must be filed. Later in the day, the charges and payments received from each patient will be posted onto a ledger card. Monthly, a copy of each ledger card is mailed to those patients responsible for making personal payments. Figure 1-8 shows Rose Altobelli's ledger card after this office visit was posted.

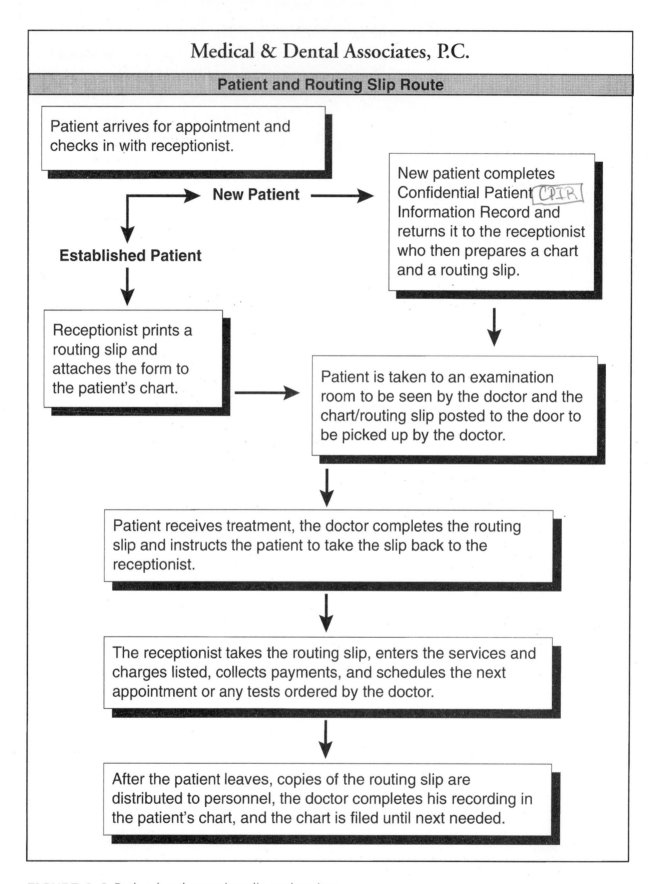

Medical & Dental Associates, P.C.

Patient and Routing Slip Route

Patient arrives for appointment and checks in with receptionist.

New Patient

Established Patient

New patient completes Confidential Patient [CPIR] Information Record and returns it to the receptionist who then prepares a chart and a routing slip.

Receptionist prints a routing slip and attaches the form to the patient's chart.

Patient is taken to an examination room to be seen by the doctor and the chart/routing slip posted to the door to be picked up by the doctor.

Patient receives treatment, the doctor completes the routing slip and instructs the patient to take the slip back to the receptionist.

The receptionist takes the routing slip, enters the services and charges listed, collects payments, and schedules the next appointment or any tests ordered by the doctor.

After the patient leaves, copies of the routing slip are distributed to personnel, the doctor completes his recording in the patient's chart, and the chart is filed until next needed.

FIGURE 1–6 Path taken by routing slip and patient

Medical & Dental Associates, P.C.

3733 Professional Drive #300
Indianapolis, IN 46260

317/123-4567
Tax ID# 99-9999999

Patient name *Rose Altobelli*

CPT-4 CODES

OFFICE SERVICES

	CODE	FEE
New patient, problem focused	99201	
New patient, expanded problem focused	99202	
New patient, detailed	(99203)	*60—*
New patient, comprehensive, mod.	99204	
New patient, comprehensive, high	99205	
Established patient, RN	99211	
Established patient, problem focused	99212	
Established patient, expanded problem	99213	
Established patient, detailed	99214	
Established patient, comprehensive	99215	
Consultation		

LABORATORY

	CODE	FEE
X-ray, chest/ribs; single view, frontal	71010	
X-ray, chest/ribs; stereo, frontal	71015	
Therapeutic injections ( )	907__	
Drugs, trays, supplies	99070	
Educational supplies, books, tapes	99071	
Urinalysis, routine, dip stick	81000	
Urine pregnancy test, visual color	81025	
Blood count, hemoglobin	85018	
Pap smear	88150	

ICD-9-CM

DIAGNOSES

Anxiety reaction	300.00
Bleeding rectal	569.3
Benign prostatic hypertrophy	600
Bronchitis, acute	466.0
Bronchitis, chronic	491.9
Cardiac arrhythmia	427.9
Chest pain	786.50
Cirrhosis of liver	571.5
Conjunctivitis, acute	372.00
Depression	300.4
Flu	487.0
Fracture–nasal, closed	802.0
Fractured tibia	891.2
Headache, vascular	794.0
Herpes zoster	053.9
Irritable bowel syndrome	(564.1)
Menopause	627.2
Myocardial infarction, unspecified	410.90
Otitis, acute	381.01
Pharyngitis, acute	462
Pneumonia	486
Sinusitis, acute	461.9
Tendonitis	726.90
Tennis elbow	726.32
Pregnancy	V22.2
Sprained ankle	842.5
Tonsillitis	474.0
Vertigo	386.0
Well child	V20.2

Bleeding hemorrhoids
455.8

CDT-2 CODES

DENTAL SERVICE

DIAGNOSTIC

	CODE	FEE
Periodic exam	00120	
Limited exam	00140	
Comprehensive exam	00150	
Extensive exam	00160	

PREVENTIVE

	CODE	FEE
Intraoral–FMX	00210	
Intraoral–PA	00220	
BW	0027_	
Single posteroanterior	00290	
Panoramic X-ray	00330	
Prophylaxis adult	01110	
Prophylaxis child	01120	
Topical fluoride	012__	

DENTAL SERVICE

RESTORATIVE

	CODE	FEE
Amalgams (decid) Tooth #_____	021__	
Amalgams (perm) Tooth #_____	021__	

CROWNS AND BRIDGES

	CODE	FEE
PFG crown	02750	
FG cast crown	02790	
3/4 gold cast crown	02810	
FC bridge pontic	06210	
Porcelain bridge ( )	062__	

OTHER PROCEDURES

DOCTOR'S STATEMENT: I certify that I personally provided the above services and that fees shown represent my usual fees

James P. Cartman, M.D.   *9/1/--*

Signature   Date

TOTAL	$	*60—*
AMOUNT PAID	$	*0*
BALANCE DUE	$	*60—*

FIGURE 1–7 Completed routing slip

Medical & Dental Associates, P.C.

3733 Professional Drive #300
Indianapolis, IN 46260
317/123-4567
Tax ID# 99-9999999

STATEMENT OF ACCOUNT

ALTOBELLI, Rose
4551 Hillside Drive
Indianapolis, IN 46238

19--

DATE	CODE	CHARGE	CREDITS PAYMENT	ADJ	CURRENT BALANCE
		BALANCE FORWARD ➡			
9/1	99203	60 00			60 00

PLEASE PAY LAST AMOUNT IN THIS COLUMN ↑

THIS IS A COPY OF YOUR ACCOUNT

FIGURE 1–8 Ledger card

EXERCISE 1

Directions: Fill in the following blanks. You may review the material within this chapter to assist you.

1. This Orientation Manual has been prepared for the new ___*patient*___

   of the office of ___*Medical & Dental, PC*___ .

2. The initials "P. C." in the name of the group stand for ___*Pro*___ .

3. There are _____ physicians and _____ dentists in our organization.

4. Ours is a "multispecialty" group and this means _____ .

5. Name the five main responsibilities of the **insurance billing specialist**:

   1. _____

   2. _____

   3. _____

   4. _____

   5. _____

6. The two-page form we use to gather information about a new patient is called the _____ .

7. All patients sign a form giving us permission to submit information to their insurance company and

   to have the insurance _____ sent directly to the doctors.

8. After patient information is gathered by the receptionist, we are able to prepare a _____

   which is attached to the patient's chart.

9. Three other names for this form are _____ , _____ ,

   and _____ .

10. After all charges and payments have been received, the receptionist prepares a _____

    showing all the dates, payments, or adjustments for services rendered.

GATHERING PATIENT INFORMATION FROM OTHER SOURCES

With patient Rose Altobelli, all the information needed to file a health insurance claim form was listed on the Confidential Patient Information Record and the routing slip. Sometimes, more information is needed than these two sources can provide. For example, patient John D. Steiner is an established patient of Dr. Linda Gregory.

Looking at the routing slip shown as Figure 1-9, we can see that Mr. Steiner received an expanded problem focused office call plus a rib belt, and an X-ray code is indicated on the form.

Unfortunately, certain key pieces of information that we will need to complete the insurance form are missing from the routing slip for this patient, including details about the diagnosis, treatment, and fees. This is not uncommon since the space available on the routing slip is limited. We now must retrieve the Steiner chart and look for greater detail.

At Medical & Dental Associates, P.C., our doctors complete a Medical Treatment Record during each patient encounter in the office and that slip is filed in the patient's chart. See Figure 1-10.

In other offices, this type of information may be dictated by the doctor and typed in the patient's chart, handwritten by the doctor onto plain paper and filed in the chart, or other commercial forms may be used as a guide to record treatment information. An accurate record of the patient encounter is extremely important to both doctor and patient. Treatment plans must be carefully undertaken and chart notes must document each step. Insurance companies and others to which the patients have given permission to examine treatment records have the right to visit the doctor and look into the charts to verify for themselves that appropriate treatment plans have taken place and are justified. If doctors do not record accurately the details of office visits and other patient interactions billed to the insurers, they risk sanctions and possible fines from the insurers and could be refused payment for specific treatments. In some cases, doctors have been dropped by insurers as recognized providers of patient care to their subscribers because of negligence in charting. The standard is, when submitting a claim to an insurance company, all information necessary to justify the treatment and subsequent charge to the patient must be present in the chart. Any changes or errors discovered in the chart must be documented and recorded as corrected. Nothing must be removed from the chart without describing each step and the rationale. Very specific steps must be taken to record accurately the chief complaints and physical examination findings leading to the diagnosis that appears on the insurance form. Doing otherwise is poor service to the patient and insufficient documentation of patient records.

In addition to the chart, we need a detailed copy of the fees charged to this patient. These can be retrieved from the ledger card. See Figure 1-11.

Once we have the Confidential Patient Information Record, the Medical Treatment Record, and the ledger card, we have a complete picture of the services rendered the patient, the fees charged for those services, and detailed descriptions of the problems that required these treatments as recorded by the treating doctor. We then have the information needed to complete a health insurance form.

GATHERING INFORMATION FROM HOSPITAL RECORDS

Our physicians and dentists also treat patients at Good Samaritan Hospital attached to our medical office complex. As the **insurance billing specialist**, you will need to gather information for billing insurance companies and others on behalf of those patients seen in the hospital in addition to those people seen in the office.

Our associates see patients at Good Samaritan under one of the following conditions:

- scheduled outpatient surgeries, treatments, or tests for our established patients

- scheduled inpatient surgeries, treatments, or tests for our established patients

- unscheduled outpatient or inpatient surgeries, treatments, or tests for established patients

- patients seen in consultation by one of our doctors

Medical & Dental Associates, P.C.

3733 Professional Drive #300
Indianapolis, IN 46260

317/123-4567
Tax ID# 99-9999999

Patient name *John Steiner*

CPT-4 CODES

OFFICE SERVICES	CODE	FEE
New patient, problem focused	99201	_____
New patient, expanded problem focused	99202	_____
New patient, detailed	99203	_____
New patient, comprehensive, mod.	99204	_____
New patient, comprehensive, high	99205	_____
Established patient, RN	99211	_____
Established patient, problem focused	99212	_____
Established patient, expanded problem	(99213)	*40—*
Established patient, detailed	99214	_____
Established patient, comprehensive	99215	_____
Consultation		_____

Rib Belt A4572

LABORATORY		
X-ray, chest/ribs; single view, frontal	71010	_____
X-ray, chest/ribs; stereo, frontal	71015	_____
Therapeutic injections ( )	907__	_____
Drugs, trays, supplies	99070	_____
Educational supplies, books, tapes	99071	_____
Urinalysis, routine, dip stick	81000	_____
Urine pregnancy test, visual color	81025	_____
Blood count, hemoglobin	85018	_____
Pap smear	88150	_____

71040

ICD-9-CM

DIAGNOSES	
Anxiety reaction	300.00
Bleeding rectal	569.3
Benign prostatic hypertrophy	600
Bronchitis, acute	466.0
Bronchitis, chronic	491.9
Cardiac arrhythmia	427.9
Chest pain	786.50
Cirrhosis of liver	571.5
Conjunctivitis, acute	372.00
Depression	300.4
Flu	487.0
Fracture–nasal, closed	802.0
Fractured tibia	891.2
Headache, vascular	794.0
Herpes zoster	053.9
Irritable bowel syndrome	564.1
Menopause	627.2
Myocardial infarction, unspecified	410.90
Otitis, acute	381.01
Pharyngitis, acute	462
Pneumonia	486
Sinusitis, acute	461.9
Tendonitis	726.90
Tennis elbow	726.32
Pregnancy	V22.2
Sprained ankle	842.5
Tonsillitis	474.0
Vertigo	386.0
Well child	V20.2

CDT-2 CODES

DENTAL SERVICE

DIAGNOSTIC	CODE	FEE
Periodic exam	00120	_____
Limited exam	00140	_____
Comprehensive exam	00150	_____
Extensive exam	00160	_____
PREVENTIVE		
Intraoral–FMX	00210	_____
Intraoral–PA	00220	_____
BW	0027_	_____
Single posteroanterior	00290	_____
Panoramic X-ray	00330	_____
Prophylaxis adult	01110	_____
Prophylaxis child	01120	_____
Topical fluoride	012__	_____

DENTAL SERVICE

RESTORATIVE	CODE	FEE
Amalgams (decid) Tooth #_____	021__	_____
Amalgams (perm) Tooth #_____	021__	_____
CROWNS AND BRIDGES		
PFG crown	02750	_____
FG cast crown	02790	_____
3/4 gold cast crown	02810	_____
FC bridge pontic	06210	_____
Porcelain bridge ( )	062__	_____
OTHER PROCEDURES		

Bill Ins!

DOCTOR'S STATEMENT: I certify that I personally provided the above services and that fees shown represent my usual fees

Dr. Linda Gregory   *9/28/--*
Signature   Date

TOTAL	$	_____
AMOUNT PAID	$	*0*
BALANCE DUE	$	_____

FIGURE 1–9 Routing slip

Medical & Dental Associates, P.C.

3733 Professional Drive #300
Indianapolis, IN 46260

317/123-4567
Tax ID# 99-9999999

MEDICAL TREATMENT RECORD

Patient *John Steiner*	Date *9/28/--*
Occupation *Ret.*	DOB Age *58*
Insurance Carrier *Bluestone Ins. Co.*	Social Security No.
Admitted Discharged	Consults
Hospital Other	Referred by: Dr.

CC: *Soreness in chest, rib cage, after falling from a tree*

Previous symptom: Yes / ⟨No⟩

First Symptom: *This AM*

Physical Examination *BP 150/90; P92 & reg; Temp. 37.2° C orally; Resp. 27, shallow*

General	
Appearance	*Pale*
HEENT	*Within normal limits*
Lungs	*Clear to P/A*
Cardiac	*NSR, no M*
ABD	*deferred*
Extremities	*Contusions rt. arm & leg*

Dx (Primary): *Closed fracture, 7th, 8th, 9th rt. ribs*

Dx (Secondary): *Contusions rt. forearm, leg*

Dx (Postoperative):

Procedures: *Exam and apply rib belt*

Complications: *None expected*

Dx testing (place of service): *X-rays rt. ribs, 2 views, AP&L, in office*

Plan: *Ret. 30 days on PRN*
OTC Pain
Meds PRN

Dr. Linda Gregory

Attending physician

FIGURE 1–10 Medical Treatment Record

Gathering Patient Information from Other Sources

Medical & Dental Associates, P.C.

3733 Professional Drive #300
Indianapolis, IN 46260
317/123-4567
Tax ID# 99-9999999

STATEMENT OF ACCOUNT

STEINER, John D.
1500 Crescent Ave.
Indianapolis, IN 46260

19--

DATE	CODE	CHARGE	CREDITS PAYMENT	ADJ	CURRENT BALANCE
		BALANCE FORWARD ⟶			0
9/28	99213	40 00			40 00
9/28	71040	68 00			108 00
9/28	A4572	40 00			148 00

PLEASE PAY LAST AMOUNT IN THIS COLUMN

THIS IS A COPY OF YOUR ACCOUNT

FIGURE 1–11 Ledger card

- emergency room encounters by our doctors resulting in outpatient or inpatient surgeries, treatments, or tests for new patients

For example, Dr. Portia routinely estimates the delivery date of her pregnant patients scheduled to deliver vaginally, but the exact date cannot be known until the mother begins to experience the pains of labor. That type of delivery and hospitalization would normally include one or two days additional overnight stay, and would be considered unscheduled inpatient surgery. However, if the patient needs a Caesarean-section (C-section) delivery, including four to five days postpartum inpatient hospital care, that date will be set ahead of time, qualifying as a scheduled inpatient surgery. Scheduled outpatient treatments or surgeries are planned for minimally invasive or treatments or tests, or for procedures not requiring an overnight stay and extended patient observation. Also, our physicians take turns serving on an office rotation schedule for emergency room calls or for after-hour care of patients. This means if an established patient in the practice has some type of mishap that requires a trip to the emergency room, our doctor on duty during that rotation will be called and will direct the treatment of the patient, including visiting the patient in the emergency room if necessary, or conferring with the emergency room physician to determine if hospitalization is required.

As part of their admission privileges to Good Samaritan Hospital, our doctors take turns being available (also referred to as "on-call") on a rotating basis for the treatment of new patients arriving in the emergency room who require the skills of our physicians' specialty. Therefore, it is clear that the **insurance billing specialist** must be prepared to gather billing or admission information taken at the hospital by hospital employees and treatment information dictated by our associates and sent to our office for inclusion in the patient's chart. This may include a telephone call to the Medical Records Department of the hospital or to the emergency room for help in getting the necessary billing information. It is not unusual to need to make these calls and hospital personnel are usually very cooperative in giving out the appropriate patient information over the telephone to our office so that you are not delayed in processing your claims.

Figure 1-12 is a copy of the Operative Report dictated by Dr. Portia describing an emergency procedure performed on a 28-year-old female who came to the emergency room at Good Samaritan Hospital at a time when Dr. Portia was on call. Carefully read the Operative Report but do not expect to understand all the medical terms used there. As you read it, highlight the words you will later look up in your medical dictionary. With time and practice, you will gradually become comfortable reading hospital reports.

Remember: no one is expecting you to understand all these terms and new words right away! You are in the process of learning a great deal about your new job as **insurance billing specialist**. You will have plenty of time to get used to the way the doctors dictate their hospital records. Notice the Operative Report provides a wealth of information including the diagnosis and procedure as well the general background surrounding the problem.

EMERGENCY ROOM PATIENT INFORMATION

Good Samaritan Hospital also sent Dr. Portia a copy of the Emergency Room Patient Information taken from Ms. Ferraro when she presented herself to the hospital emergency room. See Figure 1-13.

With this information, our receptionist is able to create a patient chart and a ledger card. After Dr. Portia has confirmed the treatment and fees, you will be able to prepare an insurance form for the services rendered to this patient even though she was not seen in the office and does not have a Confidential Patient Information Record on file.

Another way of gathering patient information for insurance form filing includes the patient chart and ledger card information only.

For example, patient Donald Ebner was seen in the office and underwent a minor procedure, then was admitted to Good Samaritan Hospital the next day because of problems emptying his bladder. There, a transurethral resection of the prostate gland or TURP was done. Since Mr. Ebner is an established patient, the **insurance billing specialist** will be able

GOOD SAMARITAN HOSPITAL

Indianapolis, IN

OPERATIVE REPORT

Dictated 07/12/-- by Dr. Portia   PATIENT: Sara E. Ferraro
Transcribed 07/13/-- by SC   ACCOUNT NO: B3445228

DATE OF SURGERY   07/11/--

DIAGNOSIS: Incomplete Abortion

PROCEDURE: Dilation and Curettage

The patient is a 28-year-old para I, gravida 2 Caucasian female whose last menstrual period was 05/04/--. The patient presented herself to the emergency ward with cramping and bleeding, denying the passage of tissue and admitting that she was probably pregnant.

Examination in the emergency ward showed some cervix passing through a dilated cervical os. An IV Pitocin was placed and the patient was ready for surgery.

The patient was brought to surgery and given general anesthesia. She was placed in a modified lithotomy position and had an inside/outside vaginal prep and draped in the usual manner for pelvic surgery.

The examination indicated a uterus which was approximately 7 to 8 weeks gestational size. The cervical os was dilated to approximately 3 to 4 cm with necrotic tissue passing through the os itself.

A ring clamp was used to rid the uterus of the products. The uterine cavity was then curetted with a sharp curet until clean. The uterus sounded to 9 cm. The uterine cavity was smooth. There appeared to be no indication of infection but the patient was still given 2 grams Kefzol because of her being a patient of high risk population.

The bleeding was well controlled with the Pitocin. The residual blood was removed from the vagina. The patient was allowed to awaken and taken to recovery. She maintained normal vital signs throughout the procedure. There was no complication. The needle, sponge, and apparatus count was complete at the end of the surgery.

She will be followed on an outpatient basis.

Jane R. Portia, M.D.

"My name may be mechanically affixed by using the passkey."

FIGURE 1–12 Operative Report

Good Samaritan Hospital

1212 West 88th Street • Indianapolis, IN 46260 • 317/555-1212

EMERGENCY ROOM PATIENT INFORMATION

Date 07/11/--	Time 0915	Account B3445228

Patient Name Sara E. Ferraro **Address** 235 Marshall

City Indpls.	State IN	Zip 46283

Telephone No. (317) 555-1288 **Date of Birth** 06/09/-- ⨯M F

Responsible party name and address, if different than above

Insurance company name and address Community Cross; 125 N. State; NY 10000

ID number M613807816	Group number

Insured name Sara E. Ferraro	SS# 613-80-7816

Nature of complaints Severe abdominal pain with vaginal bleeding, nausea and

vomiting

I do hereby agree to be responsible for any charges resulting from this visit in the event my insurance company denies payment of benefits. I agree to authorize payment for any insurance benefits directly to Good Samaritan Hospital, 1212 West 88th Street, Indianapolis, IN, 46260.

Signature of patient or guardian *Sara E. Ferraro*

Name	Sara E. Ferraro

Date	07/11/--

FIGURE 1–13 Emergency Room Patient Information Record

to file a claim for this surgery using the CPIR in the chart and the ledger card showing the exact date, surgery, and fee. Figures 1-14 and 1-15 show those two records.

Of course, if an operative report is available to the **insurance billing specialist**, reading this will further explain the procedure and rule out any complications or difficulties that can affect the way the insurance form is completed. Reading it will also expand your knowledge and understanding of the work done by your doctors. Take the time to look up words that are new to you and make notes of those words and terms you use most frequently.

Whether or not you have an operative report, if the ledger card shows Mr. Ebner was charged the normal fee for a TURP as outlined on the Master Fee Schedule (See Chapter 15), then the **insurance billing specialist** may proceed to file the claim. It is very important that the **insurance billing specialist** ask questions of the office manager or the physician if there is any doubt about the services rendered or the fees charged. These professionals will welcome your questions and your attention to learning to do your job correctly. **Do not guess** about services or fees or any other aspect of your job! There is no such thing as a dumb question in the medical office!

Medical & Dental Associates, P.C.

3733 Professional Drive #300   317/123-4567
Indianapolis, IN 46260   Tax ID# 99-9999999

CONFIDENTIAL PATIENT INFORMATION RECORD

(please print)

Patient Name *Donald Ebner*

Address *6018 Orchard Lane*

Blgtn, IN 47437-1237

Telephone *(812) 555-1044*

Birthdate *12/15/--*   Age *52*

Sex *M*   Marital Status *W*

Social Security No. *132-60-8001*

Responsible Party (if other than patient)

Relationship to patient

Address

Patient Employer *Self*

Address *Ebner Gallery*

Sunset Lane

Blgtn, IN 47437-1237

Telephone *(812) 555-5067*

Occupation *Artist*

Primary insured date of birth *12/15/--*

Secondary insured date of birth

Third insured date of birth

Fourth insured date of birth

(Please use the back of the form to write information about the

third and fourth insured parties, if applicable.)

INSURANCE INFORMATION

Primary insured

Subscriber

Address

Telephone

Employer *U.S. Navy, Ret.*

Address *VA Station #558*

Job/Union No.

Subscriber's SS# *132-8001*

Relationship to patient *Self*

Insurance *CHAMPUS*

Address *BC/BS of IN*

POB 33, IN 47411

Policy No.

Subscriber ID No. *132-60-8001*

Group Name/No. *U.S.N. (Gr. 9) Ret.*

Effective date *10-10-94*

Expiration date —

Secondary insured

Subscriber

Address

Telephone

Employer

Address

Job/Union No.

Subscriber's SS#

Relationship to patient

Insurance

Address

Policy No.

Subscriber ID No.

Group Name/No.

Effective date

Expiration date

FIGURE 1–14 Confidential Patient Information Record

Medical & Dental Associates, P.C.

3733 Professional Drive #300
Indianapolis, IN 46260
317/123-4567
Tax ID# 99-9999999

STATEMENT OF ACCOUNT

EBNER, DONALD
6018 Orchard Lane
Bloomington, IN 47437-1237

19--

DATE	CODE	CHARGE		CREDITS PAYMENT	ADJ		CURRENT BALANCE	
BALANCE FORWARD ➡							0	
3/11	52000	200	00				200	00
3/12	52601	1800	00				2000	00

PLEASE PAY LAST AMOUNT IN THIS COLUMN ↑

THIS IS A COPY OF YOUR ACCOUNT

FIGURE 1–15 Ledger card

EXERCISE 2

Directions: Fill in the following blanks. You may review the material within this chapter to assist you.

1. An "established patient" is one we have treated in the practice within the past _____ years; a "new patient" is one we have _____ .

2. Our associates complete a _____ for each patient encounter in the office. In other offices, this information may be _____ by the doctor and typed in the patient's chart or handwritten by the doctor on white paper and filed, or a commercial form may be used as a guide.

3. A ledger card is a record of the _____ charged and the _____ rendered as well as the balance due.

4. Our associates admit patients to _____ Hospital under one of the following conditions:

   a. _____

   _____

   b. _____

   _____

   c. _____

   _____

   d. _____

   _____

   e. _____

   _____

5. The **insurance billing specialist** must be prepared to gather insurance billing information for patients seen in the office or at the hospital through the following methods:

a. _____

_____

b. _____

_____

c. _____

_____

d. _____

_____

e. _____

_____

6. If the **insurance billing specialist** is in doubt about services rendered or fees charged, ask the

_____ or _____ for clarification in

order to maximize correct reimbursement from the insurance company or insurer.

REVIEW QUESTIONS FOR DISCUSSION

You come into the office early Monday morning after Dr. Gregory was on call at Good Samaritan Hospital all weekend. Several notes are on your desk about four new patients the doctor saw in the hospital and some treatments that were rendered. The doctor indicated she admitted two of these patients to the hospital and would see them today on rounds and the third would be coming into the office at 2:00 P.M. this afternoon for an appointment to see her. The fourth new patient was treated at the hospital, discharged, and sent home.

1. What steps would you take to see if an insurance claim needed to be submitted for the patient discharged and sent home from the hospital?

2. How would you gather information about the two new patients admitted to the hospital?

3. What would you do about the patient coming into the office this afternoon? What if the patient fails to show up for the 2:00 P.M. appointment?

4. If four established patients had been seen in the hospital over the weekend instead of four new patients, what might you have done differently?

Chapter Two

INTRODUCTION TO DIAGNOSTIC CODING

OBJECTIVES   After completing your study of this chapter, you will be able to

- tell how and when the ICD-9-CM system began
- understand the three tabular sections of the ICD-9-CM code book
- explain how to use ICD-9-CM to code diseases, symptoms, and conditions
- use the Neoplasm table correctly

POWER WORDS

bilateral   Affecting both sides of the body.

diagnosis   The term used to indicate the medical name of the disease or condition of the patient.

HCFA (Health Care Financing Administration)   The governmental agency that oversees the Medicare program and the part of state Medicaid programs to which federal money has been allocated.

HCFA-1500 (hick-fah fifteen hundred)   The abbreviated term used to describe the generic insurance form completed and submitted to Medicare and most other carriers for reimbursement.

ICD-9-CM (International Classification of Diseases, 9th Revision, Clinical Modification, Fifth Edition)   The title of the numerical system used to explain the diagnosis or symptom of the patient or reason for seeking treatment; it is applied to the routing slip, to the patient's office chart, and to the insurance form.

medical necessity   To show that the procedure or treatment administered to a patient is appropriate in light of the diagnosis, symptom, or condition stated in the patient's chart.

Medicare   Federally financed health insurance coverage administered in each state by contracted insurance carriers for those 65 and older, for the blind, for those with end-stage renal disease, and for those with certain other disabilities.

morphology	The study of the size, shape, and origin of a specimen, plant, or animal; in coding, this number is used to help us find the correct column in the Neoplasm table.
unilateral	Affecting one side only.
World Health Organization (WHO)	An international organization devoted to the improvement of human health and the study of the worldwide spread of disease; located in Geneva, Switzerland.

WHAT ARE ICD-9-CM CODES?

More than seventy years ago, the World Health Organization established a numerical system that it used to record information about the spread of diseases around the world and the deadly effects on the population. About 1950, the U.S. Public Health Service and the Veterans Administration tested the use of a version of the WHO system to help them store and retrieve medical information related to patient care within the nation's hospitals.

By 1959, the International Classification of Diseases for hospital record keeping was developed. Further study and revision followed, and since January, 1979, the International Classification of Diseases, 9th Revision, Clinical Modification, has been used by hospitals, physicians, and other health care providers as a means of communicating medical information as well as statistical gathering. The addition of the words "Clinical Modification" referred specifically to adding details for establishing a diagnosis and not just for hospital record keeping.

Use of this new coding system gradually spread to the offices of practicing physicians and passage of the Medicare Catastrophic Coverage Act of 1988 made using these codes mandatory when billing government agencies (in most cases) beginning June 1, 1989. Today, Medicare is the standard-bearer for the insurance industry because of the large numbers of people with Medicare coverage. The tendency is for private insurance companies to follow the leadership provided by Medicare in nearly all areas, including the design and completion of the generic insurance form called the HCFA-1500, as well as in the establishment of reimbursement rules and regulations.

WHAT IS THE DIAGNOSIS?

In order to complete an insurance form for reimbursement, the **insurance billing specialist** must know why medical treatment was necessary: What was the problem that brought the patient to the doctor for treatment? The term for this is the diagnosis.

The doctor establishes the diagnosis after gathering a pertinent patient history, listening to the specific complaints of the patient, and performing an examination of the area(s) affected. Sometimes, additional tests will be needed, such as X-rays or urine tests or blood tests, before a definitive diagnosis can be established. Often, the doctor cannot figure out the diagnosis until after more complicated testing is done.

For example, when Ms. Altobelli completed her Confidential Patient Information Record, she indicated she was having some problems with hemorrhoids and other minor digestive ills. We know she was examined and treated by Dr. Cartman. Figure 2-1 is a copy of that part of the routing slip showing the diagnosis as determined by Dr. Cartman. You will notice a certain preprinted number in the far right column has been circled. Another diagnosis has been handwritten and the code added. The preprinted numbers in the far right column are called ICD-9-CM codes.

The diagnoses most often used in our office are preprinted on the routing slips so that each doctor may mark the routing slip more quickly. However, very often the code needed by the doctor is not preprinted on the form. In this case, the doctor will write the diagnosis on the routing slip and the **insurance billing specialist** will need to look up the correct code in the ICD-9-CM reference book. If the doctor has memorized the code, s/he may add it for you as is the case here. Also, when the doctor performs surgeries or other treatments at the hospital, an office routing slip is not used to get that information to the **insurance billing specialist**. (See Chapter 1). Again, it is necessary for the **insurance billing specialist** to know how to use the ICD-9-CM coding book to locate diagnoses so that the insurance claim may be completed and mailed quickly. We have other staff members who are expert in the area of coding—you are not expected to master that skill at this early stage of your new career. We know this will come with time and practice. Your task is to begin to learn how to find the correct diagnostic code you need by using the ICD-9-CM manual.

HOW TO USE THE ICD-9-CM MANUAL

To use the ICD-9-CM manual correctly, the **insurance billing specialist** must first understand how the book is put together. There are three sections (called "volumes") within the single ICD-9-CM reference, and various publishers combine these three volumes in different ways. For the most part:

- Volume 1 is Diseases: Tabular List Classification of Diseases listed in Categories 001–999

- Volume 2 is Diseases: Alphabetical Index

- Volume 3 is Procedures: Tabular List and Alphabetic Index; not used in the physician's office

Because Volume Three is not used in the physician's office but is used only for hospital inpatient coding by hospital employees, we will concentrate on Volumes One and Two in this manual.

Medical & Dental Associates, P.C.

3733 Professional Drive #300
Indianapolis, IN 46260

317/123-4567
Tax ID# 99-9999999

Patient name *Rose Altobelli*

CPT-4 CODES

OFFICE SERVICES	CODE	FEE
New patient, problem focused	99201	
New patient, expanded problem focused	99202	
New patient, detailed	(99203)	60—
New patient, comprehensive, mod.	99204	
New patient, comprehensive, high	99205	
Established patient, RN	99211	
Established patient, problem focused	99212	
Established patient, expanded problem	99213	
Established patient, detailed	99214	
Established patient, comprehensive	99215	
Consultation		

LABORATORY	CODE	FEE
X-ray, chest/ribs; single view, frontal	71010	
X-ray, chest/ribs; stereo, frontal	71015	
Therapeutic injections ( )	907__	
Drugs, trays, supplies	99070	
Educational supplies, books, tapes	99071	
Urinalysis, routine, dip stick	81000	
Urine pregnancy test, visual color	81025	
Blood count, hemoglobin	85018	
Pap smear	88150	

ICD-9-CM

DIAGNOSES	
Anxiety reaction	300.00
Bleeding rectal	569.3
Benign prostatic hypertrophy	600
Bronchitis, acute	466.0
Bronchitis, chronic	491.9
Cardiac arrhythmia	427.9
Chest pain	786.50
Cirrhosis of liver	571.5
Conjunctivitis, acute	372.00
Depression	300.4
Flu	487.0
Fracture–nasal, closed	802.0
Fractured tibia	891.2
Headache, vascular	794.0
Herpes zoster	053.9
Irritable bowel syndrome	(564.1)
Menopause	627.2
Myocardial infarction, unspecified	410.90
Otitis, acute	381.01
Pharyngitis, acute	462
Pneumonia	486
Sinusitis, acute	461.9
Tendonitis	726.90
Tennis elbow	726.32
Pregnancy	V22.2
Sprained ankle	842.5
Tonsillitis	474.0
Vertigo	386.0
Well child	V20.2

Bleeding hemorrhoids
455.8

CDT-2 CODES

DENTAL SERVICE

DIAGNOSTIC	CODE	FEE
Periodic exam	00120	
Limited exam	00140	
Comprehensive exam	00150	
Extensive exam	00160	
PREVENTIVE		
Intraoral–FMX	00210	
Intraoral–PA	00220	
BW	0027_	
Single posteroanterior	00290	
Panoramic X-ray	00330	
Prophylaxis adult	01110	
Prophylaxis child	01120	
Topical fluoride	012__	

DENTAL SERVICE

RESTORATIVE	CODE	FEE
Amalgams (decid) Tooth #_____	021__	
Amalgams (perm) Tooth #_____	021__	
CROWNS AND BRIDGES		
PFG crown	02750	
FG cast crown	02790	
3/4 gold cast crown	02810	
FC bridge pontic	06210	
Porcelain bridge ( )	062__	
OTHER PROCEDURES		

DOCTOR'S STATEMENT: I certify that I personally provided the above services and that fees shown represent my usual fees

James P. Cartman, M.D.   *9/1/--*

Signature   Date

TOTAL	$	60—
AMOUNT PAID	$	0
BALANCE DUE	$	60—

FIGURE 2–1 Highlighted ICD-9-CM codes

How to Use the ICD-9-CM Manual

EXERCISE 1

Directions: Begin to familiarize yourself with the reference by looking through the Tabular List of diseases in your ICD-9-CM coding manual. Locate the following numbered categories and code ranges in your manual. Write the page number where each category first appears:

		Code Range	Page Number
1.	Infectious and Parasitic Diseases	001 to 139	1-34
2.	Neoplasms	140 to 239	35-62
3.	Endocrine, Nutritional, and Metabolic Diseases, and Immunity Disorders	240 to 279	63-77
4.	Diseases of the Blood and Blood-Forming Organs	280 to 289	79-86
5.	Mental Disorders	290 to 319	87-102
6.	Diseases of the Nervous System and Sense Organs	320 to 389	103-144
7.	Diseases of the Circulatory System	390 to 459	145-168
8.	Diseases of the Respiratory System	460 to 519	169-180
9.	Diseases of the Digestive System	520 to 579	181-204
10.	Diseases of the Genitourinary System	580 to 629	205-223
11.	Complications of Pregnancy, Childbirth, and the Puerperium	630 to 676	225-240
12.	Diseases of the Skin and Subcutaneous Tissue	680 to 709	241-250
13.	Diseases of the Musculoskeletal System and Connective Tissue	710 to 739	251-270
14.	Congenital Anomalies	740 to 759	271-288
15.	Certain Conditions Originating in the Perinatal Period	760 to 779	289-298
16.	Symptoms, Signs, and Ill-Defined Conditions	780 to 799	299-312
17.	Injury and Poisoning	800 to 999	313-366

Other parts of this tabular section may include sections called V-Codes, E-Codes and E-Code Index, Morphology of Neoplasms, Glossary of Mental Disorders, concluding with a List of Three-Digit Categories. These sections will be described in later discussions.

HOW TO USE VOLUMES I AND II OF ICD-9-CM

To further acquaint you with this manual, locate the Diseases of the Digestive System, and turn to the page you listed. Notice the bold printing at the top of the page "Diseases of the Digestive System (520-579)." This means the part of the classification located between numbers 520 and 579 includes descriptions of diseases of the digestive system. To test this, look up number 536.8 and see if you can find a notation about "indigestion," a very common stomach problem. Notice number 536 is highlighted or otherwise marked or printed in some special way to make it stand out. The exact special marking depends upon the preferences of the publisher of your reference book. There are many companies who publish this information.

☞ The **insurance billing specialist** must remember that when a three-digit number (like 536) is highlighted or marked in a special way by the publisher, this is a very important signal that this three-digit number may not be used without adding a decimal point to the right of the number and at least one more digit to the right of the decimal point. This is called *coding to the highest degree of specificity.*

Therefore, 536 may never be used alone, but either 536.0, 536.1, 536.2, 536.3, 536.8, or 536.9 must be selected. The category number 536 and the explanation next to it becomes a kind of headline separating one number group from the next.

Now look at the headline or header number 550, inguinal hernia. Here we see a different situation. The special marking or highlighting is present as with 536, and also another marking, perhaps a number 5 within a circle. Again, the marking itself depends upon the publisher.

☞ This very special second marking means the **insurance billing specialist** must now use the three digit number 550, and add a decimal point with *two* additional numbers to the right! This is called *coding to the fifth digit*; three digits or numbers to the left of the decimal point and two to the right.

Therefore, we cannot use code 550 by itself under *any* circumstances because to do so would violate the rule that we must code to the highest degree of specificity. Instead, we must find two digits to the right of the decimal point. Let's find the fourth digit first, the one just to the right of the decimal point. The code 550.0 is defined as Inguinal hernia with gangrene. This diagnosis says nothing about gangrene. Therefore, 550.0 is not correct for inguinal hernia. Code 550.1 is for hernia and obstruction, which is not what we need. However, code 550.9 is correct because it is for inguinal hernia without mention of obstruction or gangrene. Underneath that listing is another that shows inguinal hernia NOS, which stands for Not Otherwise Specified.

☞ The NOS statement means this diagnosis does not give enough information to allow the selection of another subdivision within the category.

Where is the fifth digit located? There is an entry under the header for 550 that states:

"the following fifth-digit subclassification is for use with category 550:

    0 unilateral or unspecified (not specified as recurrent)

        Unilateral NOS

    1 unilateral or unspecified, recurrent

    2 bilateral (not specified as recurrent)

        Bilateral NOS

    3 bilateral, recurrent

We have selected 550.9. Now we *must add one of the four numbers shown above* to add to the right of the .9 to satisfy the requirement of a five-digit code. Which one we select depends entirely upon the particular medical problem that we are working to code. If we stick to our diagnosis of inguinal hernia and know nothing else, the correct fifth digit is 0. Therefore, the code for the diagnosis inguinal hernia is 550.90. Staying with the category 550, how would we code the diagnosis of recurrent unilateral inguinal hernia?

We would begin with the three-digit number 550. We would look at the three choices listed and the description of each one to select code 550.9 and then we would read about the fifth-digit choices and settle for the complete code 550.91.

There is a third possibility to determine whether to use a three-digit, a fourth-digit, or a fifth-digit code.

Suppose we wished to code this diagnosis: chronic hepatitis.

☞ *Remember,* you have not yet learned to code correctly on your own through the Index. We are only examining the Tabular List to become more acquainted with the book.

Look at code 571.40 in this Tabular List. It states, "chronic hepatitis, unspecified," meaning no other information is given. Also notice code 571.4 states "chronic hepatitis " which matches our diagnosis exactly. Which code is the correct one to use, 571.4 or 571.41? Once you recall the rule of coding to the highest degree of specificity, you will know that:

☞ If a fifth-digit coding opportunity exists, that fifth-digit code must be used in the same way that a fourth-digit coding opportunity overrides three digit codes every time.

This is very consistent and very important coding rule!

EXERCISE 2

Directions: Staying within the digestive system code range of 520-579, find the following answers:

1. What is the headline or header for category 523?

2. May code 523 be used alone? Why or why not?

3. What are the fourth-digit choices for code 523?

4. Look at code 524.0 and notice the codes listed beneath. What are the fifth-digit choices?

5. When will you use code 524 or 524.0?

6. Find code 531, Gastric ulcer. What special markings are present?

7. Will you ever use code 531 by itself? Why or why not?

8. Staying with category 531, what is the code for acute gastric ulcer with perforation and obstruction?

CODING CORRECTLY USING THE INDEX OF DISEASES

Now that you have examined some of the categories of the Tabular List and the very important rule of coding to the highest degree of specificity, let's examine how to find a code correctly using both the Tabular List and the Index of Diseases, Volumes I and II.

Refer once again to the routing sheet on Rose Altobelli. Notice that Dr. Cartman indicated her diagnoses were:

1. bleeding hemorrhoids with code 455.8 handwritten

2. irritable bowel syndrome with the circled code 564.1

Let us double-check the accuracy of these codes by using Volumes I and II.

Step 1. Open the Index of Diseases and look for the word "Hemorrhoids." Note it is printed in **bold-face type**. This tells you the word "Hemorrhoids" is a main term. Subterms are indented two spaces to the right under the main terms. This is where you look for the descriptive term, "bleeding." In coding, the **insurance billing specialist** must identify the main term for the disease you are trying to locate, and then the subterm under that. If you had tried to find bleeding hemorrhoids by first looking up the word "bleeding" and then the subterm "hemorrhoids," your manual would have sent you back to the main term "hemorrhoids."

Step 2. Further indented under Hemorrhoids, bleeding, is this information:

NEC 455.8

external 455.5

internal 455.2

It is unknown if the patient's hemorrhoids are external or internal and when looking for codes,

☛ Never make assumptions about diagnoses nor code beyond the scope of the diagnostic statement given to you.

Therefore, you may consider the NEC 455.8 code. NEC stands for Not Elsewhere Classifiable (in the coding book) and is used in situations like this one in which there is not enough information to know if the bleeding hemorrhoids are external or internal. But we cannot assume this is the code you *really* want until it is confirmed in the Tabular List.

Step 3. With this working code number of 455.8, turn to the Tabular List and hunt for the 455 section to verify that 455.8 is the code you want to use. Notice the number 455 has the special marking to show it may not be used alone. This is the signal that we *must* use one of the codes printed beneath 455, add a decimal point, and find one or two digits to the right of the decimal point. Underneath the main term, 455 Hemorrhoids, notice there are words to describe what is included in this code and what is excluded. *Always look at these lines, especially the excludes box.* By "excludes" the manual is saying that if the patient has hemorrhoids because she is pregnant or if they developed during childbirth or the puerperium (shortly after childbirth), go to code 671.8. In other words, the book is giving you a very important direction about finding the right code. Dr. Cartman said nothing about Ms. Altobelli having these hemorrhoids as a result of those situations, so we are safe in proceeding to look at the codes in the 455 section.

Step 4: Look at all the codes between 455 and 456 to be sure that 455.8, as suggested by the Index of Diseases, is the most appropriate code to use. Notice 455.0, 455.1, 455.2 all describe internal hemorrhoid problems and codes 455.3, 455.4, 455.5 all describe external hemorrhoid problems. We know we cannot use one of these codes. The code 455.6 states Unspecified hemorrhoids without mention of other complications. By "Unspecified," the code means we do not know if the hemorrhoids are internal or external. But we cannot use code 455.6 because the coding statement for Ms. Altobelli stated "bleeding" hemorrhoids and that is considered a complication. We cannot use code 455.7 because the diagnosis for Ms. Altobelli mentioned nothing about "thrombosed" hemorrhoids. Code 455.8 definitely describes the diagnosis as follows:

455.8 Unspecified hemorrhoids with other complication

Hemorrhoids, unspecified whether internal or external

bleeding

prolapsed

strangulated

ulcerated

Look also at code 455.9, just to be sure this is not the code we need to use. It is not, because the diagnostic statement said nothing about skin tags.

Code 455.8 is the only code we can use from this section that fits the diagnosis given by Dr. Cartman. In other coding searches for a different patient, there could be more than one correct code from a category, but that is not true for Ms. Altobelli.

Now let's double-check the second diagnosis for Ms. Altobelli, irritable bowel syndrome with code 564.1 marked. Shall we look up the word "irritable", the word "bowel," or the word "syndrome" in the Index to Diseases? We can rule out the word "bowel" right away because the Index to Diseases is not listed by body part or organ (except in the Neoplasm table), and "bowel" is a body part of the digestive system. If you *do* look up the term "bowel," you will be told to go elsewhere and look up the condition (which means problem). So, there is no harm done!

The main term to look up is either "irritable" or "syndrome," and both will suggest the same code number, 564.1. As a beginner to coding, do not be afraid to look up all the terms and conditions of the patient until you begin to get a feel for the main terms.

If we choose "irritable," we will be sent to "irritability" and indented under that main term, we find "bowel (syndrome)" with the code number 564.1. Turn to the Tabular List and find category 564. Notice it is marked to show we cannot use only three digits. Examine the whole section even after you look at 564.1 to decide if that is the correct code. It will serve you well later to establish good habits from the beginning. Too many beginners just go to the one code they think is correct without looking at the entire category, and too often they select the wrong code because of this.

In summary, then, to code correctly a diagnosis, condition, or symptom, the **insurance billing specialist** must:

1. look in the Index to Diseases and find the main term
2. find the subterm
3. locate the suggested code number
4. look in the Tabular List to confirm the suggested number
5. find the correct category in the Tabular List
6. look for special markings indicating the need for a fourth or fifth digit
7. read and follow inclusion or exclusion statements or any special directions
8. look over *all* choices in the section, and
9. *make your selection!*

☞ *The **insurance billing specialist** may never, never stop with a code from the Index to Diseases!* The coder must always look up the suggested number in the Tabular List to confirm that the suggested code is correct.

Do not allow yourself to get lazy and "forget" to confirm the code in the Tabular List. Many, many times, the code you finally select will be different than the one suggested in the Index to Diseases and if you forget to confirm that number, you will be coding incorrectly. It may help to think of the Index to Diseases as a kind of street map: it may give you directions to the neighborhood you want to look at in the Tabular List, but only the Tabular List will get you to the right house! More mistakes happen in coding by "forgetting" to use the Tabular List than through any other single cause. Later, you will have a coding problem that will show you exactly how this can happen.

EXERCISE 3

Directions: Look up each diagnosis in the Index of Diseases, find the suggested code number, and then confirm it in the Tabular List. If you do not understand the definitions of these words and terms, please use your medical dictionary to look them up.

1. Constipation, simple   564.00

2. Tennis elbow   726.32

3. Cirrhosis of the liver, alcoholic   571.2

4. Hyaline membrane disease   769

5. Hypoacidity, gastric   _____

6. Retinitis   _____

7. Claw foot, acquired   _____

8. Sprained elbow   _____

9. Tension headache   _____

10. Claustrophobia   _____

11. Bronchitis   _____

12. Anorexia nervosa   _____

13. Senility   _____

14. Caloric malnutrition   _____

15. Mumps   _____

EXERCISE 4

Directions: Look up the following diagnoses in the Index of Diseases and confirm the suggested code in the Tabular List.

1. Diabetes mellitus, type II, uncontrolled _____

2. Aneurysm of the splenic artery _____

3. Congenital blindness, bilateral _____

4. Cleft palate with cleft lip _____

5. Separation anxiety _____

6. Mumps hepatitis _____

7. PAT _____

8. Cardiac arrest _____

9. Polycystic kidney disease _____

10. Hypospadias, female _____

11. Genital syphilis, primary _____

12. Schizophrenia simplex, chronic _____

13. Petit mal status epilepsy _____

14. Chronic peptic ulcer with bleeding _____

15. Hematuria _____

The **insurance billing specialist** may use more than one code to correctly code some diagnoses. In fact, you must use as many codes as are appropriate for the diagnoses presented to you. Other diagnoses look as though they will require two codes but once you examine the Index, and confirm the suggested code in the Tabular Listing, you will see that one code includes two diagnoses. The following exercises will give you practice at single and multiple coding.

EXERCISE 5

Directions: Find the correct codes for the diagnoses listed below. Search the Index of Diseases and confirm each suggested code in the Tabular List before moving on to the second diagnosis in each statement. Remember to use your medical dictionary to find the definitions for words you may not know.

1. Bladder inertia with urinary incontinence   ———————

2. Acute suppurative peritonitis with pancolitis   ———————

3. Nausea with vomiting and fever   ———————

4. Acute ethmoidal and sphenoidal sinusitis   ———————

5. Closed dislocation of the fifth cervical spine and open dislocation of the foot   ———————

6. Diverticulitis with diverticulosis of the small intestine   ———————

7. Adolescent misery and unhappiness disorder   ———————

8. Type I, uncontrolled diabetes with ketoacidosis   ———————

9. Fetal blood loss from ruptured cord   ———————

10. Cerebral contusion with open intracranial wound and loss of consciousness   ———————

11. Sprained deltoid ligament of the ankle with sprained Achilles tendon   ———————

12. Acute renal failure with acute tubular necrosis   ———————

13. Illegally induced abortion complicated by shock   ———————

14. Diffuse cellulitis of the buttock and hip   ———————

15. Polydactyly of fingers and toes   ———————

16. Late anemia due to isoimmunization   ———————

17. Obsessive-compulsive disorder   ———————

18. Adjustment disorder with work inhibition   ———————

19. Acute myocardial infarction of inferoposterior wall   ———————

20. Foreign body in the bladder and urethra   ———————

CODING NEOPLASMS—PART I

Neoplasms are new tissue growths and may be located anywhere inside or outside the body. Be careful not to assume that the word "neoplasm" means cancerous growth, because it certainly does not! The word "neoplasm" provides a much broader range of definition, everything from tumor, to mass, to new growth-benign, to new growth-malignant.

Coding neoplasms is different from the coding you have done so far and deserves special attention. First, find the Neoplasm tables in the Index to Diseases in the "N" area of the book. As you look through this section, you will see page after page of columns of numbers. Coding neoplasms is different from earlier coding exercises because this section of the code book lists body areas on the left side of each page. If you look through the Index to Diseases outside the Neoplasm section, you will see the book is arranged alphabetically by disease or symptom or disease name or condition. Only in the Neoplasm section of the Index do you find body areas listed exclusively.

Across the top of each page are the titles of the columns. Notice the general title, "Malignant" and under that umbrella title, three columns titled "Primary," "Secondary," and "Ca in situ."

Malignant neoplasms are the cancerous ones and there are many different types. The term "cancer" means that the tissue is growing and replicating or du-plicating itself at a very rapid rate that is out of control. Carcinoma in situ is a type of cancer that may grow as rapidly as the others, but does not invade neighboring cells. "In situ" means within or at the site. So this carcinoma is one that may grow rapidly, as do some other invasive tumors, but is well-encapsulated and does not grow or "metastasize" into neighboring cells or spread to other areas of the body through the blood or lymph channels. Therefore, if the diagnostic statement you are trying to code says "carcinoma in situ of the urinary bladder" you will code that diagnosis using the Neoplasm section of the Index of Diseases, look up the body site under the letter "b" for bladder, then go to the third column under "Ca in situ" and locate code 233.7. Of course, you would not stop here! Go to that part of the Tabular List and find 233.7. The listing is 233.7 Bladder and the name of the category is 233 Carcinoma in situ of breast and genitourinary system. Look at the codes on the previous page and below 233.7 to be certain this is the code you want.

☛ Neoplasm tables are used to list solid tumors only. Nonsolid tumors such as leukemia travel through the body lymph channels. These are malignant, but will be located in the Index to Diseases and not in the Neoplasm tables.

To help introduce you to the Neoplasm tables, find the code for the following diagnostic statements within the table and verify your selection in the Tabular List.

EXERCISE 6

Directions: Code the diagnostic statements and answer questions as requested:

1. Ca in situ of the true vocal cords   231.0

2. Ca in situ of the appendix   230.3

3. Ca in situ of the male breast   233.0

4. Ca in situ of the descending colon   230.4

5. Ca in situ of the liver   230.8

6. Did you notice you were finding the code within a very small range of numbers
   in the Tabular List?   yes

7. What is the range of codes in the Tabular List for Carcinoma in situ?   _____

8. List the number and title of each header under the classification Carcinoma in situ.
   These headers will begin farthest to the left margin of each page.

   _____

   _____

   _____

9. Do any of these codes require using a fifth digit?   NO

10. Do any of these codes require only three digits?   NO

11. Is there another Carcinoma in situ section in the Tabular List?   _____

Return to the Index of Diseases, Neoplasm tables, now that you understand how to locate carcinoma in situ.

Notice the other two malignant columns—Primary and Secondary. The primary column means the neoplasm originated or began at the body site listed, and the secondary site column means the neoplasm spread to another place. Both columns work the same way as the carcinoma in situ column when you are trying to code.

☞ In coding a malignancy that does not state "primary" or "secondary" or "ca in situ," and does not tell the **insurance billing specialist** whether the body site is primary or secondary, and does not mention any spreading, *you may assume it is a primary site.*

For example, the diagnostic statement "Carcinoma of the lung" without any further description would be coded 162.9. However, if the statement was "Carcinoma of the lung secondary to carcinoma of the liver," this problem would need two codes to fully describe it, with the primary site listed first. The answer would be 155.0 (liver, primary malignancy) and 197.0 (lung, secondary malignancy). There are other words used to describe a primary and a secondary malignancy, such as "spread to" or "metastasized to or from" or "mets" for short. Therefore, our problem would mean the same if it said:

Carcinoma of the liver with metastasis to the lung

or

Metastasis to the lung from the liver

or

Carcinoma spread to the lung from the liver

or

Carcinoma of the liver, with invasion into the lung

All four statements would be coded the same with the primary site always listed first when it is known.

Sometimes the primary or secondary site is not known or has not yet been confirmed with a pathology report. Fortunately, we have a code number (199.1) that is used to mean "unknown primary site" or "unknown secondary site." In this application, the **insurance billing specialist** must never place this unknown code first even if the primary site is unknown! In other words, the **insurance billing specialist** first lists what *is* known and then lists what *is not* known. Example: "Secondary carcinoma of the lung, primary site unknown" is coded 197.0 and then 199.1. Since the number for the secondary site is 197.0, it is listed first because we *always* list what we know first; then the unknown code 199.1 to show we do not yet know where this malignancy came from.

EXERCISE 7

Directions: Code the following diagnostic statements using the Index to Diseases first under Neoplasms, and then the Tabular List for confirmation:

1. Carcinoma of the tongue surface, dorsal   _____

2. Primary malignancy of the kidney with metastasis to the peritoneum   _____

3. Secondary carcinoma of the retina, primary site unknown   _____

4. Ca of the pineal gland   _____

5. Ca of the bronchus from the larynx   _____

6. Ca of connective tissue   _____

7. Ca to the uterus from the ovary   _____

8. Ca to the ovary from the uterus   _____

9. Pharyngeal tonsil malignancy   _____

10. Carcinoma of the prostate gland   _____

The remaining three columns of the Neoplasm table are for tumors that are Benign, or not malignant; Uncertain Behavior, meaning on the borderline between benign and malignant; Unspecified, or not stated exactly into which category the neoplasm should be placed. Those three columns are treated the same way as the first three. In every case, the **insurance billing specialist** is not responsible to determine whether a neoplasm is malignant, benign, or anything else. This information will be provided in the patient's chart or on a pathology report or otherwise marked by the physician. *Never guess* about coding neoplasms or any other area; instead, *ask* your office manager or physician.

CODING NEOPLASMS—PART II

Finding the correct column in the Neoplasm table also is different from your previous experiences and can be tricky! There is more than one way to get to the correct code:

Step 1. Look up the diagnostic statement in the Index to Diseases; i.e., find "adenocarcinoma, renal cell." Under the heading "Adenocarcinoma" locate "renal cell." There, you see the entry "renal cell (M8312/3) 189.0." You may want to look up "adenocarcinoma" in your medical dictionary to understand that it is a carcinoma or malignancy with a specific cell structure.

Step 2. Next to "renal cell" is the morphology number M8312/3. We do not apply these numbers to insurance forms or use them in ways they are used in hospitals. (For more information about the Morphology of Neoplasms, read that section located behind the Tabular List of your ICD-9-CM book.) We *are* interested in the number located to the right of the slash. This number indicates the behavior of the neoplasm we are examining.

☛ We are able to learn which column of the Neoplasm table to use if we know the morphology behavior number of the neoplasm we wish to code.

For example, /0 behavior number means the neoplasm is benign. We look in the benign column to find the code we need according to the body site. The rest of these behavior numbers are as follows:

/1 Uncertain whether benign or malignant

   Borderline malignancy

/2 Carcinoma in situ

/3 Malignant, primary site

/6 Malignant, metastatic site

   Secondary site

/9 Unspecified

Looking again at "adenocarcinoma, renal cell (M8312/3) 189.0," we now see that the behavior number indicates that this is a malignancy, primary site.

Step 3. Do we need to find the body site and look for the code in the Neoplasm table? No, we do not, because the code number 189.0 is located next to the listing in the Index to Diseases.

Step 4. Locate 189.0 in the Tabular List and you will see the listing:

> Kidney, except pelvis; Kidney NOS; Kidney parenchyma.

Step 5. To double-check this 189.0 code answer, look into the Neoplasm table, under Kidney, and look in the primary malignancy column. The number 189.0 is there. In summary:

☛ The code number may be listed in the Index to Diseases, in the Neoplasm table, or both. Once you know the behavior code of the neoplasm, you know which column to look under in the Neoplasm Table.

When coding diagnostic statements, don't forget to put the codes in the correct order and use 199.1 when appropriate. Also, remember you may *always* find the code you need by looking in the Index first under the main term, then going directly to the Tabular List to confirm the code; or by going to the Neoplasm table to the body site first and then to the Tabular List. The difference with Neoplasm coding is that sometimes you can go directly to the Neoplasm table before confirming your choice in the Tabular List and this is a very rare shortcut.

☛ *Caution:* If you do not fully understand the behavior of the kind of neoplasm you are trying to code, be sure to avoid any shortcut and go first to the Index of Diseases.

For example, consider this coding problem: melanoma, female breast. Can you go to the Neoplasm Table first, find "female breast," and select the correct code? No! If you look for the answer under "female breast" you will be looking at the wrong body site. Melanoma is a cancer of the skin. Look up "skin" in the Neoplasm table, and then find the listing "melanoma." Essentially, the Neoplasm table sends you back to the Index of Diseases. In addition, how do you know if the melanoma is primary or secondary or

Ca in situ if you go directly to the Neoplasm table to find "melanoma, female breast?" You must go *first* to the Index of Diseases, look up "Melanoma, female breast, 172.5." The morphology number is listed next to the Melanoma heading and /3 means it is a primary malignancy. But code 172.5 in the Tabular List is clearly the correct choice.

☞ As a beginning coder, play it safe and *first* check the main term in the Index to Diseases!

If the Index states "see Neoplasm, by site, malignant" or "see Neoplasm, by site, in situ," or anything else, you will know you may proceed safely to the Neoplasm table and you have been told which column to use!

OTHER NEOPLASM CODING RULES

Other coding rules regarding Neoplasms include:

☞ If a primary malignancy site has been removed surgically but the malignancy is said to be recurrent at another site, code that other site as a secondary malignancy.

☞ If two sites of malignancy are mentioned without determining which one is primary or secondary, code both sites as secondary and add the 199.1 code.

☞ When malignancies appear at locations that are very close together or overlap, and the point of origin cannot be determined, this is called a "contiguous" malignancy and the fourth digit of .8 must be used.

☞ It is possible to have more than one primary site as well as multiple secondary sites. Certain body sites are coded as secondary sites when the morphology type is not stated or the only known code is 199.1! These sites are: bone, brain, diaphragm, heart, liver (often a primary site), lymph nodes, mediastinum, meninges, peritoneum, pleura, retroperitoneum, spinal cord, or sites classifiable to 195.

☞ Code 199.0, carcinomatosis, may be used as the primary diagnosis in that very rare diagnostic event where the malignancy is very widespread throughout the body and no other information is documented.

EXERCISE 8

Diagnosis: Code the following diagnostic statements.

1. Abdominal mass   *789.3*

2. Carcinosarcoma of fallopian tube

3. Stomach malignancy with metastasis   *230.2*

4. Colon melanosis

5. Leiomyoma

6. Ca in situ, cervix

7. Plasma cell sarcoma

8. Metastasis to ankle bone from cervical uteri

9. Cancer of the salivary gland

10. Tumor of the tooth socket, #16, uncertain behavior

11. Benign prostatic hypertrophy

12. Growth on eyelid, right

13. Metastasis to meninges

14. Reticulosarcoma

15. Neurofibromatosis

REVIEW QUESTIONS FOR DISCUSSION

1. Why is correct and accurate ICD-9-CM coding important?

2. Who is responsible for determining the diagnosis for each patient?

3. Can the **insurance billing specialist** file an insurance claim before all the tests are back and a diagnosis established?

4. Why must you use both Volume One and Volume Two to code accurately?

5. What would happen if you used only the Index of Diseases?

6. Did you miss problem #7, Exercise 8, because you did not confirm the code in the Tabular List? When were you warned to look out for this possibility?

7. If the correct code is established at the time of the office visit, can you use that code again for a later visit?

8. Describe the many definitions of the word "neoplasm."

9. Why isn't "leukemia" listed in the Neoplasm table?

10. In what order should Neoplasm codes be listed?

Chapter Three

E-CODES, V-CODES, LATE EFFECT CODES, AND HYPERTENSION TABLE

OBJECTIVES   After completing your study of this chapter, you will be able to

- define E-Codes and the Table of Drugs and Chemicals
- describe Late Effect codes and when they should be used
- determine when to apply V-Codes
- understand how to use the Hypertension Tables

POWER WORDS

adverse effect   May result after a drug or medicinal substance; although correctly prescribed and correctly taken by the patient, causes a negative reaction within the patient.

E-Codes   Used to describe adverse effects of drugs and chemicals, injury and accident causes, and environmental factors resulting in disease or injury.

hypertension table   Used in coding hypertension as either the cause of disease (primary) or effect of disease (secondary), and the nature of the hypertension (benign, malignant, or unspecified).

Late Effect Codes   Used to document residual conditions that develop following the acute phase of another illness or injury.

V-Codes   Used in those situations when the patient encounters the health care system without a specific illness, disease, or diagnosis; or for treatment of a specific on-going disease; or to describe a condition or historical fact that might influence the treatment of the patient.

WHAT ARE E-CODES AND HOW ARE THEY USED?

E-Codes are used in several different ways, as stated in the opening paragraphs of the E-Code Section of your ICD-9-CM book. This section is called the "Supplementary Classification of External Causes of Injury and Poisoning (E800-E999)." The **insurance billing specialist** may choose to think of "E" as standing for "external." These codes begin with the letter "E" and are followed by either three whole numbers, or three numbers to the left of the decimal point and one number to the right. The same rule of coding to the highest degree of specificity applies here.

- ☞ E-Codes are used to explain the situation surrounding injury or sickness resulting from an external cause;

- ☞ and/or to explain poisoning sources;

- ☞ and/or adverse effects of medicines or other substances.

To demonstrate this idea of external sources of illness, imagine yourself at home, seated in front of your television set, watching a favorite program, with a beverage and the remote control nearby. Assume your home is located next to a very busy railroad track and as you are comfortably relaxing in your favorite chair, you hear the sound of an approaching train.

Suddenly, a series of loud crashes and scraping sounds tells you the train has derailed not far from your house! Through your window, you notice a menacing yellow cloud rising from the wreckage and floating in your direction. Soon the cloud is over your roof, and you begin to cough deeply and experience burning eyes and pains in your chest. *This is an E-Code situation!*

If you told this story to your doctor, depending upon your physical condition, she or he might diagnose you initially with chest pain (786.50), pulmonary congestion (514), and painful eyes (379.93) *due to* exposure to an unknown chemical substance (989.9, E866.9) following a train derailment near home (E802.8), although the codes would not necessarily be in this order. Find those two E-Codes and code 989.9 in your ICD-9-CM reference and take the time to examine other parts of this section. Some situations described are very funny!

Note, also, there is an E-Code Index separate from the Index to Diseases. To find the E-Code you need in coding situations, look there first. The following exercise will give you practice in finding E-Codes to describe the circumstances surrounding an illness or injury. To use the E-Code index, look up the word or term that describes the situation, such as "derailment." In this index, neither the body area nor the disease is listed. E-Codes are located under very colorful terms, such as accident, explosion, shooting, sting, poisoning.

EXERCISE 1

Directions: Locate the correct E-Code for the following statements using the E-Code Index first, then refer to the E-Code section of the Tabular List to confirm your selection.

1. Motor vehicle traffic accident involving collision with another vehicle (a bus) _____

2. Dog bite _____

3. Tidal wave caused by earthquake _____

4. Assault by a letter bomb _____

5. Exhaustion due to excessive exercise _____

Two codes will be needed for the following exercises: the first code to describe the sickness, injury or condition using Volumes I & II, and the second code from the Index to External Causes and E-Code section to state the circumstances surrounding the problem.

6. Heat stroke due to excessive outdoor exposure _____

7. Knee abrasion due to fall from bicycle _____

8. Unconsciousness due to blow to head _____

9. Third-degree burn, left shoulder, following residential fire _____

10. Sprained neck after fall into manhole _____

HOW TO USE THE TABLE OF DRUGS AND CHEMICALS

Turn to Section Two of your ICD-9-CM manual titled "Alphabetic Index to Poisoning and External Causes of Adverse Effects of Drugs and Other Chemical Substances, Table of Drugs and Chemicals." After reading the first page of this Section, the **insurance billing specialist** will see there is a correlation between codes 960 to 989 in the Tabular List and the numbers shown under the column heading "Poisoning" on each page of the Table. The codes listed between 960 and 979 refer to poisoning by drugs, chemicals, and other medicinal substances. Codes 980 to 989 refer to the toxic effects of substances that are predominately non-medicinal. Each code number is described in greater detail in the Tabular List.

☞ The difficulty of knowing when to apply the codes between 960 and 989 lies in determining whether the illness or condition that developed after consumption of the substance was a poisoning or an adverse effect.

In coding discussions, the word "poisoning" is used to mean the condition following the wrong or incorrect usage of a drug or substance (whether deliberate or accidental), and the term "adverse effect" is used to mean the problem that developed after the proper use of medication or drugs appropriately prescribed.

To code an adverse effect, list the condition that resulted from the offending substance, then the E-Code in the Therapeutic Use column of the Table of Drugs and Chemicals because the patient took the correct medication in the correct dosage as correctly prescribed.

When coding a poisoning effect within the diagnostic statement, the **insurance billing specialist** will use one of the codes from the Poisoning column of the Table of Drugs and Chemicals to identify which chemical or drug was responsible, the condition, and the E-Code to show *how* the poisoning took place. Coding situations may require that you show the poisoning was accidental, a documented suicide attempt, an assault by another party, or an undetermined or unknown source of poisoning.

For example, to code the statement "poisoning by accidental overdose of penicillin":

- look first for penicillin in the Table of Drugs and Chemicals
- select the poisoning code next to the drug under the Poison column heading
- add the selected and verified E-Code for penicillin under the Accident column heading of the Table of Drugs and Chemicals.

If your answer is 960.0 and E-856, you are exactly correct!

If the statement had said "severe gastritis due to accidental overdose of penicillin" the **insurance billing specialist** would:

- first code the poison code for penicillin from the Table of Drugs and Chemicals
- then the gastritis code from the Index to Diseases and verified in the Tabular List
- then the E-Code from the Accident column of the Table of Drugs and Chemicals.

But if the statement had said, "gastritis due to hypersensitivity to penicillin,"

- code the gastritis from the Index of Disease and verified in the Tabular List;
- then find the E-Code from the Therapeutic Use column of the Table on the penicillin line.

The reason for coding a drug reaction (referred to in the above problem as a hypersensitivity) under the Therapeutic Use column and not referring to any poisoning, is because the drug was properly prescribed by the doctor and taken as directed by the patient. It would not be correct or appropriate to code that the doctor had poisoned the patient! There are times when a patient may deliberately try to harm himself with a drug overdose and that situation must be coded as a poisoning. However, if the doctor correctly prescribes a medication and the patient takes it correctly but has a bad reaction to the drug, that is considered an Adverse Effect or allergic reaction and *not* considered a poisoning by the doctor or the patient.

In summary, code each statement using the following guidelines to determine the order in which the codes appear and which codes to use:

	Poison		Adverse Effect
1.	Poison Code	1.	Diagnosis, Condition, Symptom
2.	Diagnosis, Condition, Symptom	2.	E-Code for the substance the patient had the reaction to
3.	E-Code to explain how the substance was ingested or absorbed by the patient		

EXERCISE 2

Directions: Find the correct codes for the following statements:

1. Accidental poisoning by consuming noxious mushrooms

   988.1, E865.5

2. Suicide attempt by ingestion of lye

   983.2, E864.2

3. Tinnitus following accidental overdose of aspirin

   _____

4. Coma following accidental consumption of beverage laced with snake venom

   _____

5. Insomnia due to hypersensitivity to antidepressant

   _____

6. Spasms due to allergic reaction to antihistamine, taken as prescribed

   _____

7. Body rash following prescribed dosage of sulfur ointment

   _____

8. Anosmia following accidental injection of boric acid

   _____

388.30

LATE EFFECT CODES

When a new problem or condition develops within the patient after the acute phase of another problem has passed, this new problem is called the late effect or residual effect. For example, following a severe burn, the patient may develop scarring that impedes the movement or the normal function of the burned area. This kind of scarring problem happens only because of the terrible burn. If the patient had not experienced the fire and subsequent burn, the scarring would not have appeared. Scarring following a burn is a frequent occurrence. Therefore, the scarring is considered the late effect or residual effect following the burn healing.

Likewise, suppose our burn victim also had suffered a broken humerus during his attempt to escape the fire. He might be treated for the broken bone and have a proper healing without further difficulties. He might also be treated for the broken bone and have problems healing. Perhaps the fracture site refuses to mend or a malunion develops at the site of the break. A poor healing or a malunion would be considered a residual effect or late effect of the bone fracture. Again, the problem of malunion or of poor healing would not have developed without the occurrence of the broken bone.

Time is not a factor in establishing the late effect. A late effect can show up immediately as with a stroke victim who cannot speak because of the cerebral vascular accident, or it may not become apparent until a much later date, as with a patient who suffered brain damage following the life-saving pharmaceutical treatment of a deadly brain infection. In other words, while time is not a factor in applying the late effect code, the original condition must have passed the most acute phase and be well into healing or resolution before the late effect may be coded. If another condition occurs while the patient is in the acute phase of his illness, this other condition is called a complication or co-morbidity and is coded just like any other medical problem.

Coding late effects requires two codes: first, the *late effect* and then the *cause*. For example, hemiplegia due to cerebral vascular accident is coded 342.9 for hemiplegia and 438 as the late effect of the CVA. This order of listing effect first and then cause must be followed *except* for those instances when the coding book tells you to do otherwise. Those instructions always take precedence over the usual ways of coding.

To locate the correct late effect code for the problem you are trying to code, look up the term Late Effect in the Alphabetic Index to Disease. Under that heading, find the condition and follow the Index instructions to the code. There is no one listing of Late Effect codes in the Tabular Section; those codes are in various locations throughout your coding manual. Following the instructions in your manual will direct you to the correct code.

ADDITIONAL LATE EFFECT CODING RULES

☞ A late effect code may be used alone when the coding statement does not state exactly what problem is present, but that the problem is definitely a residual effect of some other condition. For example, late effects of old amputation would be coded 997.60 only.

☞ If a problem is stated as a late effect but there is no specific late effect code in your manual for that problem, code only the presenting problem. For example, gastritis due to *Clostridium botulinum* would be coded 005.1 (to the offending substance), because there was no specific code under Late Effect in the Index of Disease.

EXERCISE 3

Directions: Code the following diagnostic statements using Volumes I and II:

1. Mild mental retardation due to spinal meningitis   _____

2. Calcification of the lung due to old respiratory tuberculosis   _____

3. Infection due to indwelling urinary catheter   _____

4. Hemiplegia due to cerebrovascular lesion   _____

5. Paraplegia   _____

6. Blindness due to a previous case of trachoma   _____

7. Hepatitis due to using a contaminated needle   _____

8. Joint ankylosis due to old injury   _____

WHAT ARE V-CODES AND HOW ARE THEY USED?

The V-Code section of your ICD-9-CM book describes the three circumstances when V-Codes are used:

☞ When an individual without symptoms or disease contacts the health care system for some specific reason, such as a healthy teenager who needs a physical examination before going to band camp, or to receive preventive vaccination or discuss a nondisease problem.

☞ When someone with a known or mending injury or disease comes into the health care system for specific treatment of this problem, such as chemotherapy treatment for malignancy.

☞ When a circumstance exists that influences the patient's health but is not, itself, a current illness or injury, such as a personal or family history of disease or the state of homelessness.

V-Codes often give added dimension to the condition of the patient or describe special circumstances that might affect the treatment of the patient. The **insurance billing specialist** will see V-Codes used in the office for health maintenance treatments, for preoperative and other specified examinations, for vaccinations, and for personal and family history data. If you were working in a hospital coding environment, you also would see V-Codes used as reasons for hospital admission for treatment of specific conditions and for documentation surrounding maternity admissions and birth outcomes.

In coding V-Codes, look first in the Index to Diseases and then confirm your options in the Tabular List as you would for a diagnostic statement. For example, in coding "family history of breast cancer," look in the Index under History, then find the subheading "family," and then "malignant neoplasm" and then "breast," female or male.

EXERCISE 4

Directions: Code the following statements using V-Codes. Remember to use first the Index of Diseases and then confirm your selection in the V-Code section of ICD-9-CM.

1. Personal history of allergy to penicillin   V14.0

2. Contraceptive counseling   V25.09

3. Exposure to AIDS virus   V01.79

4. Hearing examination, annual   V72.19

5. Medical examination prior to admission to old age home   V70.3

6. Blood-alcohol test   V70.4

7. Screening for renal disease   V81.5

8. Attention to surgical dressings   V58.30

9. Occupational maladjustment   V62.29

10. Examination of potential kidney donor   V70.8

HYPERTENSION CODING

Look in the Index to Diseases and locate "hypertension" and the table that follows this term. You will see three columns to the right of the subsections listed "Malignant," "Benign," "Unspecified." The term "malignant" may seem to refer to cancer but it does not. Instead, it is used to mean a very serious and life-threatening disease. Malignant hypertension is a grave disorder with progressive damage to veins and arteries and a poor prognosis. This problem can lead to severe damage of other body systems and even death without effective treatment. Benign hypertension is a relatively mild expression of circulatory disease and tends to be prolonged or chronic in nature. If the diagnostic statement is "hypertension" without additional description, it should be coded to the "Unspecified" column.

Hypertension is a complicated disease and, therefore, we cannot expect it to be easy to code! It can cause other problems for the patient and damage other body systems, or hypertension can be the result of other disease in the patient. It is a very common problem in this culture and very high on the list of diseases under treatment. It can be highly responsive to treatment. Many patients control their hypertension with changes in lifestyle alone while others require high doses of prescribed medications.

Looking at the hypertension tables, notice the many terms listed in parenthesis under the boldface listing, "**Hypertension, hypertensive.**" Those terms in parenthesis are called "non-essential modifiers." They are non-essential because not one of them must be present in the diagnostic statement you are trying to code in order for the **insurance billing specialist** to use a specific code. For example, to code benign hypertension, look at 401.1. Go to the Tabular List and confirm that 401.1 is correct for benign hypertension. If this is true, then all the parenthetical terms are optional and may be used if needed but are not required in order to use code 401.1. That is what is meant by "non-essential" and is true in all sections of the Index for terms in parenthesis to the right of the disease or condition or symptom.

Essential modifiers are those words listed below a boldfaced term, such as the word "with" under all

the non-essential modifiers and the subterms "heart involvement," etc. These essential modifiers must be in the diagnostic statement as you have learned in working with the ICD-9-CM manual so far.

CORRECTLY READING THE TABLE

One serious challenge in using the Hypertension Table is to read and correctly use the indented statements and subterms. Although the table is only a few pages in length, it is very easy to get lost among the subterms. For example, heart problems complicating pregnancy are found under the term "complicating pregnancy, childbirth, or the puerperium" followed by the subterm "with" and then several lines deeper into the table, the subterm "due to." Therefore, to find the diagnosis "benign hypertension complicating pregnancy due to Cushing's disease" the **insurance billing specialist** would look first for "hypertension," then for "complicating pregnancy," then look seven or eight listings farther for the subterm "due to," then several more lines down to "Cushing's disease," in order to see the number 405.19 under the benign column which then must be confirmed in the Tabular List.

To help you understand the Hypertensive Disease category, turn to codes 401 to 405.99 and examine each code. Notice the frequency of fifth digits, the involvement of renal failure, and secondary hypertension.

Look back to the Hypertension Table and notice the next subterm under "complicating pregnancy, childbirth or the puerperium." What is the subterm? It is "encephalopathy." The alphabetical listing does not resume for several lines of codes following "complicating..." Likewise, how would you code "secondary benign hypertension due to renal thrombosis?"

Go to the subterm "secondary," then to "due to," then to "renal," then "stenosis," and the number 405.11 under the benign column. Confirm in the Tabular List. Notice the Tabular List states "Renovascular," which your dictionary will reveal is another way of expressing kidney/renal and heart involvement. The terms in the Tabular List need not match your Index exactly in this section or any other. When the Index sends the **insurance billing specialist** to a specific code, and no other code in the category or vicinity appears to be a better description of the diagnosis, you may use that code.

Notice the entries under "Hypertension with heart involvement (conditions classifiable to 425.8, 428,...due to hypertension)." This means if the condition related to hypertension is classifiable to the codes listed, (i.e., 428 is heart failure) then the hypertension code you seek is in one of the three columns on that line. Therefore, in order to code "hypertension with heart failure," we know heart failure is in the 428 section. The Hypertension Table lists codes 402.00 or 402.10 or 402.90 as likely choices for that statement because the heart involvement in the diagnosis belongs to the 428 category and 428 is one of several mentioned.

The **insurance billing specialist** must be careful about the terms and their correct meanings. A high blood pressure reading does not necessarily mean the patient is hypertensive. Our blood pressures fluctuate daily and often a visit to the doctor and concern about one's health can elevate the blood pressure in a patient without true hypertension. Be alert to similar spelling, for example hypotension and hypertension mean the opposite and only one letter in each diagnosis is different.

EXERCISE 5

Directions: Use the Hypertension Table, when applicable, to code the following diagnoses. Begin your search for the correct code by consulting the Index to Diseases and confirming your choice in the Tabular List.

1. Hypertensive cardiorenal disease, malignant   404.0

2. Transient hypertension   796.2

3. Accelerated hypertension   401.0

4. Chronic hypotension   458.1

5. Essential hypertension   642.00

6. Congestive heart failure   _____

7. Hypertensive congestive heart failure   _____

8. Hypertensive renal failure, chronic   _____

REVIEW QUESTIONS FOR DISCUSSION

1. Is there a difference between a late effect and a residual effect?
2. Describe the circumstances of poisoning versus adverse effect.
3. Is "time" a factor in determining a late effect? Why or why not?
4. Show one example of a diagnosis stating hypertension as the cause of another problem, and one example of a diagnosis stating hypertension as the effect of another problem.
5. Explain the difference between hypertension and elevated blood pressure.

Chapter Four

CPT CODES

OBJECTIVES   After completing your study of this chapter, you will be able to

- use the CPT Index to locate the correct procedure code
- define modifiers
- explain bundling, unbundling, and global packaging

POWER WORDS

bundle   To combine preoperative, postoperative, and surgical services into one code and apply one fee for all services.

eponyms   Surgical procedures or diseases named after the physician who developed the procedure or identified the disease.

global package   Carries the same meaning as the bundle.

modifiers   Two-digit numbers attached to procedure codes when additional clarification or special circumstances warrant them.

Physicians' Current Procedural Terminology (CPT)   A listing of descriptive terms and codes for reporting medical services and procedures performed by doctors.

surgical package   Services combined into one code representing the appropriate combination of preoperative, surgical, and postoperative care.

unbundle   Improper coding and billing that breaks apart a surgical package (global package) and results in overcharging the third party or insured.

WHAT ARE CPT CODES?

CPT codes were developed by the American Medical Association in 1966 for the same reasons as the ICD-9-CM codes: to provide detailed terms that are consistent and eliminate confusion or misinterpretation in reporting services rendered to patients. They are five-digit numbers (without any decimal points) that sometimes use two additional numbers called modifiers. New CPT reference manuals must be purchased annually because the codes are updated each October with new additions, deletions, or changes in existing numbers. When the new coding books arrive in the office, the **insurance billing specialist** and our coding specialist must examine them to find any code changes that might specifically impact our office.

HOW ARE CPT CODES USED?

Once the doctor has determined the diagnosis and the correct ICD-9 code(s) has been assigned, the **insurance billing specialist** must locate CPT code(s) to explain what services were rendered. The doctor will mark all preprinted codes on the routing slip, but other services are handwritten and those codes must be identified and added by the **insurance billing specialist**. Most of our staff say CPT codes are easier to work with than ICD-9-CM codes, if only because there are fewer of them. This is good news!

Figure 4-1 shows a circled area of the routing slip for Ms. Altobelli after Dr. Cartman saw her and marked the correct procedure code to describe the office visit.

Since Dr. Cartman marked the correct CPT code on the routing slip, no additional research is needed to find the correct code. Our doctors mark the routing slips routinely for the level of office visit. As you can see by looking at that slip, there are several levels of office visit, depending upon the complexity of the problems presented by the patient. Those decisions are made by the doctors and documented in the patient's chart.

The routing slip for James Byers, Figure 4-2, was only partially completed by the physician. The office visit code is marked, but the doctor only named the procedure he performed. Dr. Cartman listed "I and D of simple perianal abscess." I & D is the abbreviation for incision and drainage. This fee of $85.00 was marked by the receptionist, but she did not list a CPT code. In order to complete the insurance form for this patient, the **insurance billing specialist** will need to find the CPT code for this procedure.

HOW TO LOCATE THE CORRECT CPT CODE

Your CPT manual is divided into sections, starting with Evaluation/Management (E/M) codes and Anesthesia and finishing with Radiology, Pathology, and Medicine. In between, the Surgery section comprises the bulk of the book. These sections are listed from the outside of the body to the inside of the body, and each body system listed starts at the top of the body and describes codes down to the foot of the body. The five-digit CPT codes are listed as follows:

Evaluation & Management   99201 to 99499

These are the face-to-face codes involving examination and consultation, primarily, in the office, the hospital, the nursing home, and elsewhere. *We will not be working with these codes for now.* Our doctors mark their routing sheets very efficiently. You need not begin your examination of CPT codes by working in this area. The other sections we will pass by for now include Anesthesiology, Pathology, and Medicine. Our attention will be focused on the Surgery Section, Laboratory, and the Radiology Section, since these areas are coded often in our practice.

The Surgery Section is broken into major body systems and key procedures. The numerical range follows with a very general and sparse mention of the contents of each batch of numbers. Table 4-1 contains a short list, just to give you the idea.

Medical & Dental Associates, P.C.

3733 Professional Drive #300
Indianapolis, IN 46260

317/123-4567
Tax ID# 99-9999999

Patient name   *Rose Altobelli*

CPT-4 CODES

OFFICE SERVICES	CODE	FEE
New patient, problem focused	99201	
New patient, expanded problem focused	99202	
New patient, detailed	(99203)	60—
New patient, comprehensive, mod.	99204	
New patient, comprehensive, high	99205	
Established patient, RN	99211	
Established patient, problem focused	99212	
Established patient, expanded problem	99213	
Established patient, detailed	99214	
Established patient, comprehensive	99215	
Consultation		

LABORATORY		
X-ray, chest/ribs; single view, frontal	71010	
X-ray, chest/ribs; stereo, frontal	71015	
Therapeutic injections ( )	907__	
Drugs, trays, supplies	99070	
Educational supplies, books, tapes	99071	
Urinalysis, routine, dip stick	81000	
Urine pregnancy test, visual color	81025	
Blood count, hemoglobin	85018	
Pap smear	88150	

ICD-9-CM

DIAGNOSES	
Anxiety reaction	300.00
Bleeding rectal	569.3
Benign prostatic hypertrophy	600
Bronchitis, acute	466.0
Bronchitis, chronic	491.9
Cardiac arrhythmia	427.9
Chest pain	786.50
Cirrhosis of liver	571.5
Conjunctivitis, acute	372.00
Depression	300.4
Flu	487.0
Fracture–nasal, closed	802.0
Fractured tibia	891.2
Headache, vascular	794.0
Herpes zoster	053.9
Irritable bowel syndrome	(564.1)
Menopause	627.2
Myocardial infarction, unspecified	410.90
Otitis, acute	381.01
Pharyngitis, acute	462
Pneumonia	486
Sinusitis, acute	461.9
Tendonitis	726.90
Tennis elbow	726.32
Pregnancy	V22.2
Sprained ankle	842.5
Tonsillitis	474.0
Vertigo	386.0
Well child	V20.2

Bleeding hemorrhoids
455.8

CDT-2 CODES

DENTAL SERVICE

DIAGNOSTIC	CODE	FEE
Periodic exam	00120	
Limited exam	00140	
Comprehensive exam	00150	
Extensive exam	00160	
PREVENTIVE		
Intraoral–FMX	00210	
Intraoral–PA	00220	
BW	0027_	
Single posteroanterior	00290	
Panoramic X-ray	00330	
Prophylaxis adult	01110	
Prophylaxis child	01120	
Topical fluoride	012__	

DENTAL SERVICE

RESTORATIVE	CODE	FEE
Amalgams (decid) Tooth #_____	021__	
Amalgams (perm) Tooth #_____	021__	
CROWNS AND BRIDGES		
PFG crown	02750	
FG cast crown	02790	
3/4 gold cast crown	02810	
FC bridge pontic	06210	
Porcelain bridge ( )	062__	
OTHER PROCEDURES		

DOCTOR'S STATEMENT: I certify that I personally provided the above services and that fees shown represent my usual fees

James P. Cartman, M.D.   *9/1/--*

Signature   Date

TOTAL	$	60—
AMOUNT PAID	$	0
BALANCE DUE	$	60—

FIGURE 4–1 Highlighted CPT-4 codes

Medical & Dental Associates, P.C.

3733 Professional Drive #300
Indianapolis, IN 46260

317/123-4567
Tax ID# 99-9999999

Patient name   *James Byers*

CPT-4 CODES

OFFICE SERVICES	CODE	FEE
New patient, problem focused	99201	
New patient, expanded problem focused	99202	
New patient, detailed	99203	
New patient, comprehensive, mod.	99204	
New patient, comprehensive, high	99205	
Established patient, RN	99211	
Established patient, problem focused	(99212)	*32—*
Established patient, expanded problem	99213	
Established patient, detailed	99214	
Established patient, comprehensive	99215	
Consultation		
I&D perianal abcess		*85—*

LABORATORY	CODE	FEE
X-ray, chest/ribs; single view, frontal	71010	
X-ray, chest/ribs; stereo, frontal	71015	
Therapeutic injections ( )	907__	
Drugs, trays, supplies	99070	
Educational supplies, books, tapes	99071	
Urinalysis, routine, dip stick	81000	
Urine pregnancy test, visual color	81025	
Blood count, hemoglobin	85018	
Pap smear	88150	

ICD-9-CM

DIAGNOSES	
Anxiety reaction	300.00
Bleeding rectal	569.3
Benign prostatic hypertrophy	600
Bronchitis, acute	466.0
Bronchitis, chronic	491.9
Cardiac arrhythmia	427.9
Chest pain	786.50
Cirrhosis of liver	571.5
Conjunctivitis, acute	372.00
Depression	300.4
Flu	487.0
Fracture–nasal, closed	802.0
Fractured tibia	891.2
Headache, vascular	794.0
Herpes zoster	053.9
Irritable bowel syndrome	564.1
Menopause	627.2
Myocardial infarction, unspecified	410.90
Otitis, acute	381.01
Pharyngitis, acute	462
Pneumonia	486
Sinusitis, acute	461.9
Tendonitis	726.90
Tennis elbow	726.32
Pregnancy	V22.2
Sprained ankle	842.5
Tonsillitis	474.0
Vertigo	386.0
Well child	V20.2

Perianal abcess

CDT-2 CODES

DENTAL SERVICE

DIAGNOSTIC	CODE	FEE
Periodic exam	00120	
Limited exam	00140	
Comprehensive exam	00150	
Extensive exam	00160	
PREVENTIVE		
Intraoral–FMX	00210	
Intraoral–PA	00220	
BW	0027_	
Single posteroanterior	00290	
Panoramic X-ray	00330	
Prophylaxis adult	01110	
Prophylaxis child	01120	
Topical fluoride	012__	

DENTAL SERVICE

RESTORATIVE	CODE	FEE
Amalgams (decid) Tooth #_____	021__	
Amalgams (perm) Tooth #_____	021__	
CROWNS AND BRIDGES		
PFG crown	02750	
FG cast crown	02790	
3/4 gold cast crown	02810	
FC bridge pontic	06210	
Porcelain bridge ( )	062__	
OTHER PROCEDURES		

DOCTOR'S STATEMENT: I certify that I personally provided the above services and that fees shown represent my usual fees

James P. Cartman, M.D.   *9/23/--*

Signature   Date

TOTAL	$	*117—*
AMOUNT PAID	$	*0*
BALANCE DUE	$	

FIGURE 4–2 Routing slip

Table 4–1

Integumentary System (Skin and breast and nails)	10040 to 19499
Musculoskeletal System (Muscles and bones—a large section)	20000 to 29909
Respiratory System (Lungs, breathing apparatus)	30000 to 32999
Cardiovascular System (Heart, arteries, blood vessels)	33010 to 37799
Hemic and Lymphatic Systems (Spleen, bone marrow, lymph nodes)	38100 to 38999
Mediastinum and Diaphragm (Look up these in your dictionary!)	39000 to 39599
Digestive System (Lips, mouth, esophagus [food pipe], stomach, liver, intestine, rectum, anus)	40490 to 49999
Urinary System (Kidneys, ureters, bladder, urethra)	50010 to 53899
Male Genital System (Prostate, penis, testicles)	54000 to 55980
Laparoscopy/Peritoneoscopy/Hysteroscopy (Look up these terms also!)	56300 to 56399
Female Genital System (Uterus, ovaries, vagina)	56405 to 58999
Maternity Care and Delivery (Term delivery, C-Section, abortion)	59000 to 59899
Endocrine and Nervous Systems (Ductless glands, brain, spinal cord)	60000 to 64999
Eyes (Iris, lens, cataracts)	65091 to 68899
Ears (Internal and external)	69000 to 69979
Radiology (X-ray), Whole Body, Radiation Treatment, Nuclear Medicine (isotope imaging)	70010 to 79999

EXERCISE 1

Directions: Looking at just these systems and the code ranges of each one, please write below which range you would expect to use in each situation. For example:

1. The doctor removed a fish bone from a young woman's throat.
   Answer: Range 40490 to 40999

2. The doctor assisted a young woman who gave birth to a premature baby.   56405 - 58999

3. The doctor treated a teenager with a chemical peel for severe facial acne.   10400 - 19999

4. The doctor operated on a small child who had a hole in his heart. _____

5. A middle-aged man asked the doctor to perform a vasectomy for permanent birth control. _____

6. The Physician's Assistant removed a jelly bean from a toddler's ear. _____

7. A young woman needed radiation therapy following surgery for breast cancer. _____

8. The doctor treated a woman for a collapsed lung after an auto accident. _____

9. The doctor operated on a severely fractured right leg and fractured right ankle. _____

10. The doctor performed surgery on a young swimmer with a cyst on her spinal cord. _____

11. The doctor performed surgery on a waitress with large kidney stones. _____

12. The doctor removed a piece of glass from a patient's eye. _____

13. The doctor performed surgery to remove infected tonsils from a 6-year-old child. _____

14. The doctor performed surgery to remove an inflamed appendix. _____

HOW TO DETERMINE THE MAIN TERM AND CODE

Finding the *exact* code to use within each range is very much like finding the correct ICD-9-CM code. Begin within the Index at the back of your CPT book. You will see the Index is organized by main terms.

There are four primary classes of main terms.

1. Procedure or service, i.e., Removal, Repair, Reconstruction, Placement, Incision and Drainage

2. Organ or other body site, i.e., Hip, Lung, Liver, Lip, Nail Bed

3. Condition, i.e., Abscess, Blood Clot, Cataract, Cyst, Fracture, Hemorrhage, Lesion, Miscarriage

4. Synonyms, Eponyms, and Abbreviations, i.e., there is an abbreviation in the index of STS. The entry under that states See Syphilis Test; Bricker Operation was developed by Dr. Bricker; Clagett Procedure is listed, followed by Chest Wall, Repair, Closure.

UNDERSTANDING THE INDEX

Whenever more than one code applies to a given entry, a code range is listed in the Index—much smaller than the system ranges we began examining at the beginning of this chapter. This index is telling you where to look to find the code you need. For example, if you are trying to find the code to explain that the doctor amputated a patient's foot, you would find:

Foot

Amputation..........28800, 28805

The index is telling you to look at *both* codes 28800 and 28805 to find the one you really want. The **insurance billing specialist** cannot decide which code to use until after each is carefully examined. In other words, you cannot code from the Index alone! You must go forward to the code numbers listed in the systems sections and find the correct code.

Another way codes are listed includes a greater number of possibilities. For example, if you are trying to find the code to explain that the doctor performed a diagnostic electrocardiogram monitoring test, you would find this in your index:

Cardiology

Diagnostic

Electrocardiogram

Monitoring............93224–93237

This is telling you to look at *all* the codes listed between 93224 and 93237 before deciding which code is correct. Again, the **insurance billing specialist** cannot code by only using the Index. The specific system and specific code range(s) must be looked at before the best choice can be made. It is also common to have the codes listed like this:

........93313–93314, 93350

In this situation, you must look at all three numbers before making your selection.

EXERCISE 2

Directions: Look up these index listings and write down the codes you find.
For example, Lesion
    Breast
        Excision .... <u>19120</u>

1. Acne treatment
    Abrasion .... _____

2. Eyebrow
    Repair
        Ptosis.. _____

3. Removal
    Ear Wax
        Auditory Canal, External .... _____

4. Flu Shots... _____

5. Eyelid
    Reconstruction
        Total Eyelid, Lower .... _____

6. Fitting
    Contact Lens.. _____

7. Reflex Test
    Blink Reflex .... _____

8. Urinalysis
    Pregnancy Test .... _____

9. Radiology
    Therapeutic Planning.............................. _____

10. Incision
    Bladder with Destruction......................... _____

CPT CODE INDENTATIONS

Notice the main terms have subterms indented beneath them, getting more and more indented as greater detail is listed. In going forward from the Index to find the correct code, you will see the same kind of indentation.

For example, look up this main term in the index:

Incision and Drainage

Abscess

Ovary

Vaginal Approach................58820

Now, go forward to code 58820. Notice that the code within the Female Genital System looks like this:

58820 Drainage of ovarian abscess; vaginal approach

This is the code you wanted. Congratulations!! Take special note of the location of the semicolon just before the words "vaginal approach."

☛ The placement of the semicolon is extremely important to the coder.

For example, suppose you had wanted to find the code for:

Incision and Drainage

Abscess

Ovary

Abdominal Approach........58822

Look at 58822 in your CPT manual. It is presented as an indented phrase under the listing for the 58820 code already found. What is the relationship between codes 58820 and 58822? You will observe a very important feature of CPT code listings: the basic and vital method of *finding and reading the correct code* in all sections of the book! Code 58822 is to be read in your mind as if it appeared just to the right of the semicolon in the 58820 code as follows:

58822 Drainage of ovarian abscess; abdominal approach

Apparently, the makers of this coding system decided against repeating the whole coding phrase for each code number. If they had not made that decision, there would be no indented phrases in the coding book and codes 58820 and 58822 might be printed like this:

58820 Drainage of ovarian abscess; vaginal approach

58822 Drainage of ovarian abscess; abdominal approach

Likewise, look in your manual at codes 31200 and 31201, 31205 beneath. If the developers of the coding system had decided to spell out each code, those three codes might look like this:

31200 Ethmoidectomy; intranasal, anterior

31201 Ethmoidectomy; intranasal, total

31205 Ethmoidectomy; extranasal, total

As you examine the entire coding book, imagine how thick it would be if all the indented phrases were printed with all the words to the left of the semicolon!

Some codes have lots of indented phrases beneath them and some have none. Look in your CPT book at code:

31622 Bronchoscopy; diagnostic, (flexible or rigid), with or without cell washing or brushing

There are many numbers and indented phrases beneath this code. If the **insurance billing specialist** needs to find the code for a bronchoscopy with excision of tumor, the CPT Index would send you to:

31640 with excision of tumor

The phrase by itself does not make much sense. You must read that phrase to include the term "Bronchoscopy" to the left of the semicolon next to code 31622. In your mind, you see:

31640 Bronchoscopy; with excision of tumor

Look in your Index for the code for Incision and Drainage of one carbuncle. Follow the steps below to get the correct procedure code:

Step 1. Find Incision and Drainage in the Index

Step 2. Look for carbuncle

Step 3. Identify the coding range

Step 4. Examine the choices and make your decision

There are two choices, 10060 or 10061. Go to that section in your CPT manual and examine those two choices.

Code 10060 is:

Incision and drainage of abscess (e.g., carbuncle, suppurative hidradenitis, cutaneous or subcutaneous abscess, cyst, furuncle, or paronychia); simple or single.

Code 10061 is an indented statement that is to be read as if it said:

Incision and drainage of abscess (e.g., carbuncle, suppurative hidradenitis, cutaneous or subcutaneous abscess, cyst, furuncle, or paronychia); complicated or multiple.

Both these codes mention the carbuncle and both describe an incision and drainage. Code 10060 is correct because it specifically describes a single carbuncle and that matches your coding statement. Again, the difference between those two codes is contained to the right of the semicolon. Understanding this rule is mandatory to finding the correct code.

Technically, you do not need to understand the words and terms you are coding to select the right ones, although we strongly recommend you form the habit of using the medical dictionary to build your vocabulary and avoid any possible errors. What you *must* do is look closely and match your procedural statement to the coding book. While the physician may not express exactly the same words in the same order as your coding book, the variations will be close enough to allow you to determine which statement is appropriate. With time, your vocabulary will grow and after repeated usage and some research, you will come to understand a great deal about the common procedures performed in this office as well as in the hospital.

EXERCISE 3

Directions: Locate the correct CPT code in the Index and confirm your selection in the correct system.

1. Application of finger splint, static   29130

2. Emergency endotracheal intubation   _____

3. Uvulectomy, excision of uvula   42140

4. Repair of iris, ciliary body   66680

5. Revision of arthroplasty, including removal of implant, wrist joint   _____

6. Change of cystostomy tube, complicated   _____

7. Biopsy, muscle, deep   _____

8. Excision of hydrocele, bilateral   _____

9. Excision of mediastinal cyst   _____

10. Excision of lesion of tongue with closure, posterior one-third   _____

11. Renal autotransplantation, reimplantation of kidney   _____

12. Lung transplant, double, with cardiopulmonary bypass   _____

13. Myringotomy including aspiration and eustachian tube inflation   _____

14. Frontal chest radiologic examination, stereo   _____

15. Partial splenectomy   _____

MULTIPLE CODES AND MODIFIERS

Sometimes it is appropriate to use more than one indented statement to fully code the procedure, or to use the unindented and indented statements together. For example, how would we code these procedures: "laryngoscopy, indirect, with removal of lesion and vocal cord injection"?

Look at codes 31505 to 31513 in your CPT manual. You know you may use 31512 and read it as if it was one complete sentence, beginning "laryngoscopy, indirect; with removal of lesion." Now add code 31513 to the answer, and the statement reads "laryngoscopy, indirect, with removal of lesion, with vocal cord injection." This is what we are looking to code. Therefore, the answer is 31512 AND 31513-51. What is -51?

The -51 is a two-digit modifier that states more than one procedure was done at the same time. The two-digit modifier may be attached to the five-digit code. Appendix A of your CPT manual lists all the numerical modifiers and the front of the Surgery Section of your CPT book lists the modifiers most commonly used with surgery codes. A second way of expressing modifiers is to add the three digits 099- in front of the two-digit modifier and create a five-digit code which is then placed on a line of the insurance form all by itself. You will practice this later in this manual.

The **insurance billing specialist** may use multiple codes to accurately describe the treatments applied to the patient. You must take special care, however, to ensure that you are not unbundling a surgical package code. In CPT surgical coding, preoperative and postoperative care is normally included with each procedure (unless otherwise stated) and one fee is set to cover all services before, during, and after an uncomplicated surgery. If complications develop and additional surgery is needed, one of several steps may be taken depending upon the situation.

LIST OF MODIFIERS

Here is a quick summary of the CPT modifiers effective in 1997:

-20 Microsurgery: This modifier indicates an operating microscope was needed during a surgery that ordinarily does not include this instrument. Documentation showing why the scope was necessary should be included.

-21 Prolonged E & M services: Used with the highest level code to show that even more time and/or a greater level of intensity was required in a specific situation.

-22 Unusual services: Applied when surgical services are more extensive or difficult due to any number of complicating factors, and higher payment is requested as a result.

-23 Unusual anesthesia: Used in those patient encounters when general anesthesia is required for procedures normally calling for no anesthesia or only local anesthesia.

-24 Unrelated E & M service by the same physician during a postoperative period: This modifier is designed to avoid the appearance of unbundling a surgical package; used in those situations where the patient develops a different medical problem requiring treatment during the post-op period of another medical problem.

-25 Significant, separately identifiable E & M service performed by the same physician on the same day as a minor surgical procedure.

-26 Professional/physician component of a service: Shows interpretation only of diagnostic tests.

-32 Mandated services: Related to consultations required by a third-party, as in a mandatory second opinion for certain anticipated surgeries.

-47 Anesthesia by surgeon: Not referring to local or topical anesthesia, but to general anesthesia administered by the surgeon.

-50 Bilateral procedure: Used when unilateral procedures or tests are administered bilaterally for those codes not otherwise stating that a procedure is bilateral. Example: bilateral nipple reconstruction would be shown as 19350 and 19350-50.

-51 Multiple surgeries by the same physician on the same day: Used only for those services that are not designated as add-on services and are not E & M codes. List the procedure codes in the order of most costly first, next most costly second, third most costly third, etc. The modifier -51 is added to all procedure codes *after* the first.

-52 Reduced services: Used when the service is less complicated than described by the code or when the service is eliminated. Documentation to explain the circumstances is required.

-53 Discontinued procedure: This modifier is used when the doctor decides on early termination of a procedure for the well-being of the patient. Attach this modifier to the procedure code that had been planned to be fully completed.

-54 Surgical care only: Used to show only surgical and pre-op care were administered to the patient with a second physician applying post-op care.

-55 Postoperative management only.

-56 Preoperative management only.

-57 Visit or consult day before or day of major surgery, when the decision for surgery was made during the visit.

-58 Staged or related procedure or service planned by the same physician to be done during the postoperative period.

-59 Distinct procedural service: Shows that a service or procedure was independent and distinct from other services performed on the same day. This is used to show true medical necessity when two procedures not usually performed together are reported.

-62 Two surgeons: Used to show the need for two surgeons and each one should use the modifier.

-66 Surgical team: Used with documentation in those situations requiring numbers of trained technicians and physicians.

-76 Repeat procedure by the same physician.

-77 Repeat procedure done by another physician than the original.

-78 Return to the operating room for a related or unrelated procedure during the postoperative period: Used to explain an unforseen complication and the subsequent surgical intervention.

-79 Unrelated procedure or service by the same physician during the postoperative period.

-80 Assistant surgeon.

-81 Minimum assistant surgeon.

-82 Assistant surgeon: Used by physician when a qualified resident surgeon is not available to assist.

-90 Reference to outside laboratory: Used when lab procedures are performed by someone other than the reporting physician.

-99 Multiple modifiers.

EXERCISE 4

Directions: Find the correct CPT code(s) and modifier(s) for the following services:

1. Bilateral removal of mammary implant material   19330-50

2. Replantation, thumb including distal tip to MP joint, complete amputation, during gallbladder post-op period, same MD   _____

3. Confirmatory consultation required by insurance company, including comprehensive history and exam and medical decision making of moderate complexity   _____

4. Brain imaging, complete study; static, interpretation only   _____

5. Excision, malignant lesion on the neck, .7 cm, surgical care only   _____

6. Repeat application of long arm splint done previously by another physician   _____

7. Individual medical psychotherapy scheduled for 45 minutes but discontinued for the well-being of the patient   _____

8. Physician assisted in the surgical procedure Craniotomy with excision of foreign body from brain; minimum assistance   _____

9. Vasectomy requiring general anesthesia, not usual   _____

10. Caesarean delivery including postpartum care and total hysterectomy   _____

REVIEW QUESTIONS FOR DISCUSSION

1. What two ways may modifiers be expressed?
2. What is the purpose of the semicolon within the description of a procedure in your CPT manual?
3. Why is it important not to unbundle a surgical package?
4. Give an example of a deliberate unbundling.
5. May modifiers be used anywhere in the CPT manual?

Chapter Five

HCPCS CODES

OBJECTIVES   After completing your study of this chapter, you will be able to

- define HCPCS codes and modifiers
- explain the format of the HCPCS book
- understand when and how to use HCPCS codes and modifiers
- define the three levels of HCPCS usage

POWER WORDS

adjudication   The process of examining insurance claims for payment.

Advanced Life Support (ALS) Ambulance Service   Includes at least one paramedic crew member and sufficient medical equipment to apply life-saving techniques.

alphanumerical codes   Begin with a letter of the alphabet and are followed by numbers, such as code J1820 found in the HCPCS manual.

Basic Life Support (BLS) Ambulance Service   Includes at least one crew member trained in first aid techniques at the Emergency Medical Technician (EMT) level but not a paramedic.

Durable Medical Equipment Regional Carriers (DMERCS)   Four regional carriers designated to process all claims for durable medical equipment when prescribed for Medicare patients.

Federal Register   The government's official publication of daily business conducted including the results of normal government transactions, enacted laws, and revisions.

Fiscal Intermediary (FI)   The insurance company adjudicating Medicare claims in each state or region.

generic name   The official chemical name assigned to a drug. A given name is licensed under its generic name and all manufacturers of the drug must list it by its generic name. However, a drug is usually marketed under a trade name chosen by the manufacturer.

HCPCS (pronounced hicks-picks) Health Care Financing Administration Common Procedure Coding System	A listing of codes and modifiers used to report supplies, injections, materials, and certain other specific services and procedures to Medicare for reimbursement following appropriate administration to the patient; codes revised yearly.
neonate	A baby from birth to four weeks of age.
prophylaxis	Preventive care.
route of administration	Term used to explain how drug or substance gets inside the body of the patient.
systemic	Affecting the entire body.

HCPCS CODE LEVELS

There are three levels of Medicare coding: National Level I, National Level II, Local Level III.

National Level I codes are all the CPT codes, except anesthesiology, published and updated annually for the AMA as discussed in Chapter 4.

National Level II codes are those we call the HCPCS codes with alphanumerical ranges of A0000 through V5999. These codes are applied to the supplies, medications, therapeutic substances, medical equipment, and certain specialized services needed by the patient. Examples include codes for wheelchairs, crutches, medications taken other than orally (except for certain immunosuppressive drugs), transportation services to and from treatment locations, artificial limbs, dental procedure codes (for Medicare patients only), blood for transfusion, and much more.

Local Level III codes are developed for each state or region by the local Medicare fiscal intermediary. These codes use alphanumerical ranges W0000 through Z9999 and might describe a given supply or medication or service as defined by a particular state or region. This classification of codes is expected to be discontinued in a few years in compliance with the National Correct Coding Primer policy aimed at national standardization. However, the **insurance billing specialist** must continue to read the monthly newsletters from the state or regional fiscal interme-

diary and note any regional changes until Local Level III codes are officially discontinued.

APPLYING HCPCS CODES

Even though HCPCS Level II National codes have been in use since 1983, many offices are not aware of these codes and/or do not use them appropriately. The **insurance billing specialist** must not shrink away from using this coding system to describe the supplies and injections used by physicians. While these codes are required to describe supplies and equipment sold or rented to Medicare patients, most other insurance carriers also recognize their use. In some cases, a specific insurance carrier may disregard or ignore or even deny HCPCS Level II or Level III codes on your claims or may send you a list of codes preferred by them alone. If this happens, you will need to adjust to those specific requirements for the affected patients.

☛ It is our policy to submit Level II and III codes when appropriate to encourage the acceptance of these codes by all insurance carriers, not just Medicare, and to aid in establishing a uniform and consistent coding policy among all insurance carriers.

Years ago, the HCFA insurance form was not recognized by a majority of insurance carriers; yet today, about 97 percent of insurance carriers accept claims submitted on this form. Therefore, we are applying Level II and III HCPCS codes consistently with the belief that eventually, these codes will be recognized and accepted as a standard in the health care industry in the same way the HCFA insurance form is now an industry standard.

Very rarely, there may be a duplication of code definitions within the three levels. If there is any confusion about which HCPCS codes to use, remember in the eyes of the Medicare FI:

☞ Local Level III codes have priority over National Levels I and II.

☞ National Level II codes have priority over National Level I.

The one exception to this rule is the HCPCS dental codes that we use when we file Medicare dental claims only. All other times, we use Current Dental Terminology, Second Edition codes published by the American Dental Association as discussed in Chapter 6. Again, when we learn with certainty that a particular insurance company consistently requires a different coding system for a specific service, we adapt to that company's requirement. Overall, we maintain a standardized coding system in our office and that approach has saved us more money in maximizing our reimbursement than it has cost us in time lost due to resubmissions.

HCPCS MANUAL FORMAT

HCPCS National II Level Medicare codes are released by the Health Care Financing Administration each November and recorded first in the Federal Register. Several private companies then publish the codes to sell to providers' offices. The exact layout of your HCPCS book is entirely dependent upon the publisher of the one you are using. However, the same basic information is included in all reputable manuals regardless of any specific features that certain publishers might prefer to include.

The heart of all HCPCS Level II books is divided into twenty sections with the supplies, services, and equipment grouped alphanumerically within each section as shown in Table 5–1.

BEGIN TO USE HCPCS MANUAL

Turn to the Index in your HCPCS National Level II Medicare code book. Looking at the Index, you will notice great similarities between this Index and the CPT Index. The HCPCS Index displays all listings alphabetically on the left side of each page with the correct alphanumeric code or code range given on the right side of the page.

☞ Again, the **insurance billing specialist** must never code from the Index, but must locate a possible code and verify that code in the Tabular section of the book.

For example, how do we find the code for an elastic bandage?

First, look in the HCPCS Index under the letter "E" and find the word "Elastic."

Second, under "Elastic," locate the indented subheading "bandage" and make a notation of the code you find.

Third, go to the alphabetical section shown by the first letter of the code and locate the code you want. It simply states "Elastic Bandage." Is this the correct code?

As with CPT codes, HCPCS codes also may be indented and must be read in the same way CPT codes are read. For example, look at code A4398. It states, "bags." We know it is dependent upon the full statement located above and to the left of the semicolon. Therefore, we read code A4398 as if it said in print, "Irrigation supply; bags."

Likewise, code A4399 is read as if it said in print, "Irrigation supply; cone/catheter." After the work you have completed with CPT codes, this will be easier for you to grasp.

Table 5–1

Transportation Services	A0000 to A0999
Chiropractic Services	A2000 to A2999
Medical and Surgical Supplies	A4000 to A4999
Miscellaneous and Experimental	A9000 to A9999
Enteral and Parenteral Therapy	B4000 to B9999
Dental Procedures (Medicare Claims Only)	D0000 to D9999
Durable Medical Equipment (DME)	E0000 to E9999
Procedures/Services Temporary	G0000 to G9999
Rehabilitative Services	H5000 to H5999
Drugs Administered Other Than Oral Method (with the exception of Immunosuppressive Drugs)	J0000 to J8999
Chemotherapy Drugs	J9000 to J9999
Temporary Codes for DMERCS	K0000 to K9999
Orthotic Procedures	L0000 to L4999
Prosthetic Procedures	L5000 to L9999
Medical Services	M0000 to M9999
Pathology and Laboratory	P0000 to P9999
Temporary Codes	Q0000 to Q0099
Diagnostic Radiology Services	R0000 to R5999
Vision Services	V0000 to V2999
Hearing Services	V5000 to V5999

EXERCISE 1

Directions: Use the Index to locate the codes for the following items and verify them in the Tabular section of your HCPCS book.

1. Syringe, sterile, 20cc or greater _____

2. Paraffin _____

3. Adhesive remover or solvent _____

4. Ambulance waiting time (ALS or BLS), one-half-hour increments _____

5. Manipulation of spine by chiropractor _____

6. Crutches, underarm, aluminum, adjustable or fixed; pair with pads, tips and handgrip _____

7. Electrodes for apnea monitor _____

8. Lancets, 1 box _____

9. Contact lens, PMMA; bifocal, per lens _____

10. Surgical trays _____

11. Red blood cells, each unit _____

12. Thoracic, rib belt; custom fabricated _____

13. Foot rest, for use with commode chair, each _____

14. Topical application of fluoride (including prophylaxis), child _____

15. Stomach tube—Levine type _____

16. Occupational therapy _____

17. Repair of prosthetic device, labor component, per 15 minutes _____

18. Hand restoration (shading and measurements included), replacement glove for above _____

19. Speech screening _____

20. Walker, wheeled, without seat _____

USING HCPCS MODIFIERS

HCPCS National Level II Modifiers serve the same general functions as CPT modifiers: they provide additional information designed to achieve accurate reimbursement and/or to assist in gathering data about health care recipients. A complete list of current HCPCS modifiers may be found in Appendix A.

While CPT modifiers are all numerical, HCPCS modifiers are either alphabetical or alphanumerical (i.e., AA or E1).

☛ CPT modifiers may be used with CPT or HCPCS codes and HCPCS modifiers may be used with HCPCS or CPT codes in any combination.

While there are only 30 CPT modifiers, there are many more HCPCS modifiers. In the front of each of the twenty sections of the HCPCS manual is a listing of those HCPCS modifiers most commonly associated with that section. This is helpful in reminding the **insurance billing specialist** to use modifiers when appropriate, but you are not restricted to any particular ones and may discover that a different modifier or two more clearly describes the special circumstances or extenuating facts. HCPCS modifiers appear next to the CPT and/or HCPCS codes on the insurance form as discussed in Chapter 4.

HCPCS REVISION LISTS

Appendix B lists a summary of the HCPCS changes in the current issue versus the previous one. Be sure to check for new codes, deleted codes, and revised codes when your new reference book arrives each year. There are always changes listed and sometimes they can be extremely important and significant to this practice.

APPLYING APPENDIX C

Appendix C is a very important tool for the **insurance billing specialist**. It presents an alphabetical listing of drugs by their generic names. When a drug is known only by the trade name or brand name, look for the brand name in the Index or in Appendix C. There, you will be directed to the generic name. Next to the generic name in Appendix C is information about the dosage; in the next column are the route(s) of administration to give the medication to the patient, if appropriate. On the far right side of the page is the HCPCS code for that drug. Go forward to the "J" section to find the correct code and the dosage amount considered to be one billing unit.

All drugs are in the "J" section. Drugs are listed by generic name in the Index without additional information about route of administration and dosage amount. Again, if a drug is known chiefly by the brand name, find that name in Appendix C and the generic name will be listed. Therefore, the **insurance billing specialist** may find drug codes under the generic or brand name in Appendix C.

Sometimes, both Appendix C and the Index may be used to be sure the correct code is located. For example, look in the Index for the drug with the brand name "Decadron." Make a note of the number listed. Go to the Tabular section and locate the code in the "J" section. How can you be sure you have the correct drug since you do not see the name "Decadron?" Look for Decadron in Appendix C and note it says "see Dexamethasone sodium phosphate," which was the phrase you saw within the definition of code J1100. In the future, you may want to save time by working just within Appendix C.

Certain abbreviations used in the route of administration column of the manual may be found in the front of Appendix C. These abbreviations include the measurement or common dosage form of the medication or substance in addition to the route of administration.

IMMUNIZATION CODES

A number of immunization codes may be found in your CPT book in the Medicine section. Those codes are used often in well-baby care, for example. Remember, HCPCS codes have priority over CPT codes in Medicare billing, especially in the case of coding statements that appear to be duplicated in both books, and with other major carriers. Therefore, look first for the drug code you want in the HCPCS book and if it is not there, consult your CPT manual.

EXERCISE 2

Directions: Locate the correct HCPCS codes for the following substances:

1. Injection, kutapressin, 2 ml   _____

2. Prednisolone, oral, per 5 mg   _____

3. Injection, tetracycline, 200 mg   _____

4. Injection, gamma globulin, IM, 9 cc   _____

5. Prescription drug, oral chemotherapy, for malignant disease   _____

6. Injection, insulin, 80 units   _____

7. Mitomycin, 30 mg   _____

8. Infusion, dextran 40, 400 ml   _____

9. Deca-Durabolin, 40 mg   _____

10. Primaxin, 250 mg   _____

11. Tetanus immune globulin, human, 200 units   _____

12. Iron dextran, 4 cc   _____

CASE STUDY ABSTRACTS

Now that you have practiced locating HCPCS codes in your manual, let's try coding a few specific situations, including the appropriate modifiers. For example:

HCPCS CASE STUDY #1

Miss H. was driving her car to work when she was struck broadside by Miss W. The police arrived and called the ABC Ambulance Service to stabilize Miss H. and take her to the nearest hospital. The ambulance service submitted a claim to Miss H.'s insurance company stating that a Basic Life Support emergency ambulance transported the patient from the accident site to the hospital five miles away. The fee of $300.00 included all services, materials, and mileage fees, along with a 15-minute wait before the patient could be transported.

How did the ABC Ambulance Service billing specialist code these fees for submission to the insurance company? What steps must be taken?

1. Locate the range of codes for Ambulance Service in your HCPCS manual. _____

2. What is the name of this section of the manual? _____

3. Read the Guidelines about this section. How many modifiers are listed? _____

4. What is the modifier for "Scene of the accident or acute event?" _____

5. What is the modifier for "Hospital?" _____

6. What is the modifier stating "Ambulance trip from the scene of the accident to a hospital?" _____

7. Turning to the Transportation Services codes, what is the code stating "Ambulance service; basic life support (BLS), non-emergency transport, supplies included, mileage separately billed"? _____

8. Is this the correct code for this case study? _____

9. What is the correct code and why? _____

10. What is the correct code with the modifier added? _____

HCPCS CASE STUDY #2

Mr. L. was at his vacation residence with his family when he became ill. Because of his history of heart disease, his wife called 911 and an Advanced Life Support (ALS) ambulance soon arrived. After examination and stabilization by the paramedics on board, it was not thought Mr. L. had a heart problem but the decision was made to transport him to the hospital for possible gallbladder surgery. This was not an emergency transport, no specialized services were rendered, and the bill for $250.00 included all supplies and mileage.

Code(s) _____

HCPCS CASE STUDY #3

A critically ill neonate was transported via ambulance from the hospital where he was born to another hospital specializing in his systemic disease.

Code(s) _____

HCPCS CASE STUDY #4

Mrs. B. was en route to the hospital in an ALS ambulance because her doctor thought she might have had another heart attack at the nursing home where she resides. This was an emergency transport and the Heartline Ambulance Service normally bills separately for disposable supplies and mileage. Unexpectedly, Mrs. B. began to show signs of a convulsive seizure and other life-threatening problems. The paramedic secured her airway with an esophageal intubation and started IV drug therapy.

Code(s) _____

REVIEW QUESTIONS FOR DISCUSSION

1. When and why are HCPCS codes used?
2. Do HCPCS codes take priority over CPT codes if there is a duplication of codes in both books? Why or why not?
3. May any health care provider use HCPCS codes?
4. How long have HCPCS codes been in common usage?
5. Do Local Level HCPCS codes precede National Level codes? Why or why not?

Chapter Six

CDT-2 DENTAL CODES

OBJECTIVES After completing your study of this chapter, you will be able to

- define CDT-2 codes
- outline the nine sections of the CDT-2 manual
- explain the twelve categories of CDT-2 codes
- understand when and how to use CDT-2 codes
- contrast the difference between CDT-2 codes and HCPCS "D" codes

POWER WORDS

accounts receivable (A/R) The amount of money left unpaid by insurance or not yet paid by any third party; the list of outstanding dollars or unpaid bills owed to our Association physicians.

American Dental Association (ADA) A nonprofit organization of dentists and dental specialists devoted to furthering the professional development of its members; to educating the public about its members and their services; and to establishing policies that ensure the highest standards of quality of care.

Council on Dental Benefit Programs A policy of uniform standards of communication through uniform coding; a division of the ADA.

Current Dental Terminology, Second Edition (CDT-2) The coding system designed by the American Dental Association for use in submitting claims to dental insurance companies for reimbursement to the dentists.

predetermination The process of submitting a proposed treatment plan to the dental insurance company for approval prior to beginning the work.

AMERICAN DENTAL ASSOCIATION CODING— CDT-2, SECOND EDITION, 1995–2000

The fourth coding system used by Medical & Dental Associates, P.C., is the American Dental Association (ADA) system, Current Dental Terminology, Second Edition, 1995 - 2000 (CDT-2), for non-Medicare claims. CDT-1 was introduced in 1991 after four years of research with information gathered from all sectors of the dental field, including insurers, by the Council on Dental Benefit Programs. It was designed to serve as a tool to accurately report services provided by dentists to their non-Medicare patients. It soon became necessary to expand the coding system and include greater specificity with the advisory that CDT-2 codes are *not* open to interpretation but are to be used exactly as described, as are all the coding systems explained to the **insurance billing specialist**.

The Second Edition of Current Dental Terminology outlines the time frame of 1995 to 2000. Whether this means a completely new dental coding system will be introduced after the year 2000 is unknown. The ADA has expressed its intention to revise and update this coding system in the same timely fashion as the other coding agencies. Therefore, we will need to be attentive to periodic coding revisions and updates within this system.

The CDT-2 code manual is divided into nine sections with twelve service and procedure categories. CDT-2 uses a five-digit numerical system identical to HCPCS "D" codes except the CDT-2 codes begin with the "0" digit instead of the letter "D". This was no accident, but contractually agreed to by both the Health Care Financing Administration, which governs the Medicare program, and the American Dental Association, which developed the CDT-2 coding system. While Medicare has no coverage for routine or preventive dental care or routine tooth or gum treatment, Medicare coverage is available for situations requiring the attention of an oral surgeon. In these cases, the oral surgeon would be required to use the HCPCS codes on the regular health care form, the HCFA-1500, or any CPT codes as appropriate. In other words, the **insurance billing specialist** would not submit any ADA claim forms or use CDT-2 codes for services rendered to the Medicare patient.

CDT-2 MANUAL LAYOUT

The first section of the CDT-2 manual includes the following list of service categories and applicable code ranges:

I.	Diagnostic	00100 to 00999
II.	Preventive	01000 to 01999
III.	Restorative	02000 to 02999
IV.	Endodontics	03000 to 03999
V.	Periodontics	04000 to 04999
VI.	Prosthodontics, removable	05000 to 05899
VII.	Maxillofacial Prosthetics	05900 to 05999
VIII.	Implant Services	06000 to 06199
IX.	Prosthodontics, fixed	06200 to 06999
X.	Oral Surgery	07000 to 07999
XI.	Orthodontics	08000 to 08999
XII.	Adjunctive General Services	09000 to 09999

The second section of the CDT-2 manual is titled "Code on Dental Procedures and Nomenclature," and lists all the codes along with detailed explanations of each one. The third section of the CDT-2 manual lists all codes without detailed descriptions and includes a summary of the additions, deletions and revisions of the 1995 codes. Section Four is a glossary of common dental terms, written for those without formal dental training, and Section Five is a glossary of terms called "Dental Benefit Terminology" defining those terms commonly used in communication with third-party insurers. Many of these terms are shared by other physicians and some are specific to the specialty of dentistry. Many terms will be introduced to the **insurance billing specialist** here and in Chapter 13.

Section Six presents a diagram of the jaw and teeth with all parts named and identified and Section Seven explains the tooth numbering system used in our office and most other dental offices. Section Eight shows the ADA dental form and explains how each line item is to be completed. This information appears on the back of all ADA forms published by the American Dental Association and some other suppliers. In Chapter 13, we will discuss these instructions in detail as we practice completing ADA forms.

Finally, Section Nine is the Index you will consult when working to locate the correct CDT-2 code to apply. As with your CPT code book, this index displays the terms in alphabetical order on the left side of the page with the code or code ranges on the right side. Note these code ranges are often abbreviated. For example, the code for fluoride, topical, is listed as 01201-05. At first glance, the -05 may appear to be some type of modifier similar to those used in CPT. This is not the case. The entry is used to mean the code is between 01201 and 01205. Next to the code number(s), the ADA manual includes page number references to guide you to the correct pages immediately. The references include the listing of the detailed definition of the code and the nondefined code.

EXERCISE 1

Directions: Using only your CDT-2 manual, please supply the answers to the following questions:

1. What is the definition of code 03110, pulp cap—direct (excluding final restoration)?

   _____

   _____

2. What is the definition of the procedure scaling?

   _____

   _____

3. What is the CDT-2 code for myotomy? _____

4. What is the definition of myotomy? _____

   _____

   _____

5. What is the definition of the term "maximum allowance"?

   _____

   _____

6. What is the difference between CDT-2 codes and HCPCS dental codes?

   _____

   _____

7. How are permanent teeth numbered?

   _____

   _____

8. How are "baby teeth" or primary teeth numbered?

_____

_____

9. What CDT-2 codes are included in the range for Anesthesia in the Orthodontics section?

_____

_____

10. Is Anesthesia listed in any other section of the CDT-2 codes?

_____

_____

11. The common term for radiograph is_____

12. How are space maintenance or passive appliances used?

_____

_____

13. What is the definition of the term "Imaging, Diagnostic"?

_____

_____

EXERCISE 2

Directions: Using your CDT-2 Index, match the following terms with the definitions listed beneath them. Place the correct letter next to the number of the definition.

a) apex   b) denture   c) decay   d) caries   e) coronal   f) cavity

g) jaw   h) bridge   i) pontic   j) avulsion   k) unerupted   l) adhesive

m) temporomandibular joint (TMJ)   n) bruxism   o) alveolar   p) splint   q) by report   r) root

s) curettage   t) pulp   u) enamel   v) plaque   x) labial   y) enamel

z) dry socket

1. _____ the lay term for carious lesions in a tooth; decomposition of tooth structure.

2. _____ a fixed (or removable) partial denture which is a prosthetic replacement of one or more missing teeth cemented or attached to the abutment teeth.

3. _____ the connecting hinge mechanism between the lower jaw and base of the skull.

4. _____ pertaining to or around the lip.

5. _____ the portion of the tooth located in the socket where it is attached to the periodontal apparatus.

6. _____ the tip or end of the root end of the tooth.

7. _____ grinding the teeth.

8. _____ referring to the bone to which a tooth is attached.

9. _____ refers to the crown or top of the tooth.

10. _____ hard calcified tissue covering dentin of the crown of tooth.

11. _____ an artificial substitute for natural teeth and adjacent tissues.

12. _____ a common name for either the maxilla or the mandible.

13. _____ the term used for the artificial tooth on a fixed partial denture (bridge).

14. _____ commonly used term for tooth decay.

15. _____ decay in tooth caused by caries; also referred to as carious lesion.

16. _____ tooth/teeth that have not penetrated into the oral cavity.

17. _____ a device used to support, protect, or immobilize oral structures that have been loosened, replanted, fractured or traumatized. Also refers to devices used in the treatment of TMJ disorders.

18. _____ separation of tooth from its socket due to trauma.

19. _____ a soft sticky substance that accumulates on teeth composed largely of bacteria and bacterial derivatives.

20. _____ any substance that joins or creates close adherence of two or more surfaces.

21. _____ the blood vessels and nerve tissue that occupy the pulp cavity of a tooth.

22. _____ a narrative description used to report a service that does not have a procedure code or is specified in a code as "by report."

23. _____ scraping or cleaning the walls of a cavity or gingival pocket.

24. _____ hard calcified tissue covering dentin of the crown of tooth.

25. _____ localized inflammation of the tooth socket following extraction due to infection or loss of blood clot; osteitis.

DENTAL PATIENT INFORMATION

The Confidential Patient Information Record, transmittal slip and ledger card for the dental patient is the same as the forms used for nondental patients. A Dental Treatment Record must be prepared for each patient such as the one in Figure 6-1 for Nancy J. Hawkins.

The receptionist or chair-side dental assistant normally begins entering information on the Dental Treatment Record as well as the dentist or dental hygienist if services are required. All office personnel providing dental care to the patient must enter information about those services onto the Dental Treatment Record. Treatment rendered and treatment needed in the future are both recorded and both kinds of information will be used by the **insurance billing specialist** to get payment for services already rendered as well as authorization for treatments still needed to be done.

The selection of the correct CDT-2 code is done either through completion of the Dental Routing Slip or through a series of steps that are followed for each service if the Dental Routing Slip has not been completed for the **insurance billing specialist.** If the Dental Routing Slip has been completed for the patient by the dentist and/or other, then completion of the ADA form may proceed. (See Chapter 13). Otherwise, the **insurance billing specialist** must follow these steps in locating the proper dental service:

☛ Review the patient's chart and determine what service was provided, including which tooth or teeth were involved and the surfaces of the tooth/teeth treated.

☛ Read the descriptions of the codes in the subdivision until the matching procedural description is found and select the correct CDT-2 code.

☛ Establish the fee for each service rendered according to the Dental Fee Schedule used in this office.

DENTAL COVERAGE PREDETERMINATION

The **insurance billing specialist** will routinely check the patient record to be certain the dental insurance carrier has been contacted and the predetermination of insurance coverage has been completed. Normally, the receptionist or other staff member is responsible for this detail. The authorization is requested by marking an ADA dental claim form for "predetermination" and completing the form, without date of service or physician signature, as shown on Figure 6-2.

This incomplete ADA form is sent to the dental insurance carrier. When the form is approved and returned to us by the dental insurance carrier, the proposed procedure can be scheduled and completed. The patient will be notified of the part of the bill, if any, the dental insurance carrier will not cover and payment arrangements will be made with the Accounts Receivable department. Once the dental work is completed, this same form will be dated and signed and resubmitted for payment.

DENTAL TREATMENT RECORD
Medical & Dental Associates, P.C.

Name Nancy J. Hawkins

Parent or Guardian —

Occupation Homemaker

Dentist Dr. Lane

Date of Exam 02/21/--

Recommended by Self

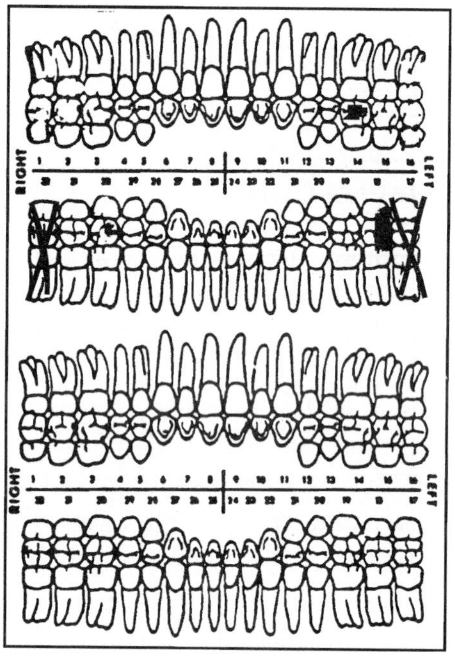

ORAL FINDINGS

Chief Complaint _____

General Physical Condition ___ Excellent ___

Condition of Teeth and Gums _____

_____

Occlusion _____

Abnormalities _____

Blood Pressure
130/90

	Hygiene	① 2 3 4
	Deposits	1 ② 3 4
	Periodontal	① 2 3 4
	Condition	

_____
_____
_____

SERVICES RENDERED

Date	Tooth	Service Rendered	Fee		Paid	Balance
01/21		Periodic Eval.	20	00		
"		Prophylaxis	25	00		
"		Bitewings—4	20	00		

DENTAL HISTORY

Date, Last Dental Visit ___ 04/03/-- ___

History of Bleeding? ___ No ___

Reaction to Anesthetic ___ No ___

Allergies? ___ No ___

Anemia? ___ No ___

Chronic Disorders-Heart? ___ No ___

Diabetes? ___ No ___

Infectious Hepatitis? ___ No ___

Nervousness? ___ No ___

Rheumatic Fever? ___ No ___

Date, Last X-rays: FMX _____

BW ___ 04/03/-- ___

Date of Models _____

FIGURE 6–1 Dental treatment record

Attending Dentist's Statement

Check one:

☐ Dentist's pre-treatment estimate

☒ Dentist's statement of actual services

Carrier name and address

THE PRUDENTIAL INSURANCE CO.
P.O. Box 999
WICKHAM, PA 19944

PATIENT SECTION

1. Patient name first m.i. last	2. Relationship to employee	3. Sex m f	4. Patient birthdate MM DD YYYY	5. If full-time student school city
Henry P. Doe	☐ self ☐ child ☐ spouse ☐ other	X	02 25 48	

6. Employee/subscriber name and mailing address	7. Employee/subscriber soc. sec. number	8. Employee/subscriber birthdate MM DD YYYY	9. Employee (company) name and address	10. Group number
1500 S. Whey Drive Hammer, IN 47422	615-28-9699	02 25 48	WWW	X2320

11. Is patient covered by another plan of benefits? Dental _____ Medical _____	12-a. Name and address of carrier(s)	12-b. Group no.(s)	13. Name and address of employer

14-a. Employee/subscriber name (if different than patient's)	14-b. Employee/subscriber soc. sec. number	14-c. Employee/subscriber birthdate MM DD YYYY	15. Relationship to patient ☐ self ☐ child ☐ spouse ☐ other

I have reviewed the following treatment plan. I authorize release of any information relating to this claim. I understand that I am responsible for all costs of dental treatment.

► _____ Date ____

Signed (Patient, or parent if minor)

I hereby authorize payment directly to the below named dentist of the group insurance benefits otherwise payable to me.

► _____ Date ____

Signed (Insured person)

DENTIST SECTION

16. Dentist name	Patrick Zunkel, DDS

17. Mailing address	3733 Professional Drive #300

City, State, Zip	Indianapolis, IN 46260

18. Dentist Soc. Sec. or T.I.N. 19. Dental licence no. 20. Dentist phone no.
99-9999999 255-1101

21. First visit date current series	22. Place of treatment Office Hosp ECF Other	23. Radiographs or models enclosed? No Yes How many?
01/03/-- X		X

24. Is treatment result of occupational illness or injury?	No	Yes	If yes, enter brief description and dates.
	X		
25. Is treatment result of auto accident?	X		
26. Other accident?	X		
27. Are any services covered by another plan?	X		

28. If prosthesis, is this initial replacement?	(If no, reason for replacement)	29. Date of prior placement

30. Is treatment for orthodontics?	X	If services already commenced enter.	Date appliances placed	Mos. treatment remaining

Identify missing teeth with "X"

FACIAL

RIGHT UPPER / PRIMARY LEFT PERMANENT

LINGUAL

LOWER / PRIMARY

LINGUAL

FACIAL

32. Remarks for unusual services

Tooth # or letter	Surface	31. Examination and treatment plan - List in order from tooth no. 1 through tooth no. 32 - Use charting system shown. Description of service (including x-rays, prophylaxis, materials used, etc.) Line No.	Date service performed Mo. Day Year	Procedure number	Fee	For administrative use only
12		1 Two Canals (Excluding		03320	320 00	
		2 Final Restoration)				
12		3 Prefabricated Post And		02954	150 00	
		4 Core In Addition To Cro				
		5 irrigation with pertide		19630	18 00	
12		6 Crown — Porcelain fused		02750	450 00	
		7 to high noble metal				
		8				
		9				
		10				
		11				
		12				
		13				
		14				
		15				

I hereby certify that the procedures as indicated by date have been completed and that the fees submitted are the actual fees I have charged and intend to collect for those procedures.

► _____ Date ____

Signed (Dentist)

Total Fee Charged	938 00
Max. Allowable	1000.00
Deductible	50.00
Carrier %	
Carrier pays	

FIGURE 6–2 Predetermination ADA Dental Form

REVIEW QUESTIONS FOR DISCUSSION

1. Explain why the dental insurance company must receive a claim form before the work is done.

2. Can the dental work proceed if the insurance company does not agree to pay for the services rendered?

3. What is the term for "baby teeth?"

Part Two

COMPLETING
INSURANCE FORMS

JOB DESCRIPTION

TITLE: Insurance Billing Specialist

IMMEDIATE SUPERVISOR: Office Manager

JOB DUTIES: Part I. To gather sufficient patient information to complete and file health insurance claims for reimbursement for services rendered by the physicians and dentists of this office. Actual patient records will be examined.

Part II. To complete the insurance forms correctly in accordance with the general requirements of most fee-for-service third-party payers. Patient records of this office will be accessed for clarification.

Part III. To adapt the insurance form completion process, as determined by specific patient records, to the general requirements of the major insurers, such as Medicare, Medicaid, Workers' Compensation, CHAMPUS, and certain other managed care insurance plans.

Part IV. To provide the references and resources necessary to complete the insurance billing process.

Part V. To furnish the forms and worksheets needed to complete all required tasks.

Chapter Seven

COMPLETING THE HCFA-1500

OBJECTIVES After completing this chapter, you will be able to

- gather the appropriate patient records needed to complete a HCFA-1500 form

- complete the top and bottom of the HCFA-1500 form for the typical medical indemnity insured

- fill in just those blocks needed to get the form processed by the insurance company

POWER WORDS

chief complaint (CC) The reason(s) the patient visits the doctor; problem or symptom.

fee-for-service Type of insurance policy outlining the benefits to be paid for each type of service normally based on the usual and customary rates (UCR) for each community.

indemnity insurance The oldest form of health insurance coverage in which the patient visits the doctor and/or hospital of choice (no gatekeeper) and benefits are paid based on the UCR.

liability insurance Provides insurance coverage in specific situations, such as automobile insurance or homeowner's insurance.

microfiche Term for making a copy of a document and storing it in miniature form on tape or film; done to save storage space while maintaining documentation.

primary diagnosis The main problem or symptom bringing the patient into the office, or the illness that is the most serious or most threatening to the well-being of the patient.

secondary diagnosis A lesser problem, but no less important in the treatment of the patient; a matter of selecting the order in which to list illnesses or diseases based upon their severity, risk, or threat to the patient.

PLEASE
DO NOT
STAPLE
IN THIS
AREA

APPROVED OMB-0938-0008

General INS Co.
101 Southway blvd
Gary, IN
48431

CARRIER

PICA — **HEALTH INSURANCE CLAIM FORM** — PICA

1. MEDICARE ☐ (Medicare #) MEDICAID ☐ (Medicaid #) CHAMPUS ☐ (Sponsor's SSN) CHAMPVA ☐ (VA File #) GROUP HEALTH PLAN ☐ (SSN or ID) FECA BLK LUNG ☐ (SSN) OTHER ☐ (ID)

1a. INSURED'S I.D. NUMBER (FOR PROGRAM IN ITEM 1): 613-07-1876

2. PATIENT'S NAME (Last Name, First Name, Middle Initial): ALTOBELLI ROSE A

3. PATIENT'S BIRTH DATE MM DD YY: 09 13 __ SEX M ☐ F ☒

4. INSURED'S NAME (Last Name, First Name, Middle Initial): ROSE ANN ALTOBELLI

5. PATIENT'S ADDRESS (No. Street): 4551 HILLSIDE DR

6. PATIENT RELATIONSHIP TO INSURED: Self ☒ Spouse ☐ Child ☐ Other ☐

7. INSURED'S ADDRESS (No. Street): SAME

CITY: INDPLS STATE: IN

8. PATIENT STATUS: Single ☒ Married ☐ Other ☐

CITY STATE

ZIP CODE: 46238 TELEPHONE (Include Area Code)

Employed ☒ Full-Time Student ☐ Part-Time Student ☐

ZIP CODE TELEPHONE (INCLUDE AREA CODE) ( )

9. OTHER INSURED'S NAME (Last Name, First Name, Middle Initial)

10. IS PATIENT'S CONDITION RELATED TO:

11. INSURED'S POLICY GROUP OR FECA NUMBER

a. OTHER INSURED'S POLICY OR GROUP NUMBER

a. EMPLOYMENT? (CURRENT OR PREVIOUS) ☐ YES ☒ NO

a. INSURED'S DATE OF BIRTH MM DD YY SEX M ☐ F ☐

b. OTHER INSURED'S DATE OF BIRTH MM DD YY SEX M ☐ F ☐

b. AUTO ACCIDENT? ☐ YES ☒ NO PLACE (State)

b. EMPLOYER'S NAME OR SCHOOL NAME: ALTOBELLI ASS

c. EMPLOYER'S NAME OR SCHOOL NAME

c. OTHER ACCIDENT? ☐ YES ☒ NO

c. INSURANCE PLAN NAME OR PROGRAM NAME

d. INSURANCE PLAN NAME OR PROGRAM NAME

10d. RESERVED FOR LOCAL USE

d. IS THERE ANOTHER HEALTH BENEFIT PLAN? ☐ YES ☒ NO *If yes,* return to and complete item 9 a – d.

READ BACK OF FORM BEFORE COMPLETING & SIGNING THIS FORM.

12. PATIENT'S OR AUTHORIZED PERSON'S SIGNATURE I authorize the release of any medical or other information necessary to process this claim. I also request payment of government benefits either to myself or to the party who accepts assignment below.

SIGNED ROSE ANN ANTOBELLI DATE 01.12.2010

13. INSURED'S OR AUTHORIZED PERSON'S SIGNATURE I authorize payment of medical benefits to the undersigned physician or supplier for services described below.

SIGNED ROSE ANN ANTOBELLI

PATIENT AND INSURED INFORMATION

FIGURE 7–1 Blank top half of HCFA-1500

FEE-FOR-SERVICE OR INDEMNITY COMPANIES

To complete an insurance form for fee-for-service or indemnity coverage, first the **insurance billing specialist** will study the top half of the HCFA-1500 and then the bottom half before going on to complete an entire form. The instructions given here are *general.* There may be variations required by some insurance carriers or in different states and those variations should be adopted when known.

The top half of the form shows spaces to complete that concern the patient and the insured; the rest of the form relates to the services rendered. Let's study the top half first, above the solid line, as Figure 7-1 shows.

To complete this form, gather the Confidential Patient Information Record, Routing Slip, and ledger card for Rose Altobelli (Record #1, Sheets 1 through 4 from Chapter 16) and Form #1 in Part V, a blank HCFA-1500 form. Complete the form using the following instructions. Remember, you are about to complete a form for a patient with fee-for-service or medical indemnity insurance. The following instructions are for that type of insurance only.

Starting at the top left corner of the upper half of the HCFA-1500 form, notice the heavy black bars and the request not to staple in the area. These bars are sometimes scanned when they are received by certain insurance companies or insurers, along with the rest of the form, and a photocopy or microfiche of the form may be made. The bars on the next form indicate a point of separation between two forms as well as the signal to the scanner to repeat the process of gathering information. Therefore, it is important not to tamper with this part of the form.

Notice the form has small numbers or letters in the upper left of each line box. The instructions given to you will describe the *minimum* work necessary to complete the form for reimbursement! It is not necessary to complete every line of the form for *most insurance companies.* If you find one that does require more completion than normal, please adapt to that request; otherwise, feel free to spend as little time as possible on each form. A few seconds or minutes saved on each form adds up to hours and days over the course of a year!

Your first instruction is to *add* information to the form that is not requested!

DO: At about the same level as the black bars, on the right side of the form, type or print the name and address of the insurance company to which you will be mailing this form. This information is on the Confidential Patient Information Record (CPIR). Adding the address here will permit you to look upon your saved copy of this form and know where it was sent. This is important to your documentation and often eases the mind of inquiring patients.

DO: Skip Box #1. You may skip this box because most indemnity insurance companies do not require that it be completed.

DO: Go to Box #1a and print the ID number of the insured.

DO: Print or type the patient's name, last name first, in Box #2.

DO: Complete Box #5, but skip the telephone number. The insurance company has it on file if they need it and we can save some seconds here.

DO: Look at Box #3 and carefully print the date of birth as 09|13|— and place an "X" in the "F" box indicating the patient is female.

Box #6 is used to show the patient's relationship to the insured: are they the same, is the patient the spouse, the child, or other? In the case of Ms. Altobelli, the patient and the insured are the same.

DO: Place an "X" in the Self square in Box #6.

Box #8 is used to show the patient's marital status and work status. For marital status, notice the "Other" square may be used for divorced or widowed patients or

to express some other relationship, such as stepchild.

DO: Since Rose is single, place an "X" in that square.

DO: Rose is employed, so place an "X" in that square, but skip the other two boxes.

They are used in those situations in which the patient is eighteen to twenty-three or twenty-four years of age, still covered by a parent's insurance, and may or may not be a student. This is not applicable for Rose.

DO: In Block #10, place an "X" in the "No" square for each of the three questions asked.

If the answer to any of these questions is yes, then the patient would not need a fee-for-service claim to be filed, but would be filing a Workers' Compensation claim, or other liability insurance form.

DO: Skip Block #10d.

It is not normally used for the filing of a first claim, but may be used to transmit information to the insurance company in other situations. You will see this later.

DO: In Block #4, print or type Rose's name again since she is the insured as well as the patient.

DO: In Block #7 you may print or type the word "same" only once and you do not need to repeat the address since the patient and the insured live at the same place. Again, skip the telephone number.

DO: Examine Block #11. It is used to list a group number as shown on the patient's CPIR. This patient does not have a group number. Go on to Block #11a.

DO: Examine Block #11a. It is completed if the insured is someone other than the patient. Since that is not the case here, go on to Block #11b.

DO: Block #11b must be completed. Again, that information is on the CPIR.

DO: Skip Block #11c because the name of the insurance company is printed at the top of the form.

DO: Block #11d is very important and must be completed.

Rose has no other insurance, according to her CPIR, and therefore place an "X" next to the "No" square. If Rose had any other insurance, then the "Yes" square would be marked along with Blocks #9 through #9d. The instructions in Block #11d direct the **insurance billing specialist** to complete those blocks when there is additional insurance coverage.

DO: Print or type "Signature on File" on the Block #12 signature line.

This line authorizes our office to release information to the insurance company so that the claim may be paid. This signature was received at the time Rose completed the CPIR. Therefore, her signature is "on file" and the **insurance billing specialist** may properly state this fact.

DO: Print or type "Signature on File" on Block #13, if the patient owes a balance on her account. This authorization line indicates the patient wants payment of the claim to be sent to our office. Unless the patient pays for all services herself and does not have a balance owed to our office, this line should be completed the same as Block #12. If the patient does not owe a bill to our office, the block may be left blank and the check will be sent to her.

DO: On the date line printed within Block #12, show the date you completed this claim form. It is not necessary to use this date line to show the date the patient's signature was collected, and the **insurance billing specialist** will be glad the

completion date was entered if the patient calls later and requests this information.

Compare the top half of your completed form with Figure 7-2.

Figure 7-3 shows the bottom half of a blank HCFA-1500. The information placed there relates to the services rendered to the patient and the health care professional who treated the patient. Let us now complete the rest of the form for patient Rose Altobelli.

DO: Skip Block #14. It may be used to show when the first symptom of the current problem appeared, or is used to show the date of an accident or injury, or the date of the last menstrual period for the pregnant patient. For Ms. Altobelli, we do not know the exact date the problem began. In these instances, leave the block blank. If the insurance company needs more information about the onset date, they will contact us or the patient.

DO: Skip Block #15. If the insurance company needs this information to process the claim (and very few do), we will be contacted by them.

DO: Skip Block #16. This is completed only when the patient is unable to work because of the condition our doctors are treating. Rose has not missed any work.

DO: Examine Block #17. If Rose had been referred by another physician, that name would be entered here. The name of the referring physician is listed only once, on the first claim form submitted.

DO: Skip Block #17a. This block is not used in indemnity insurance unless specifically requested by an insurance company.

DO: Skip Block #18. Rose was not hospitalized.

FIGURE 7–2 Completed top half of HCFA-1500

FIGURE 7–3 Blank bottom half of HCFA-1500

Figure 7-2 (top half) content:

PLEASE DO NOT STAPLE IN THIS AREA

APPROVED OMB-0938-0008

General Insurance Co.
1010 Southway Blvd.
Gary, IN 48431

CARRIER

PICA

HEALTH INSURANCE CLAIM FORM

PICA

1. MEDICARE (Medicare #) MEDICAID (Medicaid #) CHAMPUS (Sponsor's SSN) CHAMPVA (VA File #) GROUP HEALTH PLAN (SSN or ID) FECA BLK LUNG (SSN) OTHER (ID)

1a. INSURED'S I.D. NUMBER (FOR PROGRAM IN ITEM 1)
613-07-8179

2. PATIENT'S NAME (Last Name, First Name, Middle Initial)
Altobelli, Rose A.

3. PATIENT'S BIRTH DATE MM 09 DD 13 YY -- SEX M [ ] F [X]

4. INSURED'S NAME (Last Name, First Name, Middle Initial)
Altobelli, Rose A.

5. PATIENT'S ADDRESS (No. Street)
4551 Hillside Dr.

6. PATIENT RELATIONSHIP TO INSURED Self [X] Spouse [ ] Child [ ] Other [ ]

7. INSURED'S ADDRESS (No. Street)
Same

CITY Indpls. STATE IN

8. PATIENT STATUS Single [X] Married [ ] Other [ ]

CITY STATE

ZIP CODE 46238 TELEPHONE (Include Area Code)

Employed [X] Full-Time Student [ ] Part-Time Student [ ]

ZIP CODE TELEPHONE (INCLUDE AREA CODE) ( )

9. OTHER INSURED'S NAME (Last Name, First Name, Middle Initial)

10. IS PATIENT'S CONDITION RELATED TO:

11. INSURED'S POLICY GROUP OR FECA NUMBER

a. OTHER INSURED'S POLICY OR GROUP NUMBER

a. EMPLOYMENT? (CURRENT OR PREVIOUS) [ ] YES [X] NO

a. INSURED'S DATE OF BIRTH MM DD YY SEX M [ ] F [ ]

b. OTHER INSURED'S DATE OF BIRTH MM DD YY SEX M [ ] F [ ]

b. AUTO ACCIDENT? [ ] YES [X] NO PLACE (State)

b. EMPLOYER'S NAME OR SCHOOL NAME
Altobelli Assoc.

c. EMPLOYER'S NAME OR SCHOOL NAME

c. OTHER ACCIDENT? [ ] YES [X] NO

c. INSURANCE PLAN NAME OR PROGRAM NAME

d. INSURANCE PLAN NAME OR PROGRAM NAME

10d. RESERVED FOR LOCAL USE

d. IS THERE ANOTHER HEALTH BENEFIT PLAN? [ ] YES [X] NO If yes, return to and complete item 9 a – d.

READ BACK OF FORM BEFORE COMPLETING & SIGNING THIS FORM.
12. PATIENT'S OR AUTHORIZED PERSON'S SIGNATURE I authorize the release of any medical or other information necessary to process this claim. I also request payment of government benefits either to myself or to the party who accepts assignment below.
SIGNED Signature on File DATE Today

13. INSURED'S OR AUTHORIZED PERSON'S SIGNATURE I authorize payment of medical benefits to the undersigned physician or supplier for services described below.
SIGNED Signature on File

PATIENT AND INSURED INFORMATION

Figure 7-3 (bottom half) content:

17. NAME OF REFERRING PHYSICIAN OR OTHER SOURCE
JAMES P CARTMAN, MD

17a. I.D. NUMBER OF REFERRING PHYSICIAN

18. HOSPITALIZATION DATES RELATED TO CURRENT SERVICES MM DD YY FROM TO MM DD YY

19. RESERVED FOR LOCAL USE

20. OUTSIDE LAB? [ ] YES [ ] NO $ CHARGES

21. DIAGNOSIS OR NATURE OF ILLNESS OR INJURY. (RELATE ITEMS 1, 2, 3, OR 4 TO ITEM 24E BY LINE)
1. 564 .1
2. 455 .8
3. .
4. .

22. MEDICAID RESUBMISSION CODE ORIGINAL REF. NO.

23. PRIOR AUTHORIZATION NUMBER

24. A DATE(S) OF SERVICE From MM DD YY	To MM DD YY	B Place of Service	C Type of Service	D PROCEDURES, SERVICES, OR SUPPLIES (Explain Unusual Circumstances) CPT/HCPCS MODIFIER	E DIAGNOSIS CODE	F $ CHARGES	G DAYS OR UNITS	H EPSDT Family Plan	I EMG	J COB	K RESERVED FOR LOCAL USE
09 01 2010		11		99203	1, 2	60 00	1				

25. FEDERAL TAX I.D. NUMBER
99-9999999 SSN [ ] EIN [ ]

26. PATIENT'S ACCOUNT NO.

27. ACCEPT ASSIGNMENT? (For govt. claims, see back) [ ] YES [ ] NO

28. TOTAL CHARGE $ 60.00

29. AMOUNT PAID $ 0

30. BALANCE DUE $ 60.00

31. SIGNATURE OF PHYSICIAN OR SUPPLIER INCLUDING DEGREES OR CREDENTIALS (I certify that the statements on the reverse apply to this bill and are made a part thereof.)
SIGNED JAMES P CARTMAN, M.D/TDB-C DATE

32. NAME AND ADDRESS OF FACILITY WHERE SERVICES WERE RENDERED (If other than home or office)

33. PHYSICIAN'S SUPPLIER'S BILLING NAME, ADDRESS, ZIP CODE & PHONE #
JAMES P CARTMAN
3733 PROFESSIONAL DR # 300
INDIANAPOLIS, IN 46260
PIN# GRP#

(APPROVED BY AMA COUNCIL ON MEDICAL SERVICE 8/88)

PLEASE PRINT OR TYPE

FORM HCFA-1500 (U2) (12-90)
FORM OWCP-1500 FORM RRB-1500

PHYSICIAN OR SUPPLIER INFORMATION

DO: Skip Block #19. This block is not used in indemnity insurance unless specifically requested by an insurance company.

DO: Skip Block #20. This block is not used in indemnity insurance unless specifically requested by an insurance company.

DO: Place the primary and secondary ICD-9-CM diagnoses for Ms. Altobelli on lines 1 (564.1) and 2 (455.8) in Block #21.

Block #21 is very important to the **insurance billing specialist** since this is the place on the form where the diagnoses are listed. If this block of the form is not completed or is completed incorrectly, proper reimbursement is threatened or the form may be returned to you and precious time will be lost. There are four short, numbered lines with a decimal place showing.

DO: Skip Block #22. This block may be required by Medicaid, but not by indemnity insurance.

DO: Skip Block #23. This block is not used in indemnity insurance unless specifically requested by an insurance company.

Block #24 is the heart of the lower half of the form. It is subdivided into areas with capital letters A through K.

DO: Place the date of the office visit (09|01|—) under #24-A in the column marked "from."

DO: The Place of Service code for an office visit is 11. Put that number in the B column. (A complete list of Place of Service codes are located in Part IV of this text.)

DO: Skip column C. This information is not normally required by the insurance company.

DO: Use column D to list the CPT code 99203 that appears on the ledger card. No modifiers are needed, so leave the rest of that line blank.

DO: Place "1, 2" in Column E.

This column is used to refer to the diagnoses in Block #21. There is not enough room to repeat each whole ICD-9-CM number and that is not the intent of this small box. Placing "1, 2" in this box shows that both diagnoses listed in Block #21 were present and were treated at the time of this office visit. Those two numbers will be read by the claim adjudicator to mean "1.564.1 and 2.455.8" as you presented them in Block #21.

DO: In Block F place the $90.00 fee and put the number 1 in the G box to show one office visit unit. None of the remaining boxes are used for indemnity insurance unless specifically requested, but that is very rare.

As you can see, there are six lines on this HCFA-1500 and up to six services may be listed, all on the same or different days as appropriate. In the case of Ms. Altobelli, only one visit needs to be submitted to her insurance company.

DO: Go to Block #28 and list the total charge shown on this claim form.

DO: Place a "0" in Block #29 since Rose made no out-of-pocket payment.

DO: Show the balance due of $60.00 in Block #30.

This completes the patient services part of the form.

We now must give information about the doctor who treated Ms. Altobelli. In Part IV of this text/workbook, you will find a complete listing of information about the doctors in our practice that may be needed to complete insurance forms. This information includes certain provider numbers that you will need in completing claims in later chapters. The **insurance billing specialist** may sometimes get the necessary information from the routing slip copy. Look on Ms. Altobelli's routing slip and notice the Tax ID number listed at the head of the form as well as the name and address of our practice.

25. FEDERAL TAX I.D. NUMBER SSN EIN	26. PATIENT'S ACCOUNT NO.	27. ACCEPT ASSIGNMENT? (For govt. claims, see back) YES ☐ NO ☐	28. TOTAL CHARGE $ 60 00	29. AMOUNT PAID $ 0	30. BALANCE DUE $ 60 00
99-9999999 ☐ ☒					

31. SIGNATURE OF PHYSICIAN OR SUPPLIER INCLUDING DEGREES OR CREDENTIALS (I certify that the statements on the reverse apply to this bill and are made a part thereof.)	32. NAME AND ADDRESS OF FACILITY WHERE SERVICES WERE RENDERED (if other than home or office)	33. PHYSICIAN'S SUPPLIER'S BILLING NAME, ADDRESS, ZIP CODE & PHONE # James P. Cartman, M.D. 3733 Professional Drive #300 Indpls., IN 46260
SIGNED James P. Cartman, M.D./sc DATE		PIN# GRP#

(APPROVED BY AMA COUNCIL ON MEDICAL SERVICE 8/88)   *PLEASE PRINT OR TYPE*   FORM HCFA-1500 (U2) (12-90) FORM OWCP-1500   FORM RRB-1500

FIGURE 7–4 Doctor's signature with initials

DO: Place that tax ID number in Block #25 and put an "X" in the small square marked "EIN." By doing this, you are giving the insurance company the employer's federal tax ID number so that the payment coming from this claim form may be reported to the Internal Revenue Service as income to the practice. Without this number, the claim may not be adjudicated but may be returned. If that happens, more time will be lost before payment is received. EIN is the abbreviation for Employer's ID Number. If our office did not have a federal tax ID number, you could place the treating doctor's social security number in Block #25 and so indicate by marking the small square next to SSN. However, the EIN number always takes precedence over the social security number, so use the former when you have it.

DO: Skip Block #26. It is used if we have an internal numbering system for our patients, and we do not.

DO: Skip Block #27 which we will use later for other claims.

DO: Within Block #31, you may sign the doctor's name and place your initials behind that signature. Figure 7-4 shows how to do this.

You may do this because Dr. Cartman and the other physicians in this group allow the **insurance billing specialist** to take this step. Should you leave us and go to work for another doctor, be sure to get permission before taking this liberty! Do not worry about entering today's date in Block #31. There is not enough room, and you placed the date this form was completed on the top of the form in Block #12.

DO: Skip Block #32 since it is used only when services are rendered outside the office.

DO: Place the doctor's name and address in Block #33. There is no PIN (physician identification number) or GRP (group number) associated with Ms. Altobelli's insurance company, so no other information is placed in this box.

You have now completed the bottom half of the form! See Figure 7-5 and match your work to that example.

FIGURE 7–5 Completed bottom half of HCFA-1500 for Altobelli

EXERCISE 1

Remove Record #2, Sheets 1 through 4 in Chapter 16 for patient Julie Justin, and Form #2 in Part V of this text/workbook and complete the entire HCFA-1500. Compare your completed form to the one shown by your instructor.

EXERCISE 2

Pull Record #3, Sheets 1 and 2 in Chapter 16 for patient Willisse, and Form #3 from Part V to complete. Consult with your instructor before continuing.

EXERCISE 3

Remove Record #4, Sheets 1 and 2, for patient Hammpton in Chapter 16, and Form #4 in Part V. Consult your instructor before continuing after you have completed the form.

PATIENT NOT THE INSURED

When the patient is *not* the insured, a few changes are needed to complete the top of the form, but none are needed in the bottom part of the HCFA-1500. For example, patient Richard O. Roberts, Jr., is a patient of Dr. Beckermann's. Locate Record #5, Sheets 1 and 2, in Chapter 16, and Form #5 in Part V. Let us look at the changes needed to complete the top half of the HCFA-1500 when the patient is a relative of the insured, but is not the same person.

DO: Enter the patient's name and address, birth date and sex in Blocks #2, #3, #5.

DO: In Block #1a , enter the "insured's" identification number. The insured is the father, Richard O. Roberts, Sr.

DO: List the father's name in Block #4.

DO: In Block #6, place an "X" in the square next to "Child" to show the parental relationship.

DO: Since the child lives with his father, the insured's address is *same* in Block #7.

DO: Block #11a is used to show the father's date of birth, since he is the insured, and his sex.

DO: The father's employer is listed in #11b.

Since there is no other insurance coverage, the remainder of the form is completed as you have done with previous cases. Check with your instructor to be sure you have completed the entire form correctly.

EXERCISE #4

Remove Record #6, Sheets 1 and 2 for patient Nicole M. Petroff from Chapter 16, and Form #6 from Part V. Complete the HCFA-1500 and follow your instructor's directive before continuing with this chapter.

EXERCISE #5

Remove Record #7, Sheets 1 and 2 for patient Blumquist from Chapter 16, and Form #7 from Part V. Complete the HCFA-1500 and follow your instructor's directions before continuing with the chapter review questions.

REVIEW QUESTIONS FOR DISCUSSION

1. Why is accurate completion of a HCFA-1500 important?
2. What information should be added to the form that is not currently requested?
3. Why is it acceptable to skip some boxes in completing the HCFA-1500?
4. What must be done before signing the name of the doctor to the insurance form?
5. What sources will the **insurance billing specialist** examine in order to complete the insurance form accurately?

Chapter Eight

COMPLETING THE HCFA-1500

OBJECTIVES After completing your study of this chapter, you will be able to

- determine the primary and secondary insurance carrier and others, as appropriate
- apply the birthday rule in completing a form for a dependent of undivorced parents
- adapt the completion of the HCFA-1500 to show payments received from other carriers
- handle parental concerns regarding payments from custodial and noncustodial parents

POWER WORDS

birthday rule Applied when nondivorced parents of a minor patient both carry insurance coverage for the child. The parent born closest to January 1 is the primary insured and the other parent is the secondary, regardless of the age of either parent. If the parents share the same date of birth, the parent whose policy has been in effect the longest becomes the primary insured and the other parent the secondary insured.

Coordination of Benefits (COB) The term used to mean the insurance companies providing coverage to the patient will not issue benefit payments greater than the amount owed to the doctor. Therefore, if the primary insurance company pays the entire amount of the bill submitted to it, the secondary insurance company will pay nothing.

Explanation of Benefits (EOB) Accompanies the insurance check issued to the doctor and the patient may also receive a similar document; information explains the payment made by the insurance company, any amounts left unpaid, and why.

primary insurance coverage Refers to the order in which insurance forms should be filed. When there is spousal coverage for patients with insurance of their own, their insurance must be filed first. After payment from the primary insurance company is received, a claim may be filed with the other insurance company if any balance is still owed.

secondary insurance
coverage

Coverage for the patient by another insurance company effective only after payment from the primary insurance company has been received.

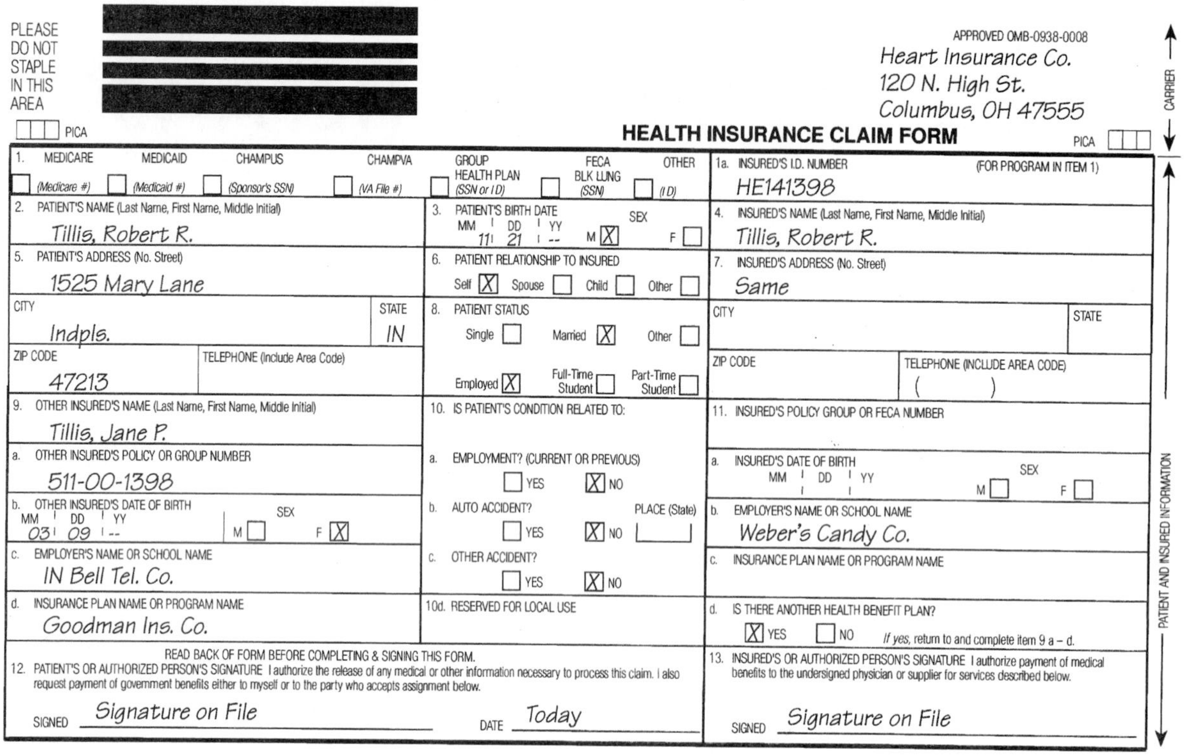

FIGURE 8–1 Completed top half of HCFA-1500 for Tillis

SPOUSAL COVERAGE

Very often, the **insurance billing specialist** will be required to file a claim for a patient with a spouse who also has insurance coverage for the patient. This is called secondary insurance coverage and cannot be filed after payment from the primary insurance company has been received.

In filing a claim for the patient with coverage by two insurance companies, the bottom half of the form is completed the same as it was for the patients in Chapter 7. However, the top half of the claim requires some changes. Locate Record #8, Sheets 1 and 2 on patient Tillis in Chapter 16, and Form #8 in Part V.

First, a claim must be submitted to the patient's insurance company and payment received before a claim may be submitted to the second company. Therefore, complete all boxes with patient information (as in Chapter 7) until you come to Block #11d.

DO: Place an "X" in the "Yes" square in Block #11d. Go to Block #9.

DO: Print or type the name of the spouse, last name first, in Block #9.

DO: In Block #9a, place the spouse's insurance ID number only. Never use this block for anything other than the insurance ID number.

DO: In Block #9b, enter the spouse's date of birth and place an "X" to indicate male or female.

DO: In Block #9c, enter the name of the employer for the spouse.

DO: In Block #9d, print or type the name of the insurance company. Figure 8-1 shows the completed top half of the form for this situation of coverage from two insurance companies.

Once payment has been received from the primary insurance company, completing another HCFA-1500 for the secondary insurance company requires minimal changes for the **insurance billing specialist**. Figure 8-2 is an example of an Explanation of Benefits letter. Remember, there is no standard format for an EOB and it seems each insurance company has its own way of delivering that information—no two EOBs look the same!

After payment has been received from the primary carrier, a claim may be filed with the secondary insurance company to try to collect payment for the balance due. The Heart Insurance Company EOB estimated that the secondary insurance carrier would pay the $72.00 balance. We must now submit a form to see if the $72.00 balance will be paid. Use Form #9 in Part V to bill to the second carrier.

DO: Print or type the name and address of the secondary insurance company at the top right of the form.

DO: Complete Blocks #2, #3, #5, #8, and #10 as before.

DO: In Block #6, show the patient relationship to insured as "Spouse."

DO: In Block #1a, place the ID number for the spouse, Jane P. Tillis.

DO: Print or type Jane's name in Block #4.

DO: Add the word "same" to Block #7 since this couple lives together.

DO: Skip Block #11 since Jane has no group number.

DO: List Jane's date of birth and sex in Block #11a.

DO: Enter Jane's employer in Block #11b.

DO: Skip Block #11c.

DO: Place an "X" in the "Yes" square in Block #11d.

DO: Complete Blocks #9 through #9d by repeating information about Robert. Remember, since we are completing this form with Jane as the insured, Robert becomes the other insured.

DO: In Block #10d, print or type the words "See Attached EOB" and don't forget to attach a copy of the form you received from the Heart Insurance Company. The Goodman Insurance Company will examine this EOB to determine what portion of the total charge has been paid by the primary insured. This information will determine what portion they will pay, if any.

DO: Complete Blocks #12 and #13 with "Signature on File."

Complete the bottom half of the HCFA-1500 with the same information that was sent to the primary insurance company except for Blocks #29 and #30.

DO: Enter the amount paid by the primary insurance company in Block #29.

DO: Enter the balance now owing in Block #30.

Compare your completed form to Figure 8-3 below.

Figure 8-4 demonstrates how several entries were posted to the ledger card for this patient.

First, the date of the consultation and the fee were posted. Next, the date the primary insurance form was filed was posted by the **insurance billing specialist**. Notice our office does not normally charge a fee for completing insurance forms. Next, the date the insurance payment was received and the amount is posted. The ledger card does not show that the secondary insurance company has been billed. Since that work has now been done, go ahead and make that entry on the ledger card for this patient.

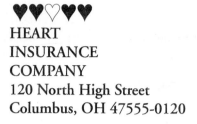

HEART
INSURANCE
COMPANY
120 North High Street
Columbus, OH 47555-0120

EXPLANATION OF BENEFITS

Patient:	*Robert R. Tillis*	Insured:	*Robert R. Tillis*
ID No:	*HE141398*	Claim No:	*6552117788900234*
Employer:	*Weber's Candy Co.*	Provider:	*James P. Cartman, M.D.*
			Medical and Dental Associates, Inc.
			3733 Professional Drive #300
			Indianapolis, IN 46260

Date of Service: *04/18/--*

Description of Service: *99245*

Amount Charged: *$200.00*

Co-Insurance: *$72.00*

Amount Paid: *$128.00*

Notes: *Benefit paid represents the Usual and Customary Rate (UCR)*
for this service.

* * * * * * * *

Benefits Paid To: *James P. Cartman, M.D.*

Amount: *$128.00*

Check No: *3229076*

FIGURE 8–2 EOB

APPROVED OMB-0938-0008

Goodman Insurance Co.
15 W. Goode Hwy.
NY, NY 10999

CARRIER

☐☐ PICA

HEALTH INSURANCE CLAIM FORM

PICA ☐☐☐

1. MEDICARE	MEDICAID	CHAMPUS	CHAMPVA	GROUP HEALTH PLAN (SSN or ID)	FECA BLK LUNG (SSN)	OTHER (ID)	1a. INSURED'S I.D. NUMBER	(FOR PROGRAM IN ITEM 1)
☐ (Medicare #)	☐ (Medicaid #)	☐ (Sponsor's SSN)	☐ (VA File #)	☐	☐	☐	511-00-1398	

2. PATIENT'S NAME (Last Name, First Name, Middle Initial)
Tillis, Robert R.

3. PATIENT'S BIRTH DATE
MM 11 DD 21 YY -- SEX M ☒ F ☐

4. INSURED'S NAME (Last Name, First Name, Middle Initial)
Tillis, Jane P.

5. PATIENT'S ADDRESS (No. Street)
1525 Mary Lane

6. PATIENT RELATIONSHIP TO INSURED
Self ☒ Spouse ☒ Child ☐ Other ☐

7. INSURED'S ADDRESS (No. Street)
Same

CITY
Indpls.
STATE
IN

8. PATIENT STATUS
Single ☐ Married ☒ Other ☐
Employed ☒ Full-Time Student ☐ Part-Time Student ☐

CITY ___ STATE ___

ZIP CODE
47213
TELEPHONE (Include Area Code)
( )

ZIP CODE ___ TELEPHONE (INCLUDE AREA CODE) ( )

9. OTHER INSURED'S NAME (Last Name, First Name, Middle Initial)
Tillis, Robert R.

10. IS PATIENT'S CONDITION RELATED TO:

11. INSURED'S POLICY GROUP OR FECA NUMBER

a. OTHER INSURED'S POLICY OR GROUP NUMBER
HE141398

a. EMPLOYMENT? (CURRENT OR PREVIOUS)
☐ YES ☒ NO

a. INSURED'S DATE OF BIRTH
MM 03 DD 09 YY -- SEX M ☐ F ☒

b. OTHER INSURED'S DATE OF BIRTH
MM 11 DD 21 YY -- SEX M ☒ F ☐

b. AUTO ACCIDENT? PLACE (State)
☐ YES ☒ NO ☐

b. EMPLOYER'S NAME OR SCHOOL NAME
IN Bell Tel. Co.

c. EMPLOYER'S NAME OR SCHOOL NAME
Weber Candy Co.

c. OTHER ACCIDENT?
☐ YES ☒ NO

c. INSURANCE PLAN NAME OR PROGRAM NAME

d. INSURANCE PLAN NAME OR PROGRAM NAME
Heart Ins. Co.

10d. RESERVED FOR LOCAL USE
See Attached EOB

d. IS THERE ANOTHER HEALTH BENEFIT PLAN?
☒ YES ☐ NO If yes, return to and complete item 9 a – d.

READ BACK OF FORM BEFORE COMPLETING & SIGNING THIS FORM.
12. PATIENT'S OR AUTHORIZED PERSON'S SIGNATURE I authorize the release of any medical or other information necessary to process this claim. I also request payment of government benefits either to myself or to the party who accepts assignment below.

SIGNED *Signature on File* DATE *Today*

13. INSURED'S OR AUTHORIZED PERSON'S SIGNATURE I authorize payment of medical benefits to the undersigned physician or supplier for services described below.

SIGNED *Signature on File*

PATIENT AND INSURED INFORMATION

14. DATE OF CURRENT: ◄ ILLNESS (First symptom) OR INJURY (Accident) OR PREGNANCY (LMP)
MM DD YY

15. IF PATIENT HAS HAD SAME OR SIMILAR ILLNESS, GIVE FIRST DATE MM DD YY

16. DATES PATIENT UNABLE TO WORK IN CURRENT OCCUPATION
FROM MM DD YY TO MM DD YY

17. NAME OF REFERRING PHYSICIAN OR OTHER SOURCE

17a. I.D. NUMBER OF REFERRING PHYSICIAN

18. HOSPITALIZATION DATES RELATED TO CURRENT SERVICES
FROM MM DD YY TO MM DD YY

19. RESERVED FOR LOCAL USE

20. OUTSIDE LAB? ☐ YES ☐ NO $ CHARGES

21. DIAGNOSIS OR NATURE OF ILLNESS OR INJURY. (RELATE ITEMS 1, 2, 3, OR 4 TO ITEM 24E BY LINE)
1. 250.5̶1 52
2. 362.01
3. ___
4. ___

22. MEDICAID RESUBMISSION CODE ___ ORIGINAL REF. NO.

23. PRIOR AUTHORIZATION NUMBER

24. A DATE(S) OF SERVICE		B Place of Service	C Type of Service	D PROCEDURES, SERVICES, OR SUPPLIES (Explain Unusual Circumstances)		E DIAGNOSIS CODE	F $ CHARGES	G DAYS OR UNITS	H EPSDT Family Plan	I EMG	J COB	K RESERVED FOR LOCAL USE
From MM DD YY	To MM DD YY			CPT/HCPCS	MODIFIER							
04 18 --		11		99245		1, 2	200 00	1				

25. FEDERAL TAX I.D. NUMBER SSN ☐ EIN ☒
99-9999999

26. PATIENT'S ACCOUNT NO.

27. ACCEPT ASSIGNMENT? (For govt. claims, see back) ☐ YES ☐ NO

28. TOTAL CHARGE $ 200 00

29. AMOUNT PAID $ 128 00

30. BALANCE DUE $ 72 00

31. SIGNATURE OF PHYSICIAN OR SUPPLIER INCLUDING DEGREES OR CREDENTIALS (I certify that the statements on the reverse apply to this bill and are made a part thereof.)
James P. Cartman, M.D./SC
SIGNED DATE

32. NAME AND ADDRESS OF FACILITY WHERE SERVICES WERE RENDERED (If other than home or office)

33. PHYSICIAN'S SUPPLIER'S BILLING NAME, ADDRESS, ZIP CODE & PHONE #
James P. Cartman, M.D.
3733 Professional Drive #300
Indpls., IN 46260
PIN# GRP#

PHYSICIAN OR SUPPLIER INFORMATION

(APPROVED BY AMA COUNCIL ON MEDICAL SERVICE 8/88)

PLEASE PRINT OR TYPE

FORM HCFA-1500 (12-90)
FORM OWCP-1500 FORM RRB-1500
FORM AMA OP050192

FIGURE 8–3 Completed secondary insurance form

Medical & Dental Associates, P.C.

3733 Professional Drive #300
Indianapolis, IN 46260
317/123-4567
Tax ID# 99-9999999

STATEMENT OF ACCOUNT

Tillis, Robert R.
1525 Mary Lane
Indpls., IN 47213

19--

DATE	CODE	CHARGE		CREDITS PAYMENT		ADJ		CURRENT BALANCE	
		BALANCE FORWARD ➡						48	00
04/18	99245	200	00					248	00
04/20	Ins. form filed	0	00					248	00
06/01	Ins. pymt			128	00			120	00

PLEASE PAY LAST AMOUNT IN THIS COLUMN ↑

THIS IS A COPY OF YOUR ACCOUNT

FIGURE 8–4 Ledger card for Tillis

Spousal Coverage

EXERCISE 1

1. Remove Record #9 for Mrs. Ai Vang, Sheets 1, 2, 3 from Chapter 16, and Form #10 from Part V.

2. Complete the form for the primary insured and make the entry onto the ledger card showing you have filed the insurance form.

3. When you have finished, remove Form #11, the EOB for payment received, and post that information to the ledger card.

4. Remove Form #12.

5. Complete Form #12 for the secondary insurance coverage.

6. Post the information to the ledger card that the secondary insurance company has been sent a form.

7. Check with your instructor before continuing with the chapter.

THE BIRTHDAY RULE

The "birthday rule" is the label used to explain which insurance carrier is primary when both parents (undivorced) have insurance to cover the child. In the "old days," the father was automatically determined to be primary and the mother was secondary. This seemed to work all right until significant numbers of women entered the workplace and bought insurance coverage for themselves and their families. At that point, another method was needed to determine who is primary and who is secondary. The birthday rule states that:

☞ the nondivorced parent whose birthday is closest to January 1 is the primary insured and the other parent the secondary insured, regardless of the age or sex of their parent.

☞ if the parents share the same date of birth, then the parent whose insurance has been in effect the longest is the primary insured and the other parent is the secondary insured.

The term nondivorced is used because the rules change when dealing with divorced parents. Again, even under the birthday rule, there is no change in completing the bottom half of the HCFA-1500 until after payment from the primary insured has been received and the second form is prepared.

Find Record #10 for patient Moyer in Chapter 16 and Form #13 in Part V. This patient is governed by the birthday rule. How shall we complete the insurance form?

DO: Complete the patient information blocks as usual.

DO: List the identification number of the primary insured parent in Block #1a.

DO: List the name of that parent, last name first, in Block #6. #4

DO: Enter the word "same" in Block #7 since the family lives at the same address.

DO: Skip down to Block #11. Enter a Group number from the patient ID information, if there is one; otherwise, leave this block blank.

DO: Enter the parent's *date of birth*, sex, and employer's name in Blocks #11a and #11b.

DO: Skip Block #11c.

DO: In Block #11d, answer "Yes" and move to Blocks #9a to 9d and complete the information about the other parent. When you are finished, your form should look like Figure 8-5.

COORDINATION OF BENEFITS

Years ago, before the advent of Coordination of Benefits (COB), both insurance companies of working married couples with coverage paid insurance claims submitted to them without asking about other insurance coverage. As a result, the patient or doctor sometimes received more money from those combined insurance payments than the doctor charged originally for the service rendered! Stories were told about patients financing vacations with insurance overpayments. This was not the intent of insurance coverage and surely added to the high cost of health care in general. After a time of observing this phenomenon, COB clauses began appearing in insurance policies and overpayments were stopped. By including a copy of the Explanation of Benefits (EOBs) to the secondary carrier, overpayments are avoided. Most insurance policies will include a clause stating that in no case will combined payments of any claim exceed 100 percent. This is another way to guarantee that all the insurance carriers work together to pay the claims within the boundaries of their policies, but not beyond the amount of the bill sent to the patient.

PLEASE
DO NOT
STAPLE
IN THIS
AREA

CARRIER

APPROVED OMB-0938-0008
Good Gold Insurance Co.
8900 W. Tree Lane
Chicago, IL 60606

| | PICA | | **HEALTH INSURANCE CLAIM FORM** | PICA | | |

1. MEDICARE MEDICAID CHAMPUS CHAMPVA	GROUP HEALTH PLAN	FECA BLK LUNG	OTHER	1a. INSURED'S I.D. NUMBER (FOR PROGRAM IN ITEM 1)
(Medicare #) (Medicaid #) (Sponsor's SSN) (VA File #)	(SSN or I D)	(SSN)	(I D)	484-91-1688

2. PATIENT'S NAME (Last Name, First Name, Middle Initial)	3. PATIENT'S BIRTH DATE / SEX	4. INSURED'S NAME (Last Name, First Name, Middle Initial)
Moyer, James X. (Jr.)	MM 09 DD 09 YY -- M [X] F [ ]	*Moyer, James X. (Sr.)*

5. PATIENT'S ADDRESS (No. Street)	6. PATIENT RELATIONSHIP TO INSURED	7. INSURED'S ADDRESS (No. Street)
15 Crowe Dr.	Self [ ] Spouse [ ] Child [X] Other [ ]	*Same*

CITY	STATE	8. PATIENT STATUS	CITY	STATE
Beechline	IN	Single [X] Married [ ] Other [ ]		

ZIP CODE	TELEPHONE (Include Area Code)		CITY / ZIP CODE	TELEPHONE (INCLUDE AREA CODE)
47888		Employed [ ] Full-Time Student [ ] Part-Time Student [ ]		( )

9. OTHER INSURED'S NAME (Last Name, First Name, Middle Initial)	10. IS PATIENT'S CONDITION RELATED TO:	11. INSURED'S POLICY GROUP OR FECA NUMBER
Moyer, Charlotte		30668

a. OTHER INSURED'S POLICY OR GROUP NUMBER	a. EMPLOYMENT? (CURRENT OR PREVIOUS)	a. INSURED'S DATE OF BIRTH / SEX
400-12-3344	[ ] YES [X] NO	MM 04 DD 10 YY -- M [X] F [ ]

b. OTHER INSURED'S DATE OF BIRTH / SEX	b. AUTO ACCIDENT? PLACE (State)	b. EMPLOYER'S NAME OR SCHOOL NAME
MM 10 DD 11 YY -- M [ ] F [X]	[ ] YES [X] NO	*North Bank*

c. EMPLOYER'S NAME OR SCHOOL NAME	c. OTHER ACCIDENT?	c. INSURANCE PLAN NAME OR PROGRAM NAME
County Tyme Co.	[ ] YES [X] NO	

d. INSURANCE PLAN NAME OR PROGRAM NAME	10d. RESERVED FOR LOCAL USE	d. IS THERE ANOTHER HEALTH BENEFIT PLAN?
Elreed Ins. Co.		[X] YES [ ] NO If yes, return to and complete item 9 a – d.

READ BACK OF FORM BEFORE COMPLETING & SIGNING THIS FORM.
12. PATIENT'S OR AUTHORIZED PERSON'S SIGNATURE I authorize the release of any medical or other information necessary to process this claim. I also request payment of government benefits either to myself or to the party who accepts assignment below.

SIGNED *Signature on File*   DATE *Today*

13. INSURED'S OR AUTHORIZED PERSON'S SIGNATURE I authorize payment of medical benefits to the undersigned physician or supplier for services described below.

SIGNED *Signature on File*

PATIENT AND INSURED INFORMATION

FIGURE 8–5 Completed top half of HCFA-1500 under the Birthday Rule

EXERCISE 2

1. Remove Record #11, Sheets 1 and 2 in Chapter 16 for patient Mobutuu, and complete Form #14 from Part V.

2. Assume that a payment for $50.00 was received from the primary insurance company.

3. Locate Form #15, Part V, the EOB for the $50.00 payment.

4. Remove Form #16, Part V, and complete the second form, adding the words "See Attached EOB" in Block 10d.

DIVORCED PARENTS

Now that you understand how to complete forms for primary and secondary insurance carriers, there is one more common situation to be explored. How does the **insurance billing specialist** complete insurance forms for single divorced parents, or divorced parents who may have remarried? Which insurance company is primary and what order should be followed? This is simpler than it may seem if the patient record is properly completed at the time the child first visited our office, and our policies explained to the custodial parent.

Our office works to serve our patients and their parents whenever we can. Completing insurance forms for them at no charge is one way of providing an important service. When parents have divorced, all sorts of feelings follow and sometimes these can create problems for the parents, the children, and even for us if we are not alert to this possibility. Very often, communication between parents is strained or nonexistent, and it is important that neither this office nor the **insurance billing specialist** be swept into the middle of any parental controversies. This is one reason why we carefully explain our billing policies to the parent accompanying the child. Frequently, the mother will bring in the child stating she has custody, as decreed by the Divorce Court, while the primary insurance coverage has been decreed by the Court to be the father's responsibility. Sometimes, the mother will bring in a copy of a court document outlining specific medical payment responsibilities assigned to the father and/or to herself. We have learned the hard way that we are not the Court and have no power to enforce any of these decrees. We explain to the custodial parent we will submit all insurance forms with the information we are given, but we will be sending our bills to her! She must then do all that she can to collect from her former husband whatever the Court has determined is his share. However, we cannot place ourselves between her and her former husband or submit any bills to him. Our policy of billing the parent who brings in the patient is clearly outlined in our Patient Policy booklet as well as our intent to help all we can by completing and submitting insurance forms. Beyond this, we can

do no more. By taking this stand, we have given back to the custodial parent the responsibility of supervising the bill by billing the other parent, who frequently claims he knows nothing about any medical treatment. This same policy is applied regardless of the sex of the custodial parent. If the child lives with the father and the mother has the primary insurance responsibility, the bill will be sent to the father.

Following this understanding, the sequencing of insurance form filing is dependent upon several questions: 1) Which parent has primary insurance responsibility? 2) Does the other natural parent have insurance coverage for the child? 3) Has either parent remarried? 4) Does the new spouse (stepparent) have insurance coverage for this child?

All this information must be gathered at the initial visit of the child. "A worst-case scenario" would be if both parents remarried and both stepparents had insurance coverage for the patient. This is highly unlikely! Most insurance policies do not include coverage for stepchildren. However, if we assumed all four adults had insurance coverage for this single child, the order of completing forms would be: 1) parent decreed by the Court with primary insurance coverage; 2) the other natural parent next; 3) the spouse of parent B; 4) the spouse of parent A.

If there is coverage by parent A, none from working parent B, but coverage by the spouse of parent B, then a claim to the insurance company of parent B must be filed anyway so that a written denial may be received. The denial of coverage would then be submitted to the company of the spouse of parent B in order to get payment from that company. All EOBs and denials must be included and special caution taken to make copies of all submissions for our records.

Obviously, all four names cannot be placed on an insurance form at the same time! Do not be concerned. Continue to complete the forms listing the parent whose insurance company has not yet been contacted, and attach all EOBs and/or denials from those that have been submitted. If full payment is received from several combined insurance companies before the later one(s) can be billed, stop filing claims! Once the claim is paid in full, no additional benefits will be forthcoming because that would violate the Coordination of Benefits rule.

EXERCISE 3

1. Complete a HCFA-1500 for patient Small using Record #12 in Part IV and Forms #17 and #18 in Part V.

2. Determine which parent has primary insurance responsibility and which has secondary insurance responsibility.

3. Assume that a payment in the amount of $25.00 was received from the primary insurance company and complete Form #19 for the secondary insurance company.

EXERCISE 4

1. Complete a HCFA-1500 for patient Bacon using Record #13, Sheets 1 through 3, Chapter 16, and Form #20 in Part V.

2. Determine the primary, secondary, and tertiary insurance carriers.

3. Assume that a payment of $40.00 was received from the primary insurance company.

4. Complete Form #21 in Part V for the second insurance carrier.

5. Assume that a payment of $15.00 was received from the second insurance company.

6. Complete Form #22 in Part V for the third insurance carrier.

REVIEW QUESTIONS FOR DISCUSSION

1. How would you handle an irate custodial mother who demands that all bills for treatment be sent to the father who is living 100 miles away?

2. Select a partner to role-play this scenario and then change places.

3. If both parents have remarried and three of the four have insurance coverage for the child, how long will it take to receive insurance payments if each insurance company takes six weeks to pay this office after the claim has been received?

4. Are denials included with EOBs? How might the wording in Block #10d be altered in order to explain the attachment of an EOB and a denial?

5. Why is it important to avoid participating in any parental conflicts?

Part Three

COMPLETING INSURANCE FORMS

JOB DESCRIPTION

TITLE: Insurance Billing Specialist

IMMEDIATE SUPERVISOR: Office Manager

JOB DUTIES: Part I. To gather sufficient patient information to complete and file health insurance claims for reimbursement for services rendered by the physicians and dentists of this office. Actual patient records will be examined

Part II. To complete the insurance forms correctly in accordance with the general requirements of most fee-for-service third-party payers. Patient records of this office will be accessed for clarification.

Part III. To adapt the insurance form completion process, as determined by specific patient records, to the general requirements of the major insurers, such as Medicare, Medicaid, Workers' Compensation, CHAMPUS, and certain other managed care insurance plans.

Part IV. To provide the references and resources necessary to complete the insurance billing process.

Part V. To furnish the forms and worksheets needed to complete all required tasks.

Chapter Nine

MEDICARE COVERAGE

OBJECTIVES   After completing this chapter, you will be able to

- define who is eligible to receive Medicare coverage and what is included
- explain how Medicare coordinates with other private and/or federal insurance coverage
- explain a PAR provider
- accurately complete a Medicare claim form under all combinations of coverage
- define Medigap and Medi-Medi

POWER WORDS

CPIN (Clinical Physician Identification Number)   A seven-digit number assigned to each member of our Medicare group. This number is to be used on each Medicare claim form in column 24K.

ESRD (end-stage renal disease)   A diagnosis indicating a very serious kidney disease that usually requires kidney transplant; special Medicare coverage is provided for those suffering from this disease.

Medicare Group Number   An identification number assigned to each group location.

Medigap   A general term referring to insurance coverage purchased by the Medicare patient to cover the 20 percent "gap" left uncovered by Medicare. Some Medigap insurers may pay for the $100 deductible as well.

UPIN (Unique Physician Identification Number)   Assigned to each Medicare provider of health care services; it appears on Block #17a of claim forms of referred patients at the time the first claim is filed.

INTRODUCTION TO MEDICARE COVERAGE

Medicare insurance coverage for the elderly was created in 1965 as Title 18 of the Social Security Act. It is administered by the Health Care Finance Administration as a national program of federal insurance coverage. It selects the fiscal intermediary (FI) in each state or area to process Medicare claims based on federal guidelines and is the single largest provider of health care benefits nationwide. Medicare Part A benefits cover home health services, inpatient hospital bed and hospice fees. The **insurance billing specialist** will file claims under Medicare Part B coverage for the doctors in our office. All instructions in this manual about completing Medicare forms will always be directed toward Part B benefits since these cover our health care providers. (Remember to check with the FI in your state to see if your Medicare instructions differ from those we are about to explore.)

Those citizens eligible for Medicare coverage include:

1. all retired persons 65 and older

2. all persons of any age who have received Social Security Disability Benefits for two years or more

3. all people on Railroad Retirement 65 and over and their spouses age 65 and older

4. spouses age 65 and older of a worker who has regularly paid into the social security program, whether the worker is retired or not

5. all workers suffering from ESRD (end-stage renal disease) who have paid social security taxes; spouses or dependent children of those who have paid social security taxes

6. donors of kidneys given to ESRD patients are covered for medical expenses related to the donation

7. those retired federal employees and their spouses age 65 and over, covered by the Civil Service Retirement System.

MEDICARE AS THE ONLY COVERAGE

Remove Form #23 from Part V and Record #14, Sheets 1 and 2, from Chapter 16 for patient O'Leary. This patient has no other coverage beyond Medicare Part A and Part B.

☛ Remember, in order for the physician to be paid for services, the patient must have Part B coverage.

This information is printed on the Medicare identification card and the receptionist can tell at once if the patient has the Part B coverage for physician's services. In this case, Mrs. O'Leary has Part B coverage and, therefore, the **insurance billing specialist** must complete a Medicare claim form. These directions are only slightly different than the work done until now. Let's take a look at each block of the HCFA-1500 and complete it for Medicare.

Top, Right Corner	Print or type the name and address of the Medicare fiscal intermediary processing Medicare claims, or other address that might appear on the Medicare card.
Block #1	Requires an "X" in the Medicare box.
Block #1A	Enter the Medicare ID number appearing on the ID card.
Blocks #2 and #5	Complete patient information as usual.
Blocks #3, #6, #8, #10	Complete patient information as usual.
Block # 4	Enter insured's name, who is also the patient in this case.
Block # 7	Enter the word "same".
Block #9	Enter the word "none" to show no insurance primary to Medicare.
Block #11 a, b, c	Skip, not applicable.

Block #11d	Place an "X" in the "No" square.
Blocks #12 and #13	Type or print "signature on file" as patient records verify and enter the date the form is completed on the date line, as usual. The top of the form changed only in the addition of the "X" in the Medicare square.
Block #14	Enter the date of the illness (if known) or accident if one took place.
Blocks #15, #16, #18	Skip.
Block #20	This is completed only if patient specimens are sent to an outside laboratory for analysis and we are billed for the results. If this is the case, show we are using an outside lab by placing an "X" in the "Yes" square and show the fee we are charged by the laboratory doing the testing. Medicare wants to compare the amount we are charged against the amount we charge the patient.
Block #17	Enter the name of the referring physician for new patients, if a doctor referred the patient, for patients seen in consultation, or one coming into our practice requiring surgery.
Block #17a	Enter the UPIN (Unique Physician Identification Number) assigned by HCFA to the referring physician. All physicians in the Medicare program are assigned one of these numbers.

Blocks #22 and #23	Skip.
Block #21	Complete as usual, indicating up to four diagnoses.
Block #24a and b	Complete as usual.
Block #24c	Skip.
Block #24d	Complete as usual.
Block #24e	Enter only one diagnostic reference number on each line of the form.
Block #24f and g	Complete as usual.
Block #24h, i, j	Skip.
Block #24k	Enter the seven-digit CPIN (Clinical Physician Identification Number) assigned to each of our Medicare group members for each doctor who treated the patient as listed on the form. In other words, Dr. Cartman may have seen the patient on one day and his CPIN number would be in Block #24k; the next day, Dr. Gregory might see the patient and then her CPIN number would be entered in Block #24k.
Block #25	Complete as usual.
Block #26	Skip.
Block #27	Place an "X" in the "Yes" block. We are participating physicians in contract with Medicare and we agree to accept the approved payment amount determined by Medicare.
Blocks #28, #29, #30, #31	Complete as usual.
Block #32	Complete only if services are provided other than the office or home.

Block #33   Complete with the name and address of the physician. Add the CPIN number of the primary doctor and the Medicare Group Number in this block. Refer to the Resources list in Chapter 15 to locate the Medicare Group Number.

In summary, in this patient case, the difference between the Medicare claim form and the fee-for-services claims completed in earlier chapters by the **insurance billing specialist** are:

1. An "X" in Block #1a.

2. The word "none" in Block #9.

3. The UPIN number in Block #17a for new patients referred for consultation or surgery.

4. Identifying only one diagnosis in Block #24e.

5. Putting the CPIN number in Block #24k.

6. Adding the CPIN and Medicare Group Number to Block #33.

Compare your completed form to the one printed in the *Teacher's Guide*.

EXERCISE 1

Remove Record #15, Sheets 1 and 2, for patient Johnson from Chapter 16, and Form #24 from Part V. This patient had visits on several days. When services for the same fee are listed for several days in a row, the **insurance billing specialist** may list the first date on column #24a and the last date under the "to" listing on the column. Add the totals together and list the sum in column #24f. List the number of days lumped together in #24g. Proceed to complete the form as directed above. *Remember,* the lumping together of services and fees is acceptable only when all the fees and services are identical.

MEDICARE AS SECONDARY COVERAGE

If the Medicare patient is working or has a working spouse with private insurance coverage for the patient, then:

☞ The private insurance coverage is primary and Medicare is secondary.

This is a real departure from your previous filing experiences. HCFA is very serious about filing for private insurance coverage first before Medicare is contacted for payment. There are stiff fines and penalties levied on the health care provider who neglects to determine if private insurance coverage is available. This information is routinely gathered at the first contact with the patient, so the **insurance billing specialist** may proceed to file claims in the correct order.

Other situations that exclude Medicare as the primary source of coverage include:

1. Workers' Compensation claims (unless denied by WC—then a copy of the denial should be included).

2. Patients eligible to receive Veterans Administration benefits as well as Medicare.

3. Any third-party coverage, such as automobile insurance or other liability insurance, that would be responsible for Medicare patient injuries.

Once the **insurance billing specialist** has determined there is other primary coverage for the Medicare patient, complete the HCFA-1500 the same as in previous cases where two insurance companies were involved, only in this case, the patient is both the insured and the patient. Since Medicare is the secondary insurer, complete Blocks #17a, #20, #24e, #24k, #27 and #33 as required by Medicare. If the primary insurance company is large enough, claims will be forwarded to Medicare for processing after the primary payment has been made. As the secondary payer, Medicare will pay its portion based on the same fee schedule it applies for primary Medicare payments. Therefore, if the private insurance company pays more on the claim than the approved Medicare amount, no additional payments will be coming from Medicare.

EXERCISE 2

1. Remove Form #25 from Part V and Record #16, Sheets 1 and 2 for patient Dawson. Complete this form.

2. Complete Form #26 from Part V based on the assumption that a payment for $20.00 was received from Medicare.

MEDICARE FEE CALCULATIONS

In 1992, Medicare significantly altered its method of payment of fees in an attempt to control escalating costs. A new system called the Resource Based Relative Value Scale (RBRVS) attempts to recognize cost of living differences in areas of the country, provider overhead expenses, and also to reimburse more equitably those providers working most directly with the patient. With this scale, it is possible to calculate exactly how much Medicare will pay for any given submitted service, so long as the service is determined to be medically necessary and appropriate. Medicare will never approve payment for any services that it deems unnecessary, experimental, or unproven as effective for the diagnosis listed.

Our physicians have signed a participating provider agreement (PAR) which means they have agreed to accept assignment on all claims submitted to Medicare. This means Medicare will determine the appropriate fee for the services submitted to them, pay 80 percent of that fee (after the patient has met the $100.00 deductible each calendar year), and our providers are required to bill the patient for the remaining approved 20 percent. If the patient has a second insurance, the 20 percent may be billed to it. Our office must then write off the difference between the amount of the fee submitted and the amount approved. We are never allowed to bill the patient for any unapproved amounts. At the same time, we are required to routinely collect the 20 percent not covered by Medicare, and if we fail to do so, we are subject to severe fines and penalties from Medicare.

For example, if we bill Medicare $500.00 for a myringotomy with tube insertion and they approve only $375.00, the account must be managed as follows:

Amount submitted by us:	$500.00	
Amount approved by Medicare:		$375.00
The difference *must* be written off:	$125.00	
Amount paid is 80% of approved:		$300.00
Unpaid 20% *must* bill patient:		$ 75.00

Medicare providers are forbidden by law to charge Medicare patients more than their usual fees.

The $500.00 fee quoted above must be the same fee charged to any patient not otherwise participating in any special contractual fee arrangement. This law is designed to avoid hiking fees for Medicare patients in order to try to recover a larger portion of the amount not approved by Medicare.

If one of our physicians believes a patient requires a service that the physician knows is not covered by Medicare, very specific steps towards patient education must be taken. Figure 9-1 shows the form which must be explained, completed, and signed by the uncovered Medicare patient before the service may be provided.

Failure to inform the patient that we know a specific service is not covered by Medicare may result in severe penalties for the physician. However, if the office unknowingly provides a service that is not covered by Medicare or a service that Medicare does not believe is medically necessary in a specific case, this action is not considered to warrant a penalty. In the case of a denied Medicare claim that is usually approved for other Medicare patients, our office may collect from the patient the portion that Medicare would have approved.

MEDICARE-MEDIGAP

Many large insurance companies offer a special policy for Medicare patients designed to pay the 20 percent of the approved amount remaining after Medicare pays its 80 percent. This type of coverage is called "Medigap" because it pays benefits on the remaining gap after Medicare processes the claim. Federal law requires that each Medicare recipient be sold only one Medigap policy at a time. Medigap is simply an umbrella term for secondary insurance held by the Medicare patient. Premiums must be paid by the patient and the cost of this kind of insurance is highly competitive in the private market.

Completing a Medicare form and showing Medigap coverage is very simple with changes required above the line only.

Block #11d — Place an "X" in the "Yes" square to indicate there is insurance in addition to Medicare.

Medical & Dental Associates, P.C.

3733 Professional Drive #300
Indianapolis, IN 46260

317/123-4567
Tax ID# 99-9999999

To All Medicare Patients:

My primary concern is to provide you with the best possible care. Medicare does not pay for all services and will only allow services which it determines to be "reasonable and necessary" as defined in the Omnibus Reconciliation Act of 1986, Section 1862(a)(1). Under this law, any procedure or service deemed medically unreasonable or unnecessary will be denied. Since I believe each scheduled visit or planned procedure is both reasonable and necessary, I am required to notify you in advance that the following services/procedures may be denied by Medicare, even though we have mutually agreed to undertake these services.

Date(s) of Planned Service(s) _____

Description   Charge

_____

_____

_____

I understand denials may be made for one or more of the following reasons:
1) Medicare does not usually pay for this many visits or treatments;
2) Medicare does not usually pay for this many services within this period of time;
3) Medicare does not usually pay for this type of service for your condition and diagnosis.

However, I believe these services are both reasonable and necessary for your condition, and I will assist you in collecting payment from Medicare. In order to do that, the law requires that you read and sign the following agreement.

I have been informed by Dr. _____ that s/he believes Medicare is likely to deny payment in my case for the services and reasons outlined above. If Medicare denies payment, I agree to be personally responsible for payment.

Beneficiary's Name _____

Medicare ID# _____

Beneficiary Signature _____

Or

Signature of Authorized Representative _____

FIGURE 9–1 Form to notify patient of lack of Medicare coverage

Block #9	Enter the word "same".
Block #9a	Print the word "Medigap" followed by the ID number of the plan as found on the ID card.
Block #9b	Print the date of birth of the patient.
Block #9c	Show an abbreviated address as follows: Street number and name; State initials only, zip code. This means the city is not listed within this block. However, the state initials and zip code will get the form to the correct location.

Block #9d	Lists the name of the Medigap company.

MEDICARE-MEDICAID

Our last scenario involves the patient with Medicare and Medicaid coverage. This is sometimes called Medi-Medi. Medicare will forward the claim to Medicaid after Medicare has processed it. Medicaid will not pay more than the 20 percent gap left by Medicare, and often pays less. In this instance, Medicaid is the insurer of last resort. Therefore, complete the form for Medicare as usual. Use Block #10d to show the Medicaid (MCD) identification number preceded by the MCD initials. No other information about Medicaid must be entered above the line. Do indicate there is additional insurance in Block #11d, but Blocks #9 through #9d may be left blank.

EXERCISE 3

Let's practice completing a Medicare-Medigap claim form. Remove Form #27 from Part V, and Record #17, Sheets 1 and 2, for patient Steinbert. Once completed, follow your teacher's instructions.

EXERCISE 4

Remove Form #28 from Part V, and Record #18, Sheets 1 and 2, for patient Styvesant. Follow your instructor's directions after completing this form.

REVIEW QUESTIONS FOR DISCUSSION

1. Why are the rules and regulations issued from HCFA regarding Medicare important to the health care provider?

2. What do you think about the law requiring our office to collect the 20 percent of approved fees left uncovered by Medicare?

3. Why do you think this law came about?

4. Is Medicare coverage the same thing as a national plan for health care coverage? What are the differences or similarities?

5. Find a partner and role-play how the **insurance billing specialist** might explain Medicare coverage to an elderly patient. Take turns in each role.

Chapter Ten

MEDICAID—WORKERS' COMPENSATION

OBJECTIVES After completing this chapter, you will be able to

- explain Medicaid as a form of health care coverage and determine who is eligible to participate
- complete Medicaid claim forms accurately
- correctly complete a Workers' Compensation First Report of Injury form
- accurately complete a Workers' Compensation health insurance claim form
- explain differences in coverage for federal employees

POWER WORDS

Aid to Families with Dependent Children (AFDC) A program of aid for young children and/or pregnant women who live in households earning below the poverty level.

Supplemental Security Income (SSI) A federally supported welfare assistance plan authorized under Title 16 of the Social Security Act that provides payments to the needy, to aged, blind, or disabled citizens.

MEDICAID

In 1965, Congress enacted Title 19 of the Social Security Act, establishing a state-federal funding partnership to provide medical coverage for people living below the poverty level. This is known today as Medicaid. Unlike Medicare, each state is permitted to set most of the rules guiding Medicaid coverage within its borders, as long as basic federal guidelines are met. There is no set percentage of federal support within each state, and no set federal dictates regarding how much in benefits are to be paid to health care providers treating Medicaid patients. In general, Medicaid payments are lower than Medicare payments in most states. Controlling Medicaid costs for each state remains an important mandate, and some states are moving towards establishing Medicaid managed care programs. While the rules vary with each state, this manual describes the Indiana Medicaid program. Should the **insurance billing specialist** elect to leave us and move to another state, particular attention will need to be paid to determine how other Medicaid programs differ. In general, the Indiana plan information required is not significantly different from those plans in many other states.

Those eligible to receive Medicaid generally include the following: 1) people covered by Supplemental Security Income (SSI), 2) recipients of Aid to Families with Dependent Children (AFDC), and 3) certain Medicare-eligible people.

As with other insurance coverage, Medicaid participants must present an identification card with a twelve-digit number. Medicaid coverage is renewed month to month. Therefore, the receptionist must certify coverage at the first visit each month. If surgery or other out-of-office or unusually expensive services are needed, the receptionist will secure a preauthorization number to affix to the insurance form in Block #23. The **insurance billing specialist** may use the HCFA-1500 for the submission of Medicaid claims. In some states, special Medicaid forms are required to be completed and the HCFA-1500 may not be used.

Once the provider has agreed to treat a Medicaid patient, the provider must accept as full payment the amount received from Medicaid and may never bill the patient for any covered services.

In order to submit the HCFA-1500 to Medicaid in Indiana, the following instructions must be followed:

1. The name and address of the state administrator where the form is to be sent must be entered at the top of the form.
2. Blocks #1, #1a, #2, #3 must be completed.
3. Blocks #4 through #9 may be skipped.
4. Block #9a is required if the recipient has other insurance coverage.
5. Skip Blocks #9b and #9c.
6. Blocks #9d and #10 are required if applicable.
7. Skip Blocks #10d, #11, #11a, and #11b.
8. Blocks #11c and #11d are required if applicable.
9. Skip Blocks #12 and #13.
10. Block #14 is required if applicable.
11. Skip Blocks #15 and #16.
12. Blocks #17 through #20 are required if applicable.
13. Block #21 is required.
14. Skip Block #22.
15. Blocks #23 through #24b are required.
16. Skip Block #24c.
17. Blocks #24d through #24g are required.
18. Blocks #24h and #24i are required if applicable.
19. Block #24j is not required.
20. Block #24k is required. Place the Medicaid Provider number of the treating provider in this space.
21. Blocks #25 through #27 are not required.
22. Blocks #28 through #33 are required. Place the Medicaid Provider number next to PIN, and the group Medicaid provider number next to GRP on the insurance form in Block #33.

The **insurance billing specialist** must file the Medicaid claim as soon as possible to avoid delay in payment. Unlike many other doctors in the city, this office *does* accept nonemergency and emergency Medicaid patients. Too often, the Medicaid patient will be refused treatment for nonemergencies by the private physician because of the very low benefits paid. This is not a reflection of ill feelings toward the human beings needing treatment, but is a sign of intense frustration and dissatisfaction with very low and very slow payments received from the bureaucracy.

EXERCISE 1

Locate Record #19, Sheets 1 and 2 in Chapter 16, for patient Higson. Use Form #29 to complete a Medicaid claim.

EXERCISE 2

Locate Record #20, Sheets 1 and 2 in Chapter 16 for patient White. Use Form #30 to complete a Medicaid claim.

EXERCISE 3

Locate Record #21, Sheets 1 and 2 in Chapter 16 for patient Woods. Use Form #31 to complete a Medicaid claim.

WORKERS' COMPENSATION INSURANCE COVERAGE

Workers' Compensation Insurance Coverage was designed to provide insurance coverage for employees injured while at work or while performing tasks away from the place of employment but assigned as normal work activity. The original intent was to hasten the return to work of the injured employees and provide them with income until they are able to return to the workplace. Premiums for this kind of insurance are paid by the employer and payments to treating physicians are considered payment in full of the injured's bill. No statements are sent to the patient *unless* the injury is determined to be non-work-related.

This is an area of insurance coverage that is ripe for abuse, and many Workers' Compensation Boards take special precautions to ensure that only the truly injured and ill receive compensation. It is not the duty of the **insurance billing specialist** to be concerned about the propriety of any given patient under Workers' Compensation or any other coverage, for that matter. Once the physician has determined the nature of the injury or illness, the **insurance billing specialist** will proceed to complete the HCFA-1500 correctly.

Federal employees also have this type of coverage, but the forms are sent to different locations depending upon the specific classification of worker; that is, whether they are coal miners, longshoremen, or harbor workers. Also, some large companies are self-insured and their claims are sent to the firm providing administration of claim processing. If you are uncertain where Workers' Compensation forms should be sent (or any other kind of claim), call the personnel department at the place of employment for the correct name and address of the processing company.

When the patient first arrives for treatment after a work injury, very specific steps must be taken. The physician must complete a First Report of Injury Form as shown in Fig. 10-1.

As you review this form, it is clear the physician is required to describe the nature of the injury, future course of treatment, and estimated return to work date. One copy of this completed form is sent to the Workers' Compensation Board, one to the processing company handling the claim for the employer, one to the employer providing the coverage, and one is kept in the patient's chart. This report must be filed quickly after the patient is seen so that the process of assigning the correct claim number and getting benefits started may begin. If the patient's condition changes, a progress report must be dictated by the physician and sent to all parties involved.

If the Workers' Compensation patient is new to the office, the normal paperwork is done and the first report is submitted. If the patient has been in the office for other treatment or requires treatment for non-work-related problems, it is very important to keep the billing records separate from the work-related bill. For example, if a new patient comes to the office for a work-related problem and then develops an upper respiratory infection or other illness that is clearly not part of the work injury, you must be careful to complete a separate insurance form for infection and one for the work injury. In this situation, the patient would be billed for non-work-related illnesses, but never for a job injury.

Remove Form #32 from Part V and Record #22, Sheets 1 through 5 for patient O'Shea from Chapter 16. The Medical Treatment Record shows Mr. O'Shea hurt his left ankle at work and came into the office for treatment. Notice on the Confidential Patient Information Record (CPIR), Mr. O'Shea also requested a test for AIDS. Complete Form #32 for his work-related problem as directed, then Form #33 for the AIDS test.

Here are the instructions for completing the Workers' Compensation Claim Form in Indiana using the HCFA-1500:

Blocks #1, #2, #3, #5	Complete as usual.
Block #1a	Enter the Workers' Compensation Claim Number, if known. If not known, check with the employer for directions.
Block #8	Only place an "X" in the square next to Employed.

Department of Labor and Industry
(612) 296-6107

PHYSICIAN'S REPORT
(The use of this form for work-related injuries is
prescribed by the State of Minnesota.)

Patient's Social Security Number	Date of Claimed Injury

Name and Address of Employer

Insurer _____

Phone Number _____

PATIENT

1. Name of Patient _____ Date of Birth _____
2. Address _____
   (Street) (City) (State) (Zip Code)

HISTORY OF INJURY OR DISEASE

3. Date of first exam for this injury by this office _____
4. Date of most recent exam _____
5. History and date of injury or disease as given by patient* _____

NATURE AND EXTENT OF INJURY OR DISEASE

6. Findings, exam, lab work, x-rays, etc.* _____
7. Preliminary diagnosis* _____
   _____ ICD-9 CODE # _____ _____ _____
8. Was the injury or disease caused, aggravated, or accelerated by the patient's alleged employment activity?
   Yes _____ No _____
9. Did this injury or disease prevent the patient from working? Yes _____ No _____
   If yes, the employee is/was:
   (A) Totally unable to work from _____ to _____
   (B) Able to return to work with restrictions from _____ to _____
   Restrictions* _____

   (C) Able to return to work without restrictions as of _____
10. Is a rehabilitation assessment recommended? Yes _____ No _____ (assessment required if patient is likely to miss at least 60 work days with an injury or 30 work days with a back injury).
11. Is permanent disability likely? Yes _____ No _____ Do not know _____.
    If yes, what percentage disability to the whole body is estimated? _____% Do not know _____.
12. Is there evidence of pre-existing or other conditions that may affect this disability? Yes _____ No _____ If yes, describe*: _____

TREATMENT

13. Is further medical care necessary? Yes _____ No _____ If yes, describe*: _____
14. If admitted to hospital for this injury, name and address of hospital _____

    Date of admission to hospital _____.
15. Has any surgery been performed? Yes _____ No _____ If so, describe*: _____
16. The patient has been or will be referred to another physician. Yes _____ No _____
    If yes, name and address of physician to whom referred _____

*Additional information or remarks may be written on the reverse side or on a separate sheet.

CERTIFICATION

17. Certified by me, a licensed _____ (give degree) physician in the State of Minnesota this _____ day
    of _____ , 19 _____

Signature of Physician _____ Address _____

Name of Physician _____

License Number of Physician _____ Phone Number (_____) _____

LI-20319-02 (11/85)

FIGURE 10–1 First Report of Injury form

| Block #10a | Place an "X" in the square next to "Yes". |
| Blocks #11b and #12 | Complete as usual. |

Skip all blocks not mentioned.

Complete all blocks *below* the black line except for the following: #17, #17a, #19, #22, #24h, i, j, k, #27, #29, #30, #33PIN, and #33GRP. Complete Blocks #18 and #32 only if the patient is hospitalized or treated somewhere other than the home or office.

EXERCISE 4

Assume Mr. O'Shea returned to see Dr. Gregory on 8/4/— and the doctor determined his diagnosis was sprain/strain lumbar spine due to strenuous lifting and carrying while gardening at home that morning. He received an expanded problem focused examination and was sent home with further home care instructions. Complete Form #33 in Part V for this office visit.

REVIEW QUESTIONS FOR DISCUSSION

1. Do you know of anyone who has had a job-related injury and received Workers' Compensation coverage and/or benefits for that injury?

2. Was that person able to return to work?

3. If Workers' Compensation denied a claim for Mr. O'Shea and he was unsuccessful at winning an appeal, how would Dr. Gregory's bill be paid?

4. Visit your local library and find out: 1) when this state mandated Workers' Compensation coverage; 2) define OSHA (Occupational Safety and Health Administration) and their responsibilities toward job safety.

5. What penalties might result from unsafe job conditions? Who would levy those penalties?

Workers' Compensation Insurance Coverage

Chapter Eleven

CHAMPUS AND CHAMPVA

OBJECTIVES   After completing this chapter, you will be able to

- define CHAMPUS and CHAMPVA

- determine when a patient is covered by one or the other

- complete the CHAMPUS/CHAMPVA form

POWER WORDS

CHAMPUS (Civilian Health and Medical Program of the Uniformed Services)   A comprehensive federal health care program for civilian spouses and dependents of those in the uniformed services, either active duty personnel or those who died while on active duty; also retired personnel, their spouses and dependents.

CHAMPVA (Civilian Health and Medical Program of the Veterans Administration)   A federal program providing civilian coverage for families of deceased or 100 percent disabled veterans killed or injured while in active military service, or for retired military personnel not eligible to receive Medicare.

sponsor   The label given the person currently in military service or retired from service in good standing.

subrogation   The provision of an insurer, such as CHAMPUS to pay for the current and immediate health care needed by the injured patient, with the intention of being reimbursed for expenses at a later date from the insurance company of the person responsible for the accident or injuries. This is always a part of automobile insurance coverage so that the injured party does not bear the expense for injuries caused by another person who also has insurance coverage, and does not experience a delay in getting the necessary care.

CHAMPUS AND CHAMPVA

The military services have traditionally provided medical and dental care for men and women on active duty as one of the benefits of being in the armed forces. Well-trained personnel are readily available to care for the sick and wounded, even in peace time. However, similar benefits were not available for the dependents and families of service people left behind until 1966. At that time, Congress created a federal program providing health insurance coverage primarily for spouses and children of men and women serving their country. This is called CHAMPUS (Civilian Health and Medical Program of the Uniformed Services). Seven years later, a similar program was established for families of servicemen who had died from service related injuries or were 100 percent disabled. This is called CHAMPVA (Civilian Health and Medical Program of the Veterans Administration).

At first, families and dependents received services under these programs on military bases and facilities only and had no benefit coverage if they wanted to see a "civilian" doctor. Over time, with the dismantling of many bases and the reduced numbers of military locations providing health care, permission was given for CHAMPUS and CHAMPVA families to receive treatment from participating civilian health care workers in their communities. Persons serving in the military (called sponsors) are not eligible to receive CHAMPVA until or unless they become permanently 100 percent disabled, or experience a verifiable emergency in an area that does not have a military facility. Retired military personnel are eligible for CHAMPUS until old enough for Medicare coverage.

CHAMPUS and CHAMPVA are defined by the government as "a service-connected benefit, not an insurance program." For the **insurance billing specialist**, the emphasis is on filing the claim form correctly, using all the identification numbers gathered by the receptionist at the time of patient registration.

☛ CHAMPUS and CHAMPVA are secondary payers to *all* other medical insurance claims or benefits except MEDICAID or CHAMPUS supplemental policies.

There are severe penalties for patients who present CHAMPUS or CHAMPVA claim information and withhold knowledge of other insurance coverage. Once retired military personnel become eligible for Medicare coverage, they are no longer covered by CHAMPUS/CHAMPVA. Therefore:

☛ The **insurance billing specialist** will never see a sponsor with both Medicare and CHAMPUS/CHAMPVA coverage.

This is often a source of confusion for patients and sometimes patient education is needed in this area.

If a patient with CHAMPUS or CHAMPVA needs treatment as a result of a personal injury caused by another, such as an automobile accident, a long form called "Statement of Personal Injury—Possible Third Party Liability Statement DD Form 2527" must be completed by patient and physician. The patient must provide this form for completion. This is completed with the expectation that the government can recover its expenses from the insurance company of the party responsible for patient injuries. This is called subrogation.

If the CHAMPUS sponsor lives within a forty-mile radius of an area that provides military based treatment facilities, preauthorization for treatment of family members outside the military system must be received—in nonemergency situations. In an emergency, the patient should be directed to the nearest hospital for life-saving care. Preauthorization for nonemergency treatment must be requested by filing a nonavailability statement the patient can get from the military treatment facility. This means the treatment needed by the patient is not available on the military base and must be received from someone in the civilian community. Our office is not located within a forty mile radius of a military treatment facility, so we do not have the challenge of having to secure the preauthorizations. However, our claims must be filed within a year of the date services are rendered, and sent to the regional carrier or to the address indicated on the insurance identification card. For additional information about CHAMPUS and CHAMPVA coverage or exclusion, contact the health benefits advisor at the nearest military facility or refer to our manual received at the time our physicians registered to become CHAMPUS/CHAMP-VA providers.

COMPLETING THE HCFA-1500 FOR CHAMPUS OR CHAMPVA

Locate Form #34 in Part V, and Record #23, Sheets 1 through 3 in Chapter 16 for a retired military man, Donald Ebner. He was first seen in the office on 3/11/— because of urinary retention due to benign prostatic hypertrophy. Dr. Cartman performed a cystourethroscopy in the office that day and determined the patient needed a transurethral resection of the prostate (TURP) which was done as an outpatient at Good Samaritan Hospital one week later.

Complete the form for a CHAMPUS or CHAMPVA participant as follows:

Block #1a	Sponsor (in this case, the patient) social security number; for CHAMPVA, use the SSN of the sponsor or the number in item 5 on the CHAMPVA authorization card.
Block #4	Sponsor's full name.
Blocks #5 and #6	As usual. You may use the APO or FPO number if the patient lives overseas.
Block #7	Mailing address for the retiree; active-duty sponsor-duty station address for the dependent of a sponsor.
Block #10	If this treatment is about an auto accident or other accident caused by a third party, print the words "see attached DD 2527" above 10a and complete the attachment.
Block #11d	Indicate if there is another insurance carrier.
Blocks #9 through #9d	Complete if applicable.
Blocks #12 and #13	Signature on File.

Below the Line:

Complete all as usual for a fee-for-service insurance form with the exception of skipping Blocks #14, #15, #16, #20, #24h, and #24j. Place the CHAMPUS PIN number in Block #33 and refer to Chapter 15 for the Type of Service Codes that CHAMPUS requires in column #24c.

The same form may be used for both the office and outpatient hospital services. Be sure to use the correct place of service code for each location.

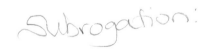
Subrogation:

REVIEW QUESTIONS FOR DISCUSSION

1. Are all physicians CHAMPUS or CHAMPVA providers?

2. Must our office keep a supply of the required forms, such as the DD2527?

3. How would you collect a bill that had been denied by CHAMPUS or CHAMPVA?

4. If a patient has Medicaid and CHAMPUS, to which would you send the first claim?

5. If a patient has CHAMPUS and the spouse has Blue Cross, Blue Shield, to which would you send the first claim?

6. When may the family seek civilian treatment within the forty-mile radius of a military facility?

Chapter Twelve

OTHER INSURANCE COVERAGE

OBJECTIVES After completing this chapter, you will be able to

- define SSI, SSDI, and other entitlement programs
- explain disability insurance coverage and who receives payment
- explain why timely completion of forms is especially important for patients applying for disability

POWER WORDS

contingency Used here as a legal term meaning one party involved in a lawsuit agrees to wait until the suit has been settled before expecting payment for services rendered. Lawyers involved in lawsuits often work on a contingency basis. If the client loses the lawsuit, the client will have to pay the legal fees out of pocket.

disability income insurance A policy that provides direct income to insured people who have fulfilled the definition of "disabled" as set by their particular policy. This may include hospitalization first followed by a number of days or weeks in which the patient is unable to work. This policy is designed to blunt the total loss of income because of disability, but does not usually provide a 100 percent match of normal income.

entitlement programs Include such government plans as Medicare, CHAMPUS, food stamps, Head Start, agricultural subsidies, and social security, in which benefits are calculated based on given formulae. This is not a welfare program in that it is not connected to poverty levels of income.

litigation A legal term meaning a civil lawsuit (or tort) has been filed and is in process of winding through the court system.

Social Security Disability Insurance (SSDI) A federally administered entitlement program—not an insurance program and not welfare. It provides direct forms of financial assistance after documentation of complete or partial disability has been proven and a waiting period has passed.

DISABILITY INSURANCE

Very often, the **insurance billing specialist** is called upon to complete other types of forms providing benefits to the patient that are not limited to paying their bills with our office. For example, millions of Americans buy commercial disability income insurance so that they may collect at least a portion of their normal income if they become disabled temporarily due to an automobile accident or severe illness, and are unable to work. This type of insurance does not take the place of the other kinds of plans the **insurance billing specialist** has studied to date. This insurance takes the form of direct payments to patients to be spent however they see fit.

Sometimes, an employer may pay all or part of the premium for disability insurance as a job benefit. The requirements for coverage vary from company to company. While there is no standard form to be completed automatically, like the HCFA-1500, you may be asked to complete one of those along with or instead of some other form. Normally, this will be spelled out very clearly by the patient's policy booklet. The patient trying to collect this benefit will bring in the necessary forms to be completed by the **insurance billing specialist** and will sometimes have great concern that the forms be completed quickly so that money can be received and bills paid!

Your concern will be to record very carefully all dates of treatment, details of onset of illness or injury, dates of inpatient and outpatient treatment, and any other information. Obviously, careful completion of these forms is of utmost concern to the patient. Your work and the documentation supporting the facts you report will determine when and how much the patient will collect, if anything. Therefore, proceed carefully and utilize the full patient chart. If any doubt or conflict seems apparent within the records of the patient, check with the office manager and/or the physician for clarification.

SOCIAL SECURITY DISABILITY INSURANCE

Another type of insurance that is extremely important to the patient is Social Security Disability Insurance (SSDI). This coverage began with the amendment to the Social Security Act to include Title 2 to provide this entitlement.

To be eligible for SSDI, one must be under age 65 and must have worked a minimum number of quarters in which Social Security taxes were withheld from one's paycheck. The actual number of quarters is dependent upon the age of the patient. Once the process of applying for SSDI begins, the patient must wait a minimum of five months before payments will be received. Nineteen months later, or a full twenty-four months after it has been determined the patient is disabled, the patient will be eligible to receive Medicare coverage and must apply for that benefit.

The criteria for disability determination is very strict and not easily attained. However, for millions, it provides an important financial base. Again, the **insurance billing specialist** will be required to complete sometimes confusing forms in a very careful and deliberate manner.

SUPPLEMENTAL SECURITY INCOME

SSI or Supplemental Security Income is a federally administered welfare program established under Title 16 of the Social Security Act. This is sometimes confused with SSDI, but it is definitely not the same program. Again, eligibility is very strictly defined and limited to needy aged, blind, and disabled persons, and to others living at or below the poverty level.

AUTO LIABILITY FORMS

Most Americans carry automobile insurance coverage in the event of an accident driving or while an authorized person with coverage is driving. As with all other insurance coverage, eventually a report or a form will be needed to explain fully the nature of the injuries and the prognosis for the patient.

Sometimes, the parties involved cannot agree upon a settlement and a lawsuit is filed. It is very important that our office avoid agreeing to postpone expecting payment on patient accounts until after any lawsuit has run its course. Too often, it takes many months or years before automobile litigation is resolved and the money is available to pay medical bills. Our office avoids this dilemma by plainly stating that we do not treat patients on a contingency basis, but do expect payment for services rendered or will set up a regular plan of affordable payments.

Normally, we file for payment first through the private health care insurance of the patient. The **insurance billing specialist** must be careful to check the correct box in Block #10 if an accident (auto or other) is the reason why the patient sought treatment in our office. If payment is received from the private insurance company, they are certain to subrogate the insurance of the party who caused the accident as explained in Chapter 11. However, their payment of our bill and of other bills amassed by the patient means the patient does not have to wait until the suit is settled before paying creditors.

OTHER INSURANCE

There are a few other programs, federal and otherwise, offering different forms of assistance to those in need. The physician is required to provide the de-tailed clinical information necessary and to answer the many questions that sometimes must be done in letter form. In every case, careful attention must be paid to accuracy in reporting dates of injury and dates treatment as well as the nature of treatment. Naturally, the **insurance billing specialist** is dedicated to careful completion of every form that passes over his or her desk. In these special cases, particular scrutiny and timeliness are required.

Please make every effort to process all claims within 24 to 48 hours of receiving them. Sometimes, others working on the records will prevent you from completing your portion of the claim as quickly as we both would like. However, once the record and/or claim form has been passed on to you for final completion, please do so quickly. This is not only a matter affecting reimbursement to our office, but often is a matter of grave financial importance to the living standard of the patient. You will sometimes receive telephone calls from anxious patients wanting to know if completed forms have left our office so that they might soon receive much-needed financial support. If you maintain your professional goal of 24 to 48 hours processing time, you will not disappoint our patients and you will soon realize that you have made an important contribution to their lives and their well-being.

REVIEW QUESTIONS FOR DISCUSSION

1. How is the coverage discussed in this chapter different from the many types of insurance described in previous chapters?

2. What forms will you complete for these patients?

3. Why is quick completion of these forms especially important?

4. What would you say to an anxious patient calling to check on the status of her liability claim form?

5. Select a partner and take turns role-playing the anxious patient and the **insurance billing specialist**.

Chapter Thirteen

COMPLETING THE ADA FORM

OBJECTIVES   After completing this chapter, you will be able to

- explain the difference in benefit payments between dental and medical insurance companies
- define ADA and explain its purpose
- complete dental insurance forms for covered patients

POWER WORDS

orthodontics   A general term meaning the application of braces or other dental appliances used to correct tooth alignment problems or adjust the bite pattern.

prosthesis   An artificial device created to replace the appearance and/or function of an original organ, limb, teeth, etc., removed or lost because of disease or trauma.

COMPLETING THE ADA FORM

After your study of HCFA-1500 medical form completion, learning to complete the Attending Dentist's Statement (ADA form) will be much easier. You will use most of the same knowledge along with a few new skills. The number of patients with dental insurance continues to grow as well as the number of private companies offering dental insurance coverage. Therefore, it is important to this office that the **insurance billing specialist** know how to complete accurately the ADA form and understand the CDT-2 and HCPCS coding systems used in form completion.

Dental insurance benefits usually are based on two components:

1. the length of time the policy has been in force, and

2. the benefit amount established by the insurance company.

Often, patients with dental insurance coverage for one year or less will find their claims paid at a lower level than patients with dental insurance in force for three years or more. Normally, after three years of coverage, dental benefits stabilize and remain constant unless the benefit plan established by the insurance company goes up or down. Also, there is usually an annual maximum benefit that will be paid for all or most services. Both the patient and the **insurance billing specialist** will want to examine the policy booklet sent to the patient to learn more about policy limitations in each case.

Routine, annual, or semiannual dental treatment, such as cleaning the teeth or taking X-rays or filling a cavity, does not usually require preauthorized approval from the dental insurance company before the work may proceed. The patient's policy booklet will clearly explain fees for these routine treatments. However, if the doctor recommends more extensive dental work, an Attending Dentists's Statement pretreatment (ADA) form must be completed and submitted if the patient wishes the work to be paid by insurance, in whole or in part. Of course, the patient may always elect to pay for dental work or any other medical treatment out-of-pocket and some of our pa-

tients do just that. Others have no dental or health insurance. Our discussion in this chapter relates to those dental patients with dental insurance and the steps to be taken to collect those benefits.

Figure 13-1 is an example of the generic Attending Dentist's Statement (ADA) dental form to be completed for preauthorization and/or payment after the work is done.

Locate Record #24, Sheets 1 through 4, in Chapter 16, for patient Nancy Hawkins, and Form #35 in Part V. Notice the Confidential Patient Information Records and ledger card are the same as those used for medical insurance patients; however, the Dental Treatment Record is very different. It contains information about dental history, oral findings, and uses a full-mouth dental illustration so that the dentist or his assistant can indicate which teeth are being attended to at the time of the examination. This form allows the kind of documentation about the dental health of the patient that the Medical Treatment Record spaces provide. It may also record specific charges and payment records, although it is not intended to replace the ledger card. Also, the transmittal sheet may be used to provide the **insurance billing specialist** with information about fees, especially in very routine cases.

Look at the Attending Dentist's Statement (ADA form) and complete each block as follows:

1. In the upper left corner of the form, place an "X" in the box to show this is a statement of actual services already rendered. If this had been an authorization for more extensive dental payment, an "X" would be placed in the box labeled Dentist's pretreatment estimate.

2. At the top of the form, next to the entry "Carrier name and address," place the name and address of the dental insurance company where this form is to be sent.

3. In Block #1, print the full name of the patient.

4. In Block #2, print the relationship of the patient to the insured.

5. In Block #3, place an "X" to show the sex of the patient.

Attending Dentist's Statement

Check one:	Carrier name and address
☐ **Dentist's pre-treatment estimate**	
☐ **Dentist's statement of actual services**	

PATIENT SECTION

1. Patient name first m.i. last	2. Relationship to employee ☐ self ☐ child ☐ spouse ☐ other	3. Sex m f	4. Patient birthdate MM DD YYYY	5. If full-time student school city

6. Employee/subscriber name and mailing address	7. Employee/subscriber soc. sec. number	8. Employee/subscriber birthdate MM DD YYYY	9. Employee (company) name and address	10. Group number

11. Is patient covered by another plan of benefits? Dental _____ Medical _____	12-a. Name and address of carrier(s)	12-b. Group no.(s)	13. Name and address of employer

14-a. Employee/subscriber name (if different than patient's)	14-b. Employee/subscriber soc. sec. number	14-c. Employee/subscriber birthdate MM DD YYYY	15. Relationship to patient ☐ self ☐ child ☐ spouse ☐ other ____

I have reviewed the following treatment plan. I authorize release of any information relating to this claim. I understand that I am responsible for all costs of dental treatment.

▶ _____
Signed (Patient, or parent if minor)   Date

I hereby authorize payment directly to the below named dentist of the group insurance benefits otherwise payable to me.

▶ _____
Signed (Insured person)   Date

DENTIST SECTION

16. Dentist name	24. Is treatment result of occupational illness or injury?	No	Yes	If yes, enter brief description and dates.
17. Mailing address	25. Is treatment result of auto accident? 26. Other accident?			
City, State, Zip	27. Are any services covered by another plan?			
18. Dentist Soc. Sec. or T.I.N. 19. Dental licence no. 20. Dentist phone no.	28. If prosthesis, is this initial replacement?		(If no, reason for replacement)	29. Date of prior placement
21. First visit date current series 22. Place of treatment Office Hosp ECF Other 23. Radiographs or models enclosed? No Yes How many? 30. Is treatment for orthodontics?			If services already commenced enter: Date appliances placed Mos. treatment remaining	

Identify missing teeth with "X"

31. Examination and treatment plan - List in order from tooth no. 1 through tooth no. 32 - Use charting system shown.

Tooth # or letter	Surface	Description of service (including x-rays, prophylaxis, materials used, etc.) Line No.	Date service performed Mo. Day Year	Procedure number	Fee	For administrative use only
		1				
		2				
		3				
		4				
		5				
		6				
		7				
		8				
		9				
		10				
		11				
		12				
		13				
		14				
		15				

32. Remarks for unusual services

I hereby certify that the procedures as indicated by date have been completed and that the fees submitted are the actual fees I have charged and intend to collect for those procedures.

▶ _____   Date _____

Signed (Dentist)

Total Fee Charged	
Max. Allowable	
Deductible	
Carrier %	
Carrier pays	

FIGURE 13–1 Attending Dentist's Statement (ADA) dental form

6. In Block #4, show the date of birth using two digits for the month, date, and year.

7. Skip Block #5. This patient is not a full-time student. When the doctors treat full time students, complete this block.

8. Place the name and address of the subscriber in Block #6.

9. Place the subscriber's insurance ID number (or if none, the social security number) in Block #7 and the subscriber's date of birth in Block #8.

10. Enter the name and address of the subscriber's employer in Block #9 and the group number in Block #10 if there is one.

11. Block #11 asks about other dental insurance. Complete it and Blocks #12a, #12b, and #13 if appropriate.

12. Blocks #14 and #15 are to be used to provide information about the subscriber when the subscriber is someone other than the patient.

13. Place "Signature on File" on the two signature lines, if appropriate, and enter the date you are completing this form on the date line.

14. Blocks #16 through #20 give information about the treating dentist.

15. Place the date of treatment in Block #21. Sometimes, complete dental treatment requires a series of visits. If this is applicable, list the date for the first visit of the series in this block.

16. Place an "X" in the correct area to show the place of treatment in Block #22.

17. Block #23 asks if X-rays or models are going to be included with this claim. Sometimes this is done so that the dental insurance company can have a clearer understanding of the necessity for treatment. X-rays may be required for claims covering certain inlays, individual crowns, fixed bridges, surgical extractions, impactions, and endodontic services. If the policy booklet requires this documentation, be sure the patient's name, social security number and dentist's name and license number are attached to a label and affixed on the model or the X-ray envelope. Staple the envelope containing the mounted and labeled X-rays to the upper right corner of the insurance form. Models should be boxed and labeled and all items sent together. If you forget to send an X-ray or a model with the ADA form, do not send it separately. Wait until you hear from the insurance company for specific instructions.

18. Blocks #24 to #26 are about any occupational or accidental cause for the treatment.

19. Block #27 is used when an appliance or dental prosthesis is placed in the patient's mouth.

20. Block #28 is completed if a prior placement had occurred.

21. Block #29 is used to show if the treatment is for orthodontics.

22. Block #30 is the part of the form where information about treatment is placed.

   A. First, place the number of the adult tooth or the letter of the primary tooth that is referred to on each line of the form. This information may be obtained from the Dental Treatment Record. It is not necessary to shade any of the teeth shown in the diagram to the left of area 30 on the ADA form if:

      1. you list the number or letter of the tooth being treated, or

      2. if the treatment is general and not directed at any specific tooth.

   B. The description of service is a very brief few words. For this patient, "Periodic Oral Exam" (code 00120) may be used on line 1, "Bitewings four films" (code 00274) for the X-rays on line 2, and "Adult Prophylaxis" (code 0110) on line 3, to show cleaning and polishing of the teeth. In other cases, refer to the descriptions next to the CDT-2 codes in your manual.

C. Next show the date of service, each CDT-2 code, and find the fee for each service in your master fee schedule. Total the fee. Enter the maximum allowable amount by the insurance company, if you know it, or leave it blank.

D. Sign the form, enter the license number of the physician and the date you completed the form.

23. Block #31 is used only if the doctor has additional information about the particular patient or some specific request. It is seldom used since most forms are self-explanatory.

Congratulations, you just completed your first dental form! Now, you need more practice at using these new skills.

EXERCISE 1

1. Locate Form #36 from Part V, and Record #25, Sheets 1 and 2 in Chapter 16, for patient Bogan. Complete this form for a general examination. Notice the patient paid $10.00 out of pocket toward the bill, but there is no place to show that on the ADA form.

2. Locate Form #37 from Part V, and Record #26, Sheets 1 and 2 in Chapter 16, for patient McCullough. Complete this form for a general examination. Notice this patient paid in full for her services. Remember, when the patient pays in full for an office visit and has no other balance due on the ledger card, *do not* sign "Signature on file" on the line authorizing payment to come to us. Without that authorization, the payment will be mailed to the patient. If the patient has a zero balance with our office, this is fully appropriate and we want payment to be sent to the patient.

EXERCISE 2

Locate Form #38 from Part V, and Record #27, Sheets 1 to 3, for patient Konklin. These records include two routing sheets. Notice on 2/15 the patient had his first stage of treatment for $104.00 and he paid $25.00 out of pocket. On 3/1, he returned to have a crown installed and the doctor applied the number #14 on both routing sheets to show which tooth received the preparation and then the gold crown. You may complete one form showing all work completed on the two different dates. Be sure to give the grand total of all fees. Do not deduct the payment made by the patient in calculating the fee. The insurance company will make the proper entries.

MEDICARE COVERAGE

Medicare does not provide dental services for its participants. However, if a Medicare patient has a disease, an accident, or trauma to the mouth that requires the services of an oral surgeon and/or other dental skills, this claim may be filed like those for any other Medicare patient—on a HCFA-1500 claim form. CPT codes may be used to describe the surgical procedures, but the CDT-2 codes may not. Instead of using the CDT-2 codes, the **insurance billing specialist** may use the HCPCS codes in the "D" section of the manual. You will quickly notice that while the CDT-2 codes begin with the number zero, the HCPCS codes begin with "D," but the remainder of the code is the same.

EXERCISE 3

Locate Form #39 in Part V, and Record #28, Sheets 1 to 3 for patient Marshall, a Medicare patient injured in an automobile accident and seen by Dr. Lane in consultation at Good Samaritan Hospital.

MEDICAID DENTAL COVERAGE

Some states provide various levels of dental insurance coverage for Medicaid patients and will direct its providers on which form to use. In our state, Medicaid coverage is available and an example of the form is shown in Figure 13–2.

This form is very similar to the standard ADA form and should pose no new challenges for the **insurance billing specialist.** Only the placement of certain boxes for information is different, but the basic data needed to complete the form may be located in the patient's record.

MEDICAID DENTAL CLAIM FORM

INDIANA STATE DEPARTMENT OF PUBLIC WELFARE
MEDICAID DEPARTMENT
P.O. BOX 68767
INDIANAPOLIS, INDIANA 46268-8767

1. PATIENT NAME

2. RELATIONSHIP TO EMPLOYEE
SELF / SPOUSE / CHILD / OTHER

3. SEX
M / F

4. PATIENT BIRTHDATE
MO / DAY / YEAR

5. IF FULL TIME STUDENT
SCHOOL — CITY

6. EMPLOYEE/SUBSCRIBER NAME
FIRST — MIDDLE — LAST

7. MEDICAID ID NO.

9. NAME OF GROUP DENTAL PROGRAM

8. EMPLOYEE/SUBSCRIBER MAILING ADDRESS

CITY, STATE, ZIP

10. EMPLOYER (COMPANY) NAME AND ADDRESS

11. GROUP NUMBER

12. LOCATION (LOCAL)

13. ARE OTHER FAMILY MEMBERS EMPLOYED?
EMPLOYEE NAME — SOC. SEC. NO.

14. NAME AND ADDRESS OF EMPLOYER IN ITEM 13

15. IS PATIENT COVERED BY ANOTHER DENTAL PLAN?
DENTAL PLAN NAME — UNION LOCAL — GROUP NO. — NAME AND ADDRESS OF CARRIER

16. REASON FOR SERVICE

____ (E) EMERGENCY (RELIEF OF PAIN)   ____ (X) INITIAL EXAM   ____ (R) ROUTINE

17. DENTIST SOC. SEC. OR TIN

18. DENTIST LICENSE NO.

19. DENTIST PHONE NO.

20. DENTIST NAME AND ADDRESS

PROVIDER CODE NUMBER

21. FIRST VISIT DATE CURRENT SERIES

22. PLACE OF TREATMENT
OFFICE / IH / OH / ECF / OTHER

23. RADIOGRAPHS OR MODELS ENCLOSED?
NO / YES / HOW MANY?

24. WAS PATIENT'S CONDITION CAUSED BY AN ACCIDENT?
NO / YES — IF YES, ENTER BRIEF DESCRIPTION AND DATE

(A) On-The-Job

(B) Vehicle

(C) Home

(Z) Other

27. ARE ANY SERVICES COVERED BY ANOTHER PLAN?
NO / YES

27A. HOSPITAL DISCHARGE DATE MO/DA/YR.

28. IF PROSTHESIS IS THIS INITIAL PLACEMENT?
NO / YES (IF NO, REASON FOR REPLACEMENT)

29. DATE OF PRIOR PLACEMENT

30. IS TREATMENT FOR ORTHODONTICS?

IF SERVICES ALREADY COMMENCED ENTER — DATE APPLIANCES PLACED — MOS TREATMENT REMAINING

IDENTIFY MISSING TEETH WITH "X"

31. EXAMINATION AND TREATMENT PLAN - LIST IN ORDER FROM TOOTH NO. 1 THROUGH TOOTH NO. 32 - USE CHARTING SYSTEM SHOWN.

FACIAL

LINGUAL

RIGHT / UPPER / LOWER — PERMANENT — PRIMARY / LEFT

LINGUAL

FACIAL

32. REMARKS FOR UNUSUAL SERVICES

TOOTH # OR LETTER	SUR-FACE	DESCRIPTION OF SERVICE (INCLUDING X-RAYS, PROPHYLAXIS, MATERIALS USED ETC.) LINE NO.	DATE SERVICE PERFORMED MO. DAY Yr.	NO. VISITS	UNITS OF SVC	PROCEDURE NUMBER	FEE	ADMINISTRATIVE USE ONLY

32. SIGNATURE OF PROVIDER (READ REVERSE SIDE PRIOR TO SIGNATURE)
I HEREBY CERTIFY THAT THE PROCEDURES HAVE BEEN COMPLETED AND THAT THE FOREGOING INFORMATION IS TRUE, ACCURATE, AND COMPLETE. I UNDERSTAND THAT PAYMENT AND SATISFACTION OF THE CLAIM WILL BE FROM FEDERAL AND STATE FUNDS, AND THAT ANY FALSE CLAIMS, STATEMENTS, OR DOCUMENTS, OR CONCEALMENT OF A MATERIAL FACT MAY BE PROSECUTED UNDER APPLICABLE FEDERAL OR STATE LAWS."

DENTIST SIGNATURE _____ DATE _____

TOTAL FEE CHARGED

LESS THIRD PARTY PAYMENT

NET CHARGE

EARLY PERIODIC SCREENING DIAGNOSIS AND TREATMENT (EPSDT)

33. Was an examination performed for the EPSDT program?

34. As a result of the screening further diagnosis and/or treatment required?

35. In the course of screening for the EPSDT program, indicate detection of:
2. Dental Problems
5. Other Problems

36. Prior Authorization Number, if applicable

378-005 (4-91)

EDS COPY

FIGURE 13–2 Blank form for Medicaid patients

EXERCISE 4

1. Locate Form #40 in Part V, and Record #29, Sheets 1 to 2, in Chapter 16, for patient James. Complete the Medicaid form for this patient.

2. Locate Form #41 in Part V, and Record #30, Sheets 1 to 2, in Chapter 16, for patient Williams. Complete this standard dental form, showing the final step in applying a porcelain crown.

REVIEW QUESTIONS FOR DISCUSSION

1. Describe the HCFA-1500 and ADA form differences.

2. How do dental insurance benefits differ from health insurance benefits?

3. What is the difference between primary and permanent teeth?

4. Do you think more people have dental insurance or medical insurance?

5. If a patient's spouse also has dental insurance that covers your patient, in what order would the two claims be filed?

Chapter Fourteen

MANAGED CARE

OBJECTIVES After you have completed your study of this chapter, you will be able to

- define Managed Care
- understand when to seek preauthorization for medical care
- secure the necessary authorization numbers and know when to use them
- understand capitation and its impact on health care distribution

POWER WORDS

aging report An Accounts Receivable listing showing the uncollected fees of each patient and dividing those fees into columns marked current, 30-days, 60-days, 90-days, 120-days-old, with a grand total of the complete amount owed. This report enables the bookkeeper and collection clerk to contact patients or insurance companies to find out why accounts are taking many months to get paid.

capitation A method of calculating prepayment to participating physicians in managed care contracts. In general, the physicians are prepaid a set fee monthly for each enrolled patient regardless of the actual number of office visits or other patient contact. The goal is to provide quality treatment to all patients without exceeding the dollar limits of the prepayments. At the end of the contract year, physicians may receive a portion of any unused cost allowances set aside by the insurance company.

preexisting condition In terms of insurance plan jargon, refers to a medical condition suffered by the patient or other potential insured before the effective date of the current insurance plan coverage.

HEALTH CARE REFORM

Concern continues to grow nationally over the large numbers of uninsured and underinsured men, women, and children, in our country. Dozens of health-care plans have been debated in congressional hearings for years, culminating in the passage of the Kassebaum-Kennedy bill in 1996. That first small step toward easing the financial catastrophe of major illness was written to allow workers to change jobs without fear of losing insurance coverage for medical conditions they or their families have on an ongoing basis. In the past, when new employees applied for insurance coverage at the new place of employment, they often found they were without insurance coverage for any medical problem that existed prior to the beginning date of new employment. This is called a preexisting condition and different insurance companies handle this provision in very separate ways.

For example, if a new employee has a child with cystic fibrosis, and if the new insurance policy requires a waiting period of one year before preexisting conditions are included in its benefit package, that would mean any treatment for that child connected to his cystic fibrosis would not be covered until one full calendar year had passed at the new place of employment. Waiting periods for coverage for preexisting conditions vary from "no" waiting period through to "no" coverage, ever! There has been no national standard. Until passage of the Kassebaum-Kennedy bill, millions of Americans were afraid to change jobs because of medical problems that had developed while currently employed that would fall under the preexisting clause of a new insurance policy. Even now, this new law does not become effective until 1998, does not include companies of all sizes, and critics claim there are many loopholes that will take years to be closed via test lawsuits.

MANAGED CARE EXAMINED

While Congress continues to search for ways to provide health care for all Americans, whether or not employed, private enterprise has come up with some ideas of its own. Many of them have been strongly supported by governmental agencies.

"Managed Care" is a catch-all phrase that implies methods of providing low to medium cost health care coverage to working employees. It is not really the "care" that is to be managed as much as the cost of the care. The ideal is to provide excellent "care" and to do so more efficiently and more cheaply than we have managed until now. In several areas, especially the western states of California, Nevada, Oregon, and Washington, state agencies have experimented with several types of plans for both employed and unemployed Americans. In these areas, managed care, which includes prepayment to physicians, hospitals, pharmacies, and others, is widely used and studied. Capitation of benefits and payments to health care providers has meant that creative yet medically safe methods have had to be developed to keep people well and out of the doctor's office.

While managed care plans continue to spread throughout the United States, they are still a small share of the insurance pie. According to a nationwide Coopers & Lybrand study, "more than 80% of patient revenue earned by group practices in 1995 was fee-for-service based. Capitation, on the other hand, accounted for barely more than 10% *(Medical Economics/December 9, 1996, p. 24).* In those western states mentioned where managed care has made the most progress, the capitation portion for groups was nearly twice the national average. Therefore, while managed care plans have not taken over the national scene, continued discussion and evaluation has affected the way private insurance companies and groups of physicians and hospitals do business. New arrangements of health care plans and groups spring up constantly, and our physicians are contacted often to participate in one group or another.

IMPACT ON INSURANCE BILLING SPECIALIST

For the **insurance billing specialist**, the question remains: How will managed care affect my responsibilities in completing insurance forms? In reality, the answer is, very little!

The physicians are certainly affected in their master fee schedule whenever they join into any contractual arrangement with any managed care plan. Business managers/office managers are affected in their responsibilities to track practice costs and income attributed to any given plan. Receptionists are affected in prequalifying potential patients to the practice to be sure our physicians are members of the various groups to which the potential patients might belong. Receptionists are also expected to collect the proper co-payment, if any, from plan members and may also need to call to verify coverage for *every* patient with any type of insurance coverage. Bookkeepers are affected in ensuring that the correct write-offs and adjustments are applied to patient accounts, or in establishing affordable payment plans for those who require this. However, as job duties are currently defined, the **insurance billing specialist** will continue to complete HCFA-1500 and ADA forms as usual with one exception:

☞ The **insurance billing specialist** must be aware of any authorization numbers that any given plan may require to be included on the form.

Normally, the receptionist acquires those numbers over the telephone or the patient brings written authorization from his primary care physician. In either case:

☞ All numbers relative to authorization or pre-authorization should be clearly marked and included with patient record documentation.

If this information is not obviously included in patient records and if there is no clear indication of participation in a managed care plan, feel free to handle the claim as if it is a fee-for-service claim, Medicare, etc., as indicated. If job descriptions change, new procedures will be clearly explained to you. Do not worry about all the initials you might hear tossed about, that is, initials meant to describe different kinds of managed care plans. Some might be well known to you and others very new or strange-sounding. It is simply important to realize that these initials refer to a kind of insurance plan that will require some sort of authorization numbers in order to get paid!

COMPUTERIZATION

As mentioned early in this manual, our office is making plans to convert to computerization to handle billing and insurance form processing, as well as several other tasks presently managed by hand. The **insurance billing specialist** may be called upon to enter the same patient information into the computer that she or he is currently applying to the insurance form, with the expected result of an insurance form generated by the computer. Instead of using ledger cards, the computer will generate detailed reports showing how much is owed by each patient and whether the dollars owed are current, 30-, 60-, 90-, or 120-days-old. This is called an aging report. It is a very useful tool in visually examining the age of each account. The goal will be to keep fees owed to us out of the 120-day column, and keep our office alert to potential collection problems.

Vast amounts of information will be available to us through computerization. We will be able to measure more easily the types of services we provide, the income attributable to each member of the health care team, and the costs of each type of health care plan our patients carry. We will be able to schedule appointments onto the computer instead of using an appointment book, and we plan to have computer terminals for access by more than one member at a time. Our work will be done more quickly and accurately. The question arises: How will computerization affect the **insurance billing specialist?** The answer depends upon the size and scope of computerization ultimately chosen by our physicians. Most importantly:

☞ You will need all the skills you have developed and nothing learned thus far will be wasted within the computerized office.

That is, one must know how to complete forms manually before switching to computer production. The **insurance billing specialist** must understand the need for the information requested as well as how to find and apply the correct codes. The exercises you have done so far would not be different if generated by a computer. Someone must enter the data needed to generate the form. This may be one of the new responsibilities of the **insurance billing specialist**. The codes, patient data, etc., would be entered. There is always the risk of system failure and the need to complete forms by hand until the system is restored. Sometimes, a special entry or form adjustment will be done faster by hand than by computer, or some piece of information missing in the computer can be added more quickly manually than by computer. As the scope of the computer system is determined, new job assignments will be developed. Rest assured, your skills will be imperative to the success of the transition to computer.

Later on, I envision computerized transmission of insurance forms. This means the data entered into the computer will be "mailed" in a sense, over the telephone wires to the insurance company of the patient or to a clearing house that then rebatches the forms from many offices and sends them to the smaller insurance companies. This process is quicker than mailing paper forms and should result in a quicker reimbursement. However, it is not foolproof. Submitting the claims by electronic transmission can be tedious. Sometimes, the demands of the clearing houses or of the receiving parties can result in many claims coming back because of minuscule errors that may have been overlooked on a paper claim. Likewise, as more offices participate in electronic claim transmission, the system slows down in response. When electronic billing first began, the time it took to send a claim and receive payment was very fast—perhaps ten days or less in comparison to the four to six weeks it often takes to be paid using a paper claim. However, as more claims pour into the system, the electronic claim transmission system often slows down to handle the increased load. Still, this method of filing claims is generally quicker.

Clearly, there will be a place in our computerized office of the future for the **insurance billing specialist**. Often, if employees wish to they may decide to learn more about all areas of the practice and take on greater responsibilities. In fact, when I first joined the practice some eight years ago, it was in the position of **insurance billing specialist**!

FINAL THOUGHTS

You have completed your orientation program and are now ready to assume the responsibilities you have prepared for through your studies. Your position of **insurance billing specialist** within the field of Health Information Management is an important and key component of the total team. You complete the successful cycle of doctor-patient-treatment reimbursement so important to the well-being of the patient and the ability of the practice to continue to serve the community. The need for affordable and competent health care will continue to grow in serving the aging population and the challenges of quick and accurate submission of claims will be needed to keep operating costs under control. If managed care continues to encroach group practices, this will only add to the demand for accuracy in your work. Your profession as an **insurance billing specialist** is important to us and the patients we serve. You will be expected to stay abreast of the developments in your field—to keep reading, attend workshops, and examine new coding books and information about Medicare and Medicaid as these come to you. None of us is ever "done" learning about our professions—not so long as we serve human beings. Be patient with yourself, know that you will make human errors from time to time, and that we will understand this.

Congratulations to you as the newest member of the team at Medical & Dental Associates, P.C.!

Part Four

REFERENCES AND RESOURCES

JOB DESCRIPTION

TITLE: Insurance Billing Specialist

IMMEDIATE SUPERVISOR: Office Manager

JOB DUTIES: Part I. To gather sufficient patient information to complete and file health insurance claims for reimbursement for services rendered by the physicians and dentists of this office. Actual patient records will be examined.

Part II. To complete the insurance forms correctly in accordance with the general requirements of most fee-for-service third-party payers. Patient records of this office will be accessed for clarification.

Part III. To adapt the insurance form completion process, as determined by specific patient records, to the general requirements of the major insurers, such as Medicare, Medicaid, Workers' Compensation, CHAMPUS, and certain other managed care insurance plans.

Part IV. To provide the references and resources necessary to complete the insurance billing process.

Part V. To furnish the forms and worksheets needed to complete all required tasks.

Chapter Fifteen

RESOURCES

INFORMATION ABOUT OUR PRACTICE AND OUR DOCTORS

Medical & Dental Associates, P.C.
3733 Professional Drive, #300
Indianapolis, Indiana 46260
317/123-4567
Tax ID#99-9999999
Medicare Group Number MDA80800
Medicaid Group Number 21886
Blue Cross/Blue Shield Group ID# 6772300
CHAMPUS Group Provider No. 7765003
Medical Indiana Group ID# 7665000
HMO of Indiana Group Provider No. 246-133389

James P. Cartman, M.D./Family Practitioner
State License No. 32118
Medicare UPIN #CAR811
Medicare CPIN #1141166
Medicaid Provider No. 219990218
Workers' Compensation Provider No. 52-33445561

Jane R Portia, M.D./Obstetrician-Gynecologist
State License No. 81990
Medicare UPIN #POR090
Medicare CPIN #3556011
Medicaid Provider No. 611935600
Workers' Compensation Provider No. 52-25574444

Harold S. Beckermann, M.D./Pediatrician
State License No. 61100
Medicare UPIN #BEC230
Medicare CPIN #1336900
Medicaid Provider No. 314677823
Workers' Compensation Provider No. 52-02236540

Linda R. Gregory, M.D./Internist-General Surgeon
State License No. 41777
Medicare UPIN #GRE334
Medicare CPIN #5553060
Medicaid Provider No. 477090032
Workers' Compensation Provider No. 52-36998850

Michael P. Lane, D.D.S./Dentist-Oral Surgeon
State License No. 333-2589
Medicare UPIN #LAN954
Medicare CPIN #1153288
Medicaid Provider No. 400972222
Workers' Compensation Provider No. 52-677115500

Patrick M. Zunkel, D.D.S./Dentist-Endodontics
State License No. 255-1101
Medicare UPIN #ZUN566
Medicare CPIN #4417922
Medicaid Provider No. 312207741
Workers' Compensation Provider No. 52-312448866

MASTER FEE SCHEDULE

CPT CODES

99201	$ 45.00	99211	$ 25.00
99202	50.00	99212	32.00
99203	60.00	99213	40.00
99204	72.00	99214	48.00
99205	90.00	99215	55.00
		99243	125.00
52000	200.00	99252	175.00
52601	1800.00		
		80050	45.00
71010	40.00	80058	12.00
71015	45.00	80059	12.00
71040	68.00	81000	10.00
73070	43.00	81025	12.00
76140	40.00	85018	13.00
		86593	12.00
90704	20.00	86687	30.00
97010	20.00	88150	20.00
A4460	8.00	J3250	10.00
A4572	40.00	J9293	10.00
J1631	38.00	L3700	45.00

DENTAL CODES

00120	20.00	01110	37.00
00220	10.00	02330	37.00
00272	12.00	02790	475.00
00274	20.00	02954	150.00
00330	40.00	03320	320.00

PLACE OF SERVICE CODES

MEDICAL INSURANCE CLAIMS

11	Office	Location where physician routinely provides health care to patients.
12	Home	Place where patient receives care in a private residence.
21	Inpatient Hospital	Facility that provides diagnostic, therapeutic, rehabilitative services to patients under the supervision of the admitting physician.
22	Outpatient Hospital	A portion of the hospital set aside for patients to be treated and sent home in fewer than 24 hours; a place for same-day surgery and discharge.
23	Emergency Room Hospital	A portion of the hospital designed specifically to treat emergency cases that walk in or arrive by ambulance; site for treatment of trauma patients.
24	Ambulatory Surgical Center	A freestanding facility where surgical and diagnostic services are provided.
25	Birthing Center	A specialized facility designed to provide services for the pregnant patient through the labor and delivery process.
26	Military Treatment Facility	A medical facility operated by one or more of the divisions of the military.
31	Skilled Nursing Facility	A nursing home or other similar environment where medical services are provided under the supervision of registered nurses with monthly monitoring by the physician; services are on a par with inpatient hospital care.

32	Nursing Facility	A facility providing rehabilitative care for the sick, disabled, or injured patient around the clock; services above the level of a custodial care facility.
33	Custodial Care Facility	A residence providing room, board, and/or other personal assistance, but does not include the presence of medical personnel on the premises.
34	Hospice	A facility providing palliative care to the terminally ill and support to family members.
41	Ambulance —land	A land vehicle specifically designed to provide emergency care and hospital transport to accident victims or those suddenly taken seriously ill.
42	Ambulance —air or water	An air or water vehicle built and equipped to provide emergency care and hospital transport to accident victims or those suddenly taken seriously ill.
99	Miscel- laneous	Other locations where medical services or equipment were provided or carried out under the instructions of a physician.

TYPE OF SERVICE CODES—CHAMPUS

1 Medical Care
2 Surgery
3 Consultation
4 DX X-ray
5 DX laboratory
6 Radiation Therapy
7 Anesthesia
8 Assist at Surgery
9 Other Medical Service
A DME Rental
B Drugs
C Ambulatory Surgery
D Hospice
E 2nd Surgical Opinion
F Maternity
G Dental
H Mental Health Care
J Disability Program

GLOSSARY

accounts receivable (A/R) — The amount of money left unpaid by insurance or not yet paid by any third party; the list of outstanding dollars or unpaid bills owed to our Association physicians.

adjudication — The process of examining insurance claims for payment.

admitting privileges — Rights extended to licensed physicians by hospital administrators so that patients may be assigned to beds within specific areas of the hospital. Hospitals are reimbursed for housing patients and physicians are responsible to oversee patient care and treatment while staying in the hospital.

Advanced Life Support (ALS) Ambulance Service — Includes at least one paramedic crew member and sufficient medical equipment to apply life-saving techniques.

adverse effect — May result after a drug or medicinal substance; although correctly prescribed and correctly taken by the patient, causes a negative reaction within the patient.

aging report — An Accounts Receivable listing showing the uncollected fees of each patient and dividing those fees into columns marked current, 30 days, 60 days, 90 days, 120 days, with a grand total of the complete amount owed. This report enables the bookkeeper and collection clerk to contact patients or insurance companies to find out why accounts are taking many months to get paid.

Aid to Families with Dependent Children (AFDC) — A program of aid for young children and/or pregnant women who live in households earning below the poverty level.

alphanumerical codes — Begin with a letter of the alphabet and are followed by numbers, such as code J1820 found in the HCPCS manual.

American Dental Association (ADA) — A nonprofit organization of dentists and dental specialists devoted to furthering the professional development of its members; to educating the public about its members and their services; and to establishing policies that ensure the highest standards of quality of care.

appeal letter   Formal request to insurers to reconsider their decision to deny a specific claim submitted by our office.

Basic Life Support (BLS) Ambulance Service   Includes at least one crew member trained in first aid techniques at the Emergency Medical Technician (EMT) level but not a paramedic.

benefits   The dollar amounts paid by the insurer for health care.

bilateral   Affecting both sides of the body.

birthday rule   Applied when nondivorced parents of a minor patient both carry insurance coverage for the child. The parent born closest to January 1 is the primary insured and the other parent is the secondary, regardless of the age of either parent. If the parents share the same date of birth, the parent whose policy has been in effect the longest becomes the primary insured and the other parent the secondary insured.

bundle   To combine preoperative, postoperative, and surgical services into one code and apply one fee for all services.

capitation   A method of calculating payment to participating physicians in managed care programs. In general, the physicians are prepaid a set fee monthly for each potential patient each year of the contract. The goal is to provide quality treatment to all patients without exceeding the prepayment amounts. At the end of the contract year, physicians may receive a portion of any unused cost allowance set aside by the insurance company.

CHAMPUS (Civilian Health and Medical Program of the Uniformed Services)   A comprehensive federal health care program for civilian spouses and dependents of those in the uniformed services, either active duty personnel or those who died while on active duty; also includes retired personnel, their spouses, and dependents.

chart, patient chart   Refers to the folder kept in the medical office or the separate one kept in the hospital medical records department containing all medical information about the patient and treatments rendered.

CHAMPVA (Civilian Health and Medical Program of the Veterans Administration)   A federal program providing civilian coverage for families of deceased or 100 percent disabled veterans killed or injured while in active military service, or for retired military personnel not eligible to receive Medicare.

chief complaint (CC)   The reason or reasons the patient seeks medical treatment; the problem or symptom.

consultation   1) A physician's request that one of his or her patients be seen by one of our associates. A written report is sent to the referring doctor after all examination has been completed; 2) A request from a patient for an examination and opinion in a situation where another doctor has rendered an opinion about the patient's condition; 3) The patient is seeking a "second opinion" from one of our associates.

contingency	Used here as a legal term meaning one party involved in a lawsuit agrees to wait until the suit has been settled before expecting payment for services rendered. Lawyers involved in lawsuits often work on a contingency basis. If the client loses the lawsuit, the client will have to pay the legal fees out of pocket.
Coordination of Benefits (COB)	The term used to mean the insurance companies providing coverage to the patient will not issue benefit payments greater than the amount owed to the doctor. Therefore, if the primary insurance company pays the entire amount of the bill submitted to it, the secondary insurance company will pay nothing.
co-payment	The part of the fee the patient is responsible to pay. Often, a dollar amount or percentage is stated on the insurance identification card as the co-payment due at the time services are rendered or prescriptions are filled.
Council on Dental Benefit Programs	A policy of uniform standards of communication through uniform dental coding; a division of the ADA.
CPIN (Clinical Physician Identification Number)	A seven-digit number assigned to each member of our Medicare group. This number is to be used on each Medicare claim form in column 24K.
Current Dental Terminology, Second Edition (CDT-2)	The coding system designed by the American Dental Association for use in submitting claims to dental insurance companies for reimbursement to the dentists.
diagnosis	The term used to indicate the medical name of the disease or condition of the patient.
disability income insurance	A policy that provides direct income to insured people who have fulfilled the definition of "disabled" as set by their particular policy. This may include hospitalization first followed by a number of days or weeks in which the patient is unable to work. This policy is designed to blunt the total loss of income because of disability, but does not usually provide a 100 percent match of normal income.
Durable Medical Equipment Regional Carriers (DMERCS)	Four regional carriers designated to process all claims for durable medical equipment when prescribed for Medicare patients.
E-Codes	Used to describe adverse effects of drugs and chemicals, injury and accident causes, and environmental factors resulting in disease or injury.
endodontics	The subspecialty within dentistry concerned with treatment of diseases of the tooth root and surrounding tissues, including root canal therapy.
entitlement programs	Include such government plans as Medicare, CHAMPUS, food stamps, Head Start, agricultural subsidies, and social security, in which benefits are calculated based on given formulae. This is not a welfare program in that it is not connected to poverty levels of income.

eponyms	Surgical procedures or diseases named after the physician who developed the procedure or identified the disease.
established patient	One who has been treated within the past three years by one of the associates in our office.
ESRD (end-stage renal disease)	A diagnosis indicating a very serious kidney disease that usually requires kidney transplant. Special Medicare coverage is provided for those suffering from this disease.
Explanation of Benefits (EOB)	A form letter accompanying the insurance check issued to the doctor that reflects the information sent to the insurance company on the insurance claim and outlines the benefit payment. The patient may receive a similar document.
family practice/ practitioner	Medical specialty that includes several branches of medicine; is usually a primary care physician in managed care contracts; trained to provide total health care to patients of all ages.
Federal Register	The government's official publication of daily business conducted including the results of normal government transactions, enacted laws, and revisions.
fee-for-service	The oldest and most common type of health insurance benefit payment plan. Payments are made based on coverage outlined in the patient's policy and benefits and are set according to the usual and customary fee standards in the community.
Fiscal Intermediary (FI)	The insurance company adjudicating Medicare claims in each state or region.
gatekeeper	Under managed care contracts, the primary care physician (PCP) overseeing the general health care and treatment plan of the enrolled patient and covered family members; the PCP determines if or when specialists should be consulted or if the patient should be hospitalized.
general surgeon	Physician trained to provide treatment of disease by manipulation and with operative methods.
generic name	The official chemical name assigned to a drug. A given drug is licensed under its generic name and all manufacturers of the drug must list it by its generic name. However, a drug is usually marketed under a trade name chosen by the manufacturer.
global package	Another term for the surgical bundle; includes pre-op, post-op, and surgery wrapped within one flat fee.
gynecology	The branch of medicine concerned with female health care, including diseases connected with sexual function and the reproductive organs. This specialty is nearly always practiced together with obstetrics.
HCFA (Health Care Financing Administration)	The governmental agency that oversees the Medicare program and the part of state Medicaid programs to which federal money has been allocated.
HCFA-1500 (hick-fah fifteen hundred)	The abbreviated term used to mean the generic insurance form completed and submitted to Medicare or other parties for reimbursement.

HCPCS (pronounced hick-picks) Health Care Financing Administration Common Procedure Coding System	A listing of codes and modifiers used to report supplies, injections, materials, and certain other specific services and procedures to Medicare for reimbursement following appropriate administration to the patient; codes are revised yearly.
health insurance	A plan or policy outlining benefits and limitations of coverage for issuing payments to health care providers in exchange for appropriate services rendered to policyholders.
hypertension table	Used in coding hypertension as either the cause of disease (primary) or effect of disease (secondary), and the nature of the hypertension (benign, malignant, or unspecified).
ICD-9-CM (International Classification of Diseases, 9th Revision, Clinical Modification, Fifth Edition)	The title of the numerical system used to explain the diagnosis or symptom of the patient or reason for seeking treatment; it is applied to the insurance form and to the patient's office chart.
indemnity insurance	The oldest form of health insurance coverage in which the patient visits the doctor and/or hospital of choice (no gatekeeper) and benefits are paid based on the usual and customary rules (UCR). Another term for fee-for-service insurance.
insurer	The insurance company or other third party providing health insurance coverage for the patient.
internal medicine	The branch of medicine concerned with the study of the internal organs, and with the medical diagnosis and treatment of disorders of these organs.
Late Effect Codes	Used to document residual conditions that develop following the acute phase of another illness or injury.
ledger card	A record of the fees, payments, and adjustments for each patient; used in manual office systems.
liability insurance	Provides insurance coverage in specific situations, such as automobile insurance or homeowner's insurance.
litigation	Legal term meaning a civil lawsuit (or tort) has been filed and is in the process of working through the legal system, perhaps going to trial.
managed care	A system of providing health care insurance coverage that stresses cost control and disease prevention. Patients are assigned to case managers within the insurance company who are responsible for review of the doctors' treatment plans and patient discharge plans.

Medicaid	A state-administered and mostly state-funded health insurance coverage with partial federal funding. In certain cases, premiums for Medicare Part B coverage are paid by the state for Medicaid recipients. Each state determines eligibility requirements and benefits for Medicaid participants.
medical necessity	To show that the procedure or treatment administered to a patient was appropriate in light of the diagnosis or symptom stated on the insurance form.
Medical Records Department	The part of the hospital containing the charts and other information about current or recently discharged patients. In some hospitals, transcribers, medical coders, and others work here.
Medicare	Federally financed health insurance coverage for those 65 and older, for the blind, for those with end-stage renal disease, and for those with certain other disabilities.
Medicare Group Number	An identification number assigned to each group location.
Medigap	A general term referring to insurance coverage purchased by the Medicare patient to cover the 20 percent "gap" left uncovered by Medicare. Some Medigap insurers may pay for the $100 deductible as well.
microfiche	Term for making a copy of a document and storing it in miniature form on tape or film; done to save storage space while maintaining documentation.
modifiers	Two-digit numbers attached to procedure codes when additional clarification or special circumstances warrant them.
morphology	The study of the size, shape, and origin of a specimen, plant, or animal; in coding, this number is used to help us find the correct column in the Neoplasm table.
multispecialty	The term for an office of several doctors with more than one branch of medicine represented. In our office, we have two dentists, one internist/general surgeon, one obstetrician/gynecologist, one pediatrician, and one family practitioner.
neonate	A baby from birth to four weeks old.
new patient	One who has never been treated by an associate in our practice, or who has not been seen in three years or more.
obstetrics	The branch of medicine concerned with pregnancy and childbirth, including care both before and after the birth of the child.
office fee schedule	A list of fees charged to patients based on the kind of service rendered; the standard fee charged by all associates.
office manager	The staff member hired to supervise the daily work produced by all office personnel. This position may include hiring and firing employees along with other responsibilities.
Operative Report	A part of the patient chart that describes a surgical procedure completed by one of our physicians, including the preoperative and postoperative diagnoses.

oral surgeon	A specialist in surgical procedures within the oral cavity including removal of teeth; a specialist in surgically reconstructing facial deformities caused by disease or severe accident.
orthodontics	A general term meaning the application of braces or other dental appliances used to correct tooth alignment problems or adjust the bite pattern.
pediatrician	Physician specializing in the treatment of children from birth to adolescence.
Physicians' Current Procedural Terminology (CPT)	A listing of descriptive terms and codes for reporting medical services and procedures performed by doctors.
post	In bookkeeping, this term means to record data to the patient financial record or account.
postpartum	The period of time from giving birth until about six weeks later.
predetermination	The process of submitting a proposed treatment plan to the insurance company for approval of payment prior to beginning the work.
pre-existing condition	In terms of insurance plan jargon, this refers to a medical condition suffered by the patient or other potential insured before the effective date of the current insurance plan coverage.
primary care physician (PCP)	In managed care contracts, the physician who first sees the patient and determines what treatment should be done, including referral to other physicians and/or hospitalization.
primary diagnosis	The main problem or symptom bringing the patient into the office, or the illness that is the most serious or most threatening to the well-being of the patient.
primary insurance	The insurer to which the medical or dental claim should first be sent for payment.
Professional Corporation (P.C.)	A legal term describing an organization of professionals who have chosen to work together in the same office space and share overhead expense and, possibly, income.
prophylaxis	Preventive care.
prosthesis	An artificial device created to replace the appearance and/or function of an original organ, limb, teeth, etc., removed or lost because of disease or trauma.
receptionist	Staff person responsible for greeting the patients, gathering current patient information, booking appointments, preparing routing forms, collecting payments, and more, depending on the size of the office.
reimbursement	In the medical office, this term most often means receiving payment from the insurance company or other third-party payer.
route of administration	Term used to explain how a drug or substance gets inside the body of the patient.
secondary diagnosis	A lesser problem, but no less important in the treatment of the patient; a matter of selecting the order in which to list illnesses or diseases based upon their severity, risk, or threat to the patient.

secondary insurance	Coverage for the patient by another insurance company effective only after payment from the primary insurance company has been received and only if benefits are available to cover the services rendered.
Social Security Disability Insurance (SSDI)	A federally administered entitlement program—not an insurance program and not welfare. It provides direct forms of financial assistance after documentation of complete or partial disability has been proven and a waiting period has passed.
sponsor	The label given the person currently in military service or retired from service in good standing.
subrogation	The provision of an insurer, such as CHAMPUS, to pay for the current and immediate health care needed by the injured patient, with the intention of being reimbursed for its expenses at a later date from the insurance company of the person responsible for the accident or injuries. This is always a part of automobile insurance coverage so that the injured party does not bear the expense for injuries caused by another person who also has insurance coverage, and does not experience a delay in getting necessary care.
subscriber	The insurance industry term for the person in whose name an insurance policy has been issued.
Supplemental Security Income (SSI)	A federally supported welfare assistance plan authorized under Title 16 of the Social Security Act that provides payments to the needy, or to aged, blind, or disabled citizens.
surgical package	Another term for global package or bundle.
systemic	Affecting the entire body.
third-party payers	The insurance company, government, or others providing insurance coverage. First-party is the patient; second-party is the provider.
unbundle	Improper coding and billing that breaks apart a surgical package and results in overcharging the third party or insured.
unilateral	Affecting one side of the body only.
UPIN (Unique Physician Identification Number)	Assigned to each Medicare provider of health care services; it appears on Block 17a of claim forms of referred patients at the time the first claim is filed.
V-Codes	Used in those situations when the patient encounters the health care system without a specific illness, disease, or diagnosis; or for treatment of a specific ongoing disease; or to describe a condition or historical fact that might influence the treatment of the patient.

Workers' Compensation	Insurance coverage provided by the employer in case of employee injury while on the job.
World Health Organization (WHO)	An international organization devoted to the improvement of human health and the study of the worldwide spread of disease; located in Geneva, Switzerland.

Chapter Sixteen

COMPLETED PATIENT INFORMATION FORMS

Medical & Dental Associates, P.C.

3733 Professional Drive #300   317/123-4567
Indianapolis, IN 46260   Tax ID# 99-9999999

CONFIDENTIAL PATIENT INFORMATION RECORD

(please print)

Patient Name	Rose Ann Altobelli	**Patient Employer**	Altobelli Assoc.
Address	4551 Hillside Dr.	Address	1200 Great Falls Rd.
	Indpls, IN 46238		Indpls, IN 46212

Telephone	(317) 555-3331
Birthdate	9/13/-- Age 32
Sex F	Marital Status S
Social Security No.	613-07-1876

Telephone   (317) 555-3400

Occupation   Financial Consultant

Responsible Party (if other than patient)

Relationship to patient

Address

Primary insured date of birth

Secondary insured date of birth

Third insured date of birth

Fourth insured date of birth

(Please use the back of the form to write information about the
third and fourth insured parties, if applicable.)

INSURANCE INFORMATION

Primary insured	Pt.	Secondary insured	
Subscriber	Pt.	Subscriber	
Address	Same	Address	
Telephone		Telephone	
Employer		Employer	
Address		Address	
Job/Union No.		Job/Union No.	
Subscriber's SS#	613-07-1876	Subscriber's SS#	
Relationship to patient		Relationship to patient	
Insurance	General Insurance Co.	Insurance	
Address	1010 Southway Blvd.	Address	
	Gary, IN 48431		
Policy No.	—	Policy No.	
Subscriber ID No.	613-07-1876	Subscriber ID No.	
Group Name/No.	—	Group Name/No.	
Effective date	4-14-95	Effective date	
Expiration date		Expiration date	

Record #1 1 of 4

176

Medical & Dental Associates, P.C.

3733 Professional Drive #300
Indianapolis, IN 46260

317/123-4567
Tax ID# 99-9999999

MEDICAL HISTORY

Patient Name *Rose Ann Altobelli*	Today's Date *9/1/--*

Are you currently in good health? *Relatively good health*

Are you under a physician's regular care at this time? *No*   If so, state reason(s) for regular treatment:

Are you currently taking prescribed medication?   If so, state brand name and dosage schedule:

No

Circle the names of the following diseases for which you have been treated:

Alcoholism	Allergies	Amenorrhea	Anemia	Arthritis
Asthma	Cancer	Colitis	Depression	Diabetes
Gingivitis	Heart Disease	Hemorrhoids	Hepatitis	Hernia
Hypertension	Hypoglycemia	Kidney Disease	Lumbago	(Migraine)
(Mononucleosis)	Periodontal Dis.	Rheumatic fever	(Rubella)	Other _____

Have you ever had prolonged bleeding? If yes, explain:

No

Have you ever had an unusual reaction to a drug, antibiotic or anesthetic, such as novocaine or penicillin?

If yes, explain: *No*

Is there any other information we should know about you or your health? *No — I'm new to the area and need a doctor*

Is there any other information we should know about previous treatments you have had? *No*

Have you ever been exposed to the HIV/AIDS virus? *No*

Purpose of the first visit *Bothered by hemorrhoids & bowel problems*

Family physician —   Who referred you to this practice? —

Authorization for Release of Medical Information to the Insurance Carrier and Assignment of Benefits to Medical & Dental Associates, P.C.

Commercial Insurance

I hereby authorize release of medical information necessary to file a claim with my insurance company and assign benefits otherwise payable to me to Medical & Dental Associates, P.C. I understand I am financially responsible for any balance due not covered by my insurance carrier or denied by my insurance carrier for lack of coverage. A copy of this signature is as valid as the original.

Signature of Patient or Legal Guardian *Rose A. Altobelli*

Medicare Insurance

Beneficiary _____ Medicare Number _____

I request that payment of authorized Medicare benefits be made either to me or on my behalf to Medical & Dental Associates, P.C. for any services furnished to me by that association. I authorize any holder of medical information about me to release to the Health Care Financing Administration and its agents any information needed to determine these benefits payable for related services.

Beneficiary Signature _____

Medicare Supplemental Insurance

Beneficiary _____ Medicare Number _____

Medigap ID Number _____

I request that payment of authorized Medigap benefits be made either to me or on my behalf to Medical & Dental Associates, P.C. for any services furnished to me by that physician. I authorize any holder of Medicare information about me to release to Medical & Dental Associates, P.C. any information needed to determine these benefits payable for related services.

Beneficiary Signature _____

Record #1 2 of 4

Medical & Dental Associates, P.C.

3733 Professional Drive #300
Indianapolis, IN 46260

317/123-4567
Tax ID# 99-9999999

Patient name *Rose Altobelli*

CPT-4 CODES

OFFICE SERVICES

	CODE	FEE
New patient, problem focused	99201	
New patient, expanded problem focused	99202	
New patient, detailed	(99203)	60—
New patient, comprehensive, mod.	99204	
New patient, comprehensive, high	99205	
Established patient, RN	99211	
Established patient, problem focused	99212	
Established patient, expanded problem	99213	
Established patient, detailed	99214	
Established patient, comprehensive	99215	
Consultation		

LABORATORY

	CODE	FEE
X-ray, chest/ribs; single view, frontal	71010	
X-ray, chest/ribs; stereo, frontal	71015	
Therapeutic injections ( )	907__	
Drugs, trays, supplies	99070	
Educational supplies, books, tapes	99071	
Urinalysis, routine, dip stick	81000	
Urine pregnancy test, visual color	81025	
Blood count, hemoglobin	85018	
Pap smear	88150	

ICD-9-CM

DIAGNOSES

Anxiety reaction	300.00
Bleeding rectal	569.3
Benign prostatic hypertrophy	600
Bronchitis, acute	466.0
Bronchitis, chronic	491.9
Cardiac arrhythmia	427.9
Chest pain	786.50
Cirrhosis of liver	571.5
Conjunctivitis, acute	372.00
Depression	300.4
Flu	487.0
Fracture–nasal, closed	802.0
Fractured tibia	891.2
Headache, vascular	794.0
Herpes zoster	053.9
Irritable bowel syndrome	(564.1)
Menopause	627.2
Myocardial infarction, unspecified	410.90
Otitis, acute	381.01
Pharyngitis, acute	462
Pneumonia	486
Sinusitis, acute	461.9
Tendonitis	726.90
Tennis elbow	726.32
Pregnancy	V22.2
Sprained ankle	842.5
Tonsillitis	474.0
Vertigo	386.0
Well child	V20.2

Bleeding hemorrhoids

CDT-2 CODES

DENTAL SERVICE

DIAGNOSTIC

	CODE	FEE
Periodic exam	00120	
Limited exam	00140	
Comprehensive exam	00150	
Extensive exam	00160	

PREVENTIVE

	CODE	FEE
Intraoral–FMX	00210	
Intraoral–PA	00220	
BW	0027_	
Single posteroanterior	00290	
Panoramic X-ray	00330	
Prophylaxis adult	01110	
Prophylaxis child	01120	
Topical fluoride	012__	

DENTAL SERVICE

RESTORATIVE

	CODE	FEE
Amalgams (decid) Tooth #_____	021__	
Amalgams (perm) Tooth #_____	021__	

CROWNS AND BRIDGES

	CODE	FEE
PFG crown	02750	
FG cast crown	02790	
3/4 gold cast crown	02810	
FC bridge pontic	06210	
Porcelain bridge ( )	062__	

OTHER PROCEDURES

DOCTOR'S STATEMENT: I certify that I personally provided the above services and that fees shown represent my usual fees

James P. Cartman, M.D.   9/1/--

Signature   Date

TOTAL	$	60—
AMOUNT PAID	$	—
BALANCE DUE	$	60—

Record #1 3 of 4

Medical & Dental Associates, P.C.

3733 Professional Drive #300
Indianapolis, IN 46260
317/123-4567
Tax ID# 99-9999999

STATEMENT OF ACCOUNT

ALTOBELLI, Rose
4551 Hillside Drive
Indianapolis, IN 46238

19--

DATE	CODE	CHARGE	CREDITS PAYMENT	ADJ	CURRENT BALANCE
BALANCE FORWARD ➡					0
09/01	99203	60 00			60 00

PLEASE PAY LAST AMOUNT IN THIS COLUMN ↑

THIS IS A COPY OF YOUR ACCOUNT

Record #1 4 of 4

Medical & Dental Associates, P.C.

3733 Professional Drive #300   317/123-4567
Indianapolis, IN 46260   Tax ID# 99-9999999

CONFIDENTIAL PATIENT INFORMATION RECORD

(please print)

Patient Name	Julie S. Justin
Address	1800 Main St.
	Greenberg, IN 47311
Telephone	(317) 555-2161
Birthdate	March 2, 19-- Age 29
Sex	F Marital Status S
Social Security No.	455-60-1562

Responsible Party (if other than patient)
—

Relationship to patient

Address

Patient Employer	KDWB Radio
Address	1 Doodle Rd.
	Greenberg, IN 47311
Telephone	(317) 555-1867
Occupation	News Broadcaster

Primary insured date of birth   3/21/--

Secondary insured date of birth   —

Third insured date of birth

Fourth insured date of birth

(Please use the back of the form to write information about the third and fourth insured parties, if applicable.)

INSURANCE INFORMATION

Primary insured	Self	
Subscriber	Self	
Address	See above	
Telephone		
Employer		
Address		
Job/Union No.		
Subscriber's SS#	455-60-1562	
Relationship to patient		
Insurance	Angel Insurance Co.	
Address	9 Sharon Lane	
	Minneapolis, MN 55415	
Policy No.	—	
Subscriber ID No.	455-60-1562	
Group Name/No.	17-6749-1254	
Effective date	12-1-95	
Expiration date	—	

Secondary insured	
Subscriber	
Address	
Telephone	
Employer	
Address	
Job/Union No.	
Subscriber's SS#	
Relationship to patient	
Insurance	
Address	
Policy No.	
Subscriber ID No.	
Group Name/No.	
Effective date	
Expiration date	

Record #2 1 of 4

Medical & Dental Associates, P.C.

3733 Professional Drive #300
Indianapolis, IN 46260

317/123-4567
Tax ID# 99-9999999

MEDICAL HISTORY

Patient Name _Julie S. Justin_	Today's Date _8/6/--_

Are you currently in good health? _Yes_

Are you under a physician's regular care at this time? | If so, state reason(s) for regular treatment:

_No_

Are you currently taking prescribed medication? | If so, state brand name and dosage schedule:

_No_

Circle the names of the following diseases for which you have been treated:

Alcoholism	(Allergies)	Amenorrhea	Anemia	Arthritis
Asthma	Cancer	Colitis	Depression	Diabetes
Gingivitis	Heart Disease	Hemorrhoids	Hepatitis	Hernia
Hypertension	Hypoglycemia	Kidney Disease	Lumbago	Migraine
Mononucleosis	Periodontal Dis.	Rheumatic fever	(Rubella)	Other _____

Have you ever had prolonged bleeding? If yes, explain: _No_

Have you ever had an unusual reaction to a drug, antibiotic or anesthetic, such as novocaine or penicillin?

If yes, explain: _No_

Is there any other information we should know about you or your health? _No_

Is there any other information we should know about previous treatments you have had? _No_

Have you ever been exposed to the HIV/AIDS virus? _No_

Purpose of the first visit _Headache, chills, ache all over_

Family physician — | Who referred you to this practice? —

Authorization for Release of Medical Information to the Insurance Carrier and Assignment of Benefits to Medical & Dental Associates, P.C.

Commercial Insurance

I hereby authorize release of medical information necessary to file a claim with my insurance company and assign benefits otherwise payable to me to Medical & Dental Associates, P.C. I understand I am financially responsible for any balance due not covered by my insurance carrier or denied by my insurance carrier for lack of coverage. A copy of this signature is as valid as the original.

Signature of Patient or Legal Guardian _Julie S. Justin_

Medicare Insurance

Beneficiary _____ Medicare Number _____

I request that payment of authorized Medicare benefits be made either to me or on my behalf to Medical & Dental Associates, P.C. for any services furnished to me by that association. I authorize any holder of medical information about me to release to the Health Care Financing Administration and its agents any information needed to determine these benefits payable for related services.

Beneficiary Signature _____

Medicare Supplemental Insurance

Beneficiary _____ Medicare Number _____

Medigap ID Number _____

I request that payment of authorized Medigap benefits be made either to me or on my behalf to Medical & Dental Associates, P.C. for any services furnished to me by that physician. I authorize any holder of Medicare information about me to release to Medical & Dental Associates, P.C. any information needed to determine these benefits payable for related services.

Beneficiary Signature _____

Record #2 2 of 4

Medical & Dental Associates, P.C.

3733 Professional Drive #300
Indianapolis, IN 46260

317/123-4567
Tax ID# 99-9999999

MEDICAL TREATMENT RECORD

Patient	*Julie S. Justin*	Date	*10/4/--*
Occupation		DOB	Age
Insurance Carrier		Social Security No.	
Admitted	Discharged	Consults	
Hospital	Other	Referred by: Dr.	

CC: *Chills, ache all over, headache*

Previous symptom: Yes / (No)

First Symptom:

Physical Examination

General	*General malaise, Temp. 101°*
Appearance	*BP 90/60, wt. 109*
HEENT	*Pharynx infected*
Lungs	*WNL*
Cardiac	*WNL*
ABD	*WNL*
Extremities	*WNL*

Dx (Primary): *Influenza*

Dx (Secondary):

Dx (Postoperative):

Procedures: *Local TX, OV, injection of Tizan, 200 mg IM*

Complications: —

Dx testing (place of service):

Plan: *Return PRN*

Linda Gregory, M.D.

Attending physician

Record #2 3 of 4

182

Medical & Dental Associates, P.C.

3733 Professional Drive #300
Indianapolis, IN 46260
317/123-4567
Tax ID# 99-9999999

STATEMENT OF ACCOUNT

JUSTIN, Julie S.
1800 Main St.
Greenberg, IN 47311

19--

| DATE | CODE | CHARGE | CREDITS | | CURRENT BALANCE |
			PAYMENT	ADJ	
		BALANCE FORWARD ⟶			46 00
10/4	99212	32 00			78 00
10/4	J3250	10 00			88 00

PLEASE PAY LAST AMOUNT IN THIS COLUMN

THIS IS A COPY OF YOUR ACCOUNT

Record #2 4 of 4

Medical & Dental Associates, P.C.

3733 Professional Drive #300   317/123-4567
Indianapolis, IN 46260   Tax ID# 99-9999999

CONFIDENTIAL PATIENT INFORMATION RECORD

(please print)

Patient Name	Tom R. Willisse	**Patient Employer**	Baker Boys Tool Co.
Address	1515 N. Merry St.	Address	8840 S. Harrah
	Temmpe, IN 46610		Temmpe, IN 46610

Telephone   (317) 555-1994

Birthdate   6/4/--   Age 31

Sex _____   Marital Status _____

Social Security No.   318-66-1499

Responsible Party (if other than patient)

Relationship to patient

Address

Telephone   (317) 555-2501

Occupation   V.P. of Sales

Primary insured date of birth   6/4/--

Secondary insured date of birth

Third insured date of birth

Fourth insured date of birth

(Please use the back of the form to write information about the third and fourth insured parties, if applicable.)

INSURANCE INFORMATION

Primary insured		Secondary insured	
Subscriber		Subscriber	
Address		Address	
Telephone		Telephone	
Employer		Employer	
Address		Address	
Job/Union No.		Job/Union No.	
Subscriber's SS#	318-66-1499	Subscriber's SS#	
Relationship to patient		Relationship to patient	
Insurance	Hart Ins. Co.	Insurance	
Address	1520 N. Main St.	Address	
	Chicago, IL 64122		
Policy No.	HA3-16689	Policy No.	
Subscriber ID No.	BAB661499	Subscriber ID No.	
Group Name/No.	—	Group Name/No.	
Effective date	8/4/90	Effective date	
Expiration date		Expiration date	

Record #3 1 of 2

184

Medical & Dental Associates, P.C.

3733 Professional Drive #300
Indianapolis, IN 46260

317/123-4567
Tax ID# 99-9999999

Patient name   *Tom Willisse*

CPT-4 CODES

OFFICE SERVICES

	CODE	FEE
New patient, problem focused	99201	
New patient, expanded problem focused	99202	
New patient, detailed	99203	
New patient, comprehensive, mod.	99204	
New patient, comprehensive, high	99205	
Established patient, RN	99211	
Established patient, problem focused	99212	✓
Established patient, expanded problem	99213	
Established patient, detailed	99214	
Established patient, comprehensive	99215	
Consultation		

LABORATORY

	CODE	FEE
X-ray, chest/ribs; single view, frontal	71010	
X-ray, chest/ribs; stereo, frontal	71015	
Therapeutic injections ( )	907__	
Drugs, trays, supplies	99070	
Educational supplies, books, tapes	99071	
Urinalysis, routine, dip stick	81000	✓
Urine pregnancy test, visual color	81025	
Blood count, hemoglobin	85018	✓
Pap smear	88150	

ICD-9-CM

DIAGNOSES

Anxiety reaction	300.00
Bleeding rectal	569.3
Benign prostatic hypertrophy	(600)
Bronchitis, acute	466.0
Bronchitis, chronic	491.9
Cardiac arrhythmia	427.9
Chest pain	786.50
Cirrhosis of liver	571.5
Conjunctivitis, acute	372.00
Depression	300.4
Flu	487.0
Fracture–nasal, closed	802.0
Fractured tibia	891.2
Headache, vascular	794.0
Herpes zoster	053.9
Irritable bowel syndrome	564.1
Menopause	627.2
Myocardial infarction, unspecified	410.90
Otitis, acute	381.01
Pharyngitis, acute	462
Pneumonia	486
Sinusitis, acute	461.9
Tendonitis	726.90
Tennis elbow	726.32
Pregnancy	V22.2
Sprained ankle	842.5
Tonsillitis	474.0
Vertigo	386.0
Well child	V20.2

CDT-2 CODES

DENTAL SERVICE

DIAGNOSTIC

	CODE	FEE
Periodic exam	00120	
Limited exam	00140	
Comprehensive exam	00150	
Extensive exam	00160	

PREVENTIVE

	CODE	FEE
Intraoral–FMX	00210	
Intraoral–PA	00220	
BW	0027_	
Single posteroanterior	00290	
Panoramic X-ray	00330	
Prophylaxis adult	01110	
Prophylaxis child	01120	
Topical fluoride	012__	

DENTAL SERVICE

RESTORATIVE

	CODE	FEE
Amalgams (decid) Tooth #_____	021__	
Amalgams (perm) Tooth #_____	021__	

CROWNS AND BRIDGES

	CODE	FEE
PFG crown	02750	
FG cast crown	02790	
3/4 gold cast crown	02810	
FC bridge pontic	06210	
Porcelain bridge ( )	062__	

OTHER PROCEDURES

DOCTOR'S STATEMENT: I certify that I personally provided the above services and that fees shown represent my usual fees

James P. Cartman, M.D.   10/15/--

Signature   Date

TOTAL	$	55—
AMOUNT PAID	$	0
BALANCE DUE	$	55—

Record #3 2 of 2

Medical & Dental Associates, P.C.

3733 Professional Drive #300   317/123-4567
Indianapolis, IN 46260   Tax ID# 99-9999999

CONFIDENTIAL PATIENT INFORMATION RECORD

(please print)

Patient Name Terry P. Hammpton	**Patient Employer** Rainbow Constr. Co.
Address 410 S. "H" St.	Address 4000 W. 10th St.
Purdie, IN 47311	Purdie, IN 47311

Telephone (317) 555-8400

Telephone (317) 555-6130

Birthdate 11/6/-- Age 28

Occupation Accountant

Sex M   Marital Status M

Social Security No. 400-13-1699

Primary insured date of birth

Responsible Party (if other than patient)

Secondary insured date of birth

Third insured date of birth

Relationship to patient

Fourth insured date of birth

Address

(Please use the back of the form to write information about the

third and fourth insured parties, if applicable.)

INSURANCE INFORMATION

Primary insured Terry	Secondary insured
Subscriber "	Subscriber
Address	Address
Telephone	Telephone
Employer	Employer
Address	Address
Job/Union No.	Job/Union No.
Subscriber's SS# 400-13-1699	Subscriber's SS#
Relationship to patient Same	Relationship to patient
Insurance Goode Mutual Ins.	Insurance
Address 1420 S. Mountain Rd.	Address
Gary, IN 49411	
Policy No.	Policy No.
Subscriber ID No. 400-13-1699	Subscriber ID No.
Group Name/No. 22310	Group Name/No.
Effective date 8/4/94	Effective date
Expiration date None	Expiration date

Record #4 1 of 2

186

Medical & Dental Associates, P.C.

3733 Professional Drive #300
Indianapolis, IN 46260

317/123-4567
Tax ID# 99-9999999

Patient name   *T. Hammpton*

CPT-4 CODES

OFFICE SERVICES	CODE	FEE
New patient, problem focused	99201	
New patient, expanded problem focused	99202	
New patient, detailed	99203	
New patient, comprehensive, mod.	99204	
New patient, comprehensive, high	99205	
Established patient, RN	99211	
Established patient, problem focused	99212	
Established patient, expanded problem	(99213)	40—
Established patient, detailed	99214	
Established patient, comprehensive	99215	
Consultation		

LABORATORY		
X-ray, chest/ribs; single view, frontal	71010	
X-ray, chest/ribs; stereo, frontal	71015	
Therapeutic injections ( )	907__	
Drugs, trays, supplies	99070	
Educational supplies, books, tapes	(99071)	5—
Urinalysis, routine, dip stick	81000	
Urine pregnancy test, visual color	81025	
Blood count, hemoglobin	85018	
Pap smear	88150	

ICD-9-CM

DIAGNOSES

Anxiety reaction	*3rd*	(300.00)
Bleeding rectal		569.3
Benign prostatic hypertrophy		600
Bronchitis, acute		466.0
Bronchitis, chronic		491.9
Cardiac arrhythmia		427.9
Chest pain	*1st*	(786.50)
Cirrhosis of liver		571.5
Conjunctivitis, acute		372.00
Depression		300.4
Flu		487.0
Fracture–nasal, closed		802.0
Fractured tibia		891.2
Headache, vascular	*2nd*	(794.0)
Herpes zoster		053.9
Irritable bowel syndrome		564.1
Menopause		627.2
Myocardial infarction, unspecified		410.90
Otitis, acute		381.01
Pharyngitis, acute		462
Pneumonia		486
Sinusitis, acute		461.9
Tendonitis		726.90
Tennis elbow		726.32
Pregnancy		V22.2
Sprained ankle		842.5
Tonsillitis		474.0
Vertigo		386.0
Well child		V20.2

CDT-2 CODES

DENTAL SERVICE

DIAGNOSTIC	CODE	FEE
Periodic exam	00120	
Limited exam	00140	
Comprehensive exam	00150	
Extensive exam	00160	
PREVENTIVE		
Intraoral–FMX	00210	
Intraoral–PA	00220	
BW	0027_	
Single posteroanterior	00290	
Panoramic X-ray	00330	
Prophylaxis adult	01110	
Prophylaxis child	01120	
Topical fluoride	012__	

DENTAL SERVICE

RESTORATIVE	CODE	FEE
Amalgams (decid) Tooth #____	021__	
Amalgams (perm) Tooth #____	021__	
CROWNS AND BRIDGES		
PFG crown	02750	
FG cast crown	02790	
3/4 gold cast crown	02810	
FC bridge pontic	06210	
Porcelain bridge ( )	062__	
OTHER PROCEDURES		

DOCTOR'S STATEMENT: I certify that I personally provided the above services and that fees shown represent my usual fees

Linda Gregory, M.D.   8/9/--

Signature   Date

TOTAL	$	45—
AMOUNT PAID	$	0
BALANCE DUE	$	45—

Record #4 2 of 2

Medical & Dental Associates, P.C.

3733 Professional Drive #300   317/123-4567
Indianapolis, IN 46260   Tax ID# 99-9999999

CONFIDENTIAL PATIENT INFORMATION RECORD

(please print)

Patient Name	Richard O. Roberts, Jr.	**Patient Employer**	Student
Address	312 Hill St.	Address	Madison Jr. High School
	Doloth, IN 46233		Mesaba Rd.
			Doloth, IN 46233
Telephone	(317) 555-0900	Telephone	(317) 555-0978 (school)
Birthdate	11/1/-- Age 13	Occupation	
Sex	M Marital Status S		
Social Security No.	320-56-6879		

Primary insured date of birth   6/5/-- (40)

Responsible Party (if other than patient)

Secondary insured date of birth   —

Third insured date of birth   —

Relationship to patient

Fourth insured date of birth   —

Address

(Please use the back of the form to write information about the third and fourth insured parties, if applicable.)

INSURANCE INFORMATION

Primary insured	Father	Secondary insured	
Subscriber	"	Subscriber	NA
Address		Address	
Telephone		Telephone	
Employer	Wall Dept. Store	Employer	
Address	21 E. Miller Mall	Address	
	Doloth, IN		
Job/Union No.	—	Job/Union No.	
Subscriber's SS#	451-03-4672	Subscriber's SS#	
Relationship to patient	FA	Relationship to patient	
Insurance	Prudential Ins. Co.	Insurance	
Address	1800 Wisconsin Blvd.	Address	
	Superior, WI 21227		
Policy No.	W4510-34672	Policy No.	
Subscriber ID No.	451034672	Subscriber ID No.	
Group Name/No.	#681745	Group Name/No.	
Effective date	10/11/90	Effective date	
Expiration date	—	Expiration date	

Record #5 1 of 2

188

Medical & Dental Associates, P.C.

3733 Professional Drive #300
Indianapolis, IN 46260

317/123-4567
Tax ID# 99-9999999

Patient name *Richard Roberts, Jr.*

CPT-4 CODES

OFFICE SERVICES

	CODE	FEE
New patient, problem focused	99201	_____
New patient, expanded problem focused	99202	_____
New patient, detailed	99203	_____
New patient, comprehensive, mod.	99204	_____
New patient, comprehensive, high	99205	_____
Established patient, RN	99211	_____
Established patient, problem focused	99212	_____
Established patient, expanded problem	(99213)	?
Established patient, detailed	99214	_____
Established patient, comprehensive	99215	_____
Consultation		_____

LABORATORY

	CODE	FEE
X-ray, chest/ribs; single view, frontal	71010	_____
X-ray, chest/ribs; stereo, frontal	71015	_____
Therapeutic injections ( )	907__	_____
Drugs, trays, supplies	99070	_____
Educational supplies, books, tapes	99071	_____
Urinalysis, routine, dip stick	81000	_____
Urine pregnancy test, visual color	81025	_____
Blood count, hemoglobin	85018	_____
Pap smear	88150	_____

ICD-9-CM

DIAGNOSES

Anxiety reaction	300.00
Bleeding rectal	569.3
Benign prostatic hypertrophy	600
Bronchitis, acute	466.0
Bronchitis, chronic	491.9
Cardiac arrhythmia	427.9
Chest pain	786.50
Cirrhosis of liver	571.5
Conjunctivitis, acute	372.00
Depression	300.4
Flu	487.0
Fracture–nasal, closed	802.0
Fractured tibia	891.2
Headache, vascular	794.0
Herpes zoster	053.9
Irritable bowel syndrome	564.1
Menopause	627.2
Myocardial infarction, unspecified	410.90
Otitis, acute	381.01
Pharyngitis, acute	462
Pneumonia	486
Sinusitis, acute	461.9
Tendonitis	726.90
Tennis elbow	726.32
Pregnancy	V22.2
Sprained ankle	842.5
Tonsillitis	474.0
Vertigo	386.0
Well child	V20.2

Acute leukemia

CDT-2 CODES

DENTAL SERVICE

DIAGNOSTIC

	CODE	FEE
Periodic exam	00120	_____
Limited exam	00140	_____
Comprehensive exam	00150	_____
Extensive exam	00160	_____

PREVENTIVE

	CODE	FEE
Intraoral–FMX	00210	_____
Intraoral–PA	00220	_____
BW	0027_	_____
Single posteroanterior	00290	_____
Panoramic X-ray	00330	_____
Prophylaxis adult	01110	_____
Prophylaxis child	01120	_____
Topical fluoride	012__	_____

DENTAL SERVICE

RESTORATIVE

	CODE	FEE
Amalgams (decid) Tooth #_____	021__	_____
Amalgams (perm) Tooth #_____	021__	_____

CROWNS AND BRIDGES

	CODE	FEE
PFG crown	02750	_____
FG cast crown	02790	_____
3/4 gold cast crown	02810	_____
FC bridge pontic	06210	_____
Porcelain bridge ( )	062__	_____

OTHER PROCEDURES

TOTAL	$	?
AMOUNT PAID	$	_____
BALANCE DUE	$	_____

DOCTOR'S STATEMENT: I certify that I personally provided the above services and that fees shown represent my usual fees

Harold S. Beckermann, M.D.   *6/3/--*

Signature   Date

Record #5 2 of 2

Medical & Dental Associates, P.C.

3733 Professional Drive #300   317/123-4567
Indianapolis, IN 46260   Tax ID# 99-9999999

CONFIDENTIAL PATIENT INFORMATION RECORD

(please print)

Patient Name	Nicole M. Petroff
Address	10 Golden Valley Rd.
	Golden Valley, IN 46411
Telephone	(812) 555-4100
Birthdate	8/31/-- Age 15
Sex	F Marital Status S
Social Security No.	382-93-3211

Patient Employer   Student
Address   Jefferson H.S.

Telephone

Occupation

Primary insured date of birth   4/2/-- (43)
Secondary insured date of birth —
Third insured date of birth —
Fourth insured date of birth —

Responsible Party (if other than patient)

     Samuel Petroff

Relationship to patient   Father

Address   Same

(Please use the back of the form to write information about the third and fourth insured parties, if applicable.)

INSURANCE INFORMATION

Primary insured	Samuel Petroff	Secondary insured	
Subscriber	Live with daughter	Subscriber	NA
Address	"	Address	
Telephone	"	Telephone	
Employer	Pillsbury Foods	Employer	
Address	Pillsbury Center	Address	
	Maples, IN 46470		
Job/Union No.	—	Job/Union No.	
Subscriber's SS#	203-00-3330	Subscriber's SS#	
Relationship to patient	Father	Relationship to patient	
Insurance	Blue Cross/Blue Shield	Insurance	
Address	Box 6433	Address	
	Gary, IN 47318		
Policy No.	—	Policy No.	
Subscriber ID No.	203003330	Subscriber ID No.	
Group Name/No.	AS240-52	Group Name/No.	
Effective date	5/14/88	Effective date	
Expiration date	None	Expiration date	

Record #6 1 of 2

190

Medical & Dental Associates, P.C.

3733 Professional Drive #300
Indianapolis, IN 46260

317/123-4567
Tax ID# 99-9999999

Patient name *Nicole Petroff*

CPT-4 CODES

OFFICE SERVICES

	CODE	FEE
New patient, problem focused	99201	_____
New patient, expanded problem focused	99202	_____
New patient, detailed	99203	_____
New patient, comprehensive, mod.	99204	_____
New patient, comprehensive, high	99205	_____
Established patient, RN	99211	_____
Established patient, problem focused	(99212)	*32—*
Established patient, expanded problem	99213	_____
Established patient, detailed	99214	_____
Established patient, comprehensive	99215	_____
Consultation		
_____		
_____		

LABORATORY

	CODE	FEE
X-ray, chest/ribs; single view, frontal	71010	_____
X-ray, chest/ribs; stereo, frontal	71015	_____
Therapeutic injections ( )	907__	_____
Drugs, trays, supplies	99070	_____
Educational supplies, books, tapes	99071	_____
Urinalysis, routine, dip stick	81000	_____
Urine pregnancy test, visual color	81025	_____
Blood count, hemoglobin	(85018)	*?*
Pap smear	88150	_____

ICD-9-CM

DIAGNOSES

Anxiety reaction	300.00
Bleeding rectal	569.3
Benign prostatic hypertrophy	600
Bronchitis, acute	466.0
Bronchitis, chronic	491.9
Cardiac arrhythmia	427.9
Chest pain	786.50
Cirrhosis of liver	571.5
Conjunctivitis, acute	372.00
Depression	300.4
Flu	487.0
Fracture–nasal, closed	802.0
Fractured tibia	891.2
Headache, vascular	794.0
Herpes zoster	053.9
Irritable bowel syndrome	564.1
Menopause	627.2
Myocardial infarction, unspecified	410.90
Otitis, acute	381.01
Pharyngitis, acute	462
Pneumonia	486
Sinusitis, acute	461.9
Tendonitis	726.90
Tennis elbow	726.32
Pregnancy	V22.2
Sprained ankle	842.5
Tonsillitis	474.0
Vertigo	386.0
Well child	V20.2

Infectious mononucleosis

CDT-2 CODES

DENTAL SERVICE

DIAGNOSTIC

	CODE	FEE
Periodic exam	00120	_____
Limited exam	00140	_____
Comprehensive exam	00150	_____
Extensive exam	00160	_____

PREVENTIVE

	CODE	FEE
Intraoral–FMX	00210	_____
Intraoral–PA	00220	_____
BW	0027_	_____
Single posteroanterior	00290	_____
Panoramic X-ray	00330	_____
Prophylaxis adult	01110	_____
Prophylaxis child	01120	_____
Topical fluoride	012__	_____

DENTAL SERVICE

RESTORATIVE

	CODE	FEE
Amalgams (decid) Tooth #_____	021__	_____
Amalgams (perm) Tooth #_____	021__	_____

CROWNS AND BRIDGES

	CODE	FEE
PFG crown	02750	_____
FG cast crown	02790	_____
3/4 gold cast crown	02810	_____
FC bridge pontic	06210	_____
Porcelain bridge ( )	062__	_____

OTHER PROCEDURES

_____		
_____		

DOCTOR'S STATEMENT: I certify that I personally provided the above services and that fees shown represent my usual fees

Harold S. Beckermann, M.D.   *10/15/--*

Signature   Date

TOTAL	$	*?*
AMOUNT PAID	$	*0*
BALANCE DUE	$	_____

Record #6 2 of 2

Medical & Dental Associates, P.C.

3733 Professional Drive #300   317/123-4567
Indianapolis, IN 46260   Tax ID# 99-9999999

CONFIDENTIAL PATIENT INFORMATION RECORD

(please print)

Patient Name Maria Blumquist

Address 4602 Betty Dr.

West Indy, IN 46200

Telephone (317) 555-3060

Birthdate 10/4/--   Age 6

Sex F   Marital Status S

Social Security No. 309-14-1688

Responsible Party (if other than patient)

Marsha Blumquist

Relationship to patient Mother

Address Same

Patient Employer

Address

Telephone

Occupation

Primary insured date of birth 3/9/-- Age 28

Secondary insured date of birth —

Third insured date of birth —

Fourth insured date of birth —

(Please use the back of the form to write information about the third and fourth insured parties, if applicable.)

INSURANCE INFORMATION

Primary insured Marsha Blumquist

Subscriber Same

Address

Telephone

Employer Petal Florists

Address 2525 W. Topiary Dr.

West Indy, IN 46208

Job/Union No.

Subscriber's SS# 341-13-6006

Relationship to patient Mother

Insurance Golden Web Ins. Co.

Address 380 N. High St.

Col, OH 36118

Policy No.

Subscriber ID No. 34113-6006-2

Group Name/No.

Effective date 10/8/93

Expiration date

Secondary insured —

Subscriber —

Address —

Telephone

Employer

Address

Job/Union No.

Subscriber's SS#

Relationship to patient

Insurance

Address

Policy No.

Subscriber ID No.

Group Name/No.

Effective date

Expiration date

Record #7 1 of 2

Medical & Dental Associates, P.C.

3733 Professional Drive #300
Indianapolis, IN 46260

317/123-4567
Tax ID# 99-9999999

Patient name *Maria Blumquist*

CPT-4 CODES

OFFICE SERVICES

	CODE	FEE
New patient, problem focused	99201	
New patient, expanded problem focused	99202	
New patient, detailed	99203	
New patient, comprehensive, mod.	(99204)	55—
New patient, comprehensive, high	99205	
Established patient, RN	99211	
Established patient, problem focused	99212	
Established patient, expanded problem	99213	
Established patient, detailed	99214	
Established patient, comprehensive	99215	
Consultation		

LABORATORY

	CODE	FEE
X-ray, chest/ribs; single view, frontal	71010	
X-ray, chest/ribs; stereo, frontal	71015	
Therapeutic injections ( )	907_	
Drugs, trays, supplies	(99070)	5—
Educational supplies, books, tapes	99071	
Urinalysis, routine, dip stick	81000	
Urine pregnancy test, visual color	81025	
Blood count, hemoglobin	85018	
Pap smear	88150	

J9293

ICD-9-CM

DIAGNOSES

Anxiety reaction	300.00
Bleeding rectal	569.3
Benign prostatic hypertrophy	600
Bronchitis, acute	466.0
Bronchitis, chronic	491.9
Cardiac arrhythmia	427.9
Chest pain	786.50
Cirrhosis of liver	571.5
Conjunctivitis, acute	372.00
Depression	300.4
Flu	487.0
Fracture–nasal, closed	802.0
Fractured tibia	891.2
Headache, vascular	794.0
Herpes zoster	053.9
Irritable bowel syndrome	564.1
Menopause	627.2
Myocardial infarction, unspecified	410.90
Otitis, acute	381.01
Pharyngitis, acute	462
Pneumonia	486
Sinusitis, acute	461.9
Tendonitis	726.90
Tennis elbow	726.32
Pregnancy	V22.2
Sprained ankle	842.5
Tonsillitis	474.0
Vertigo	386.0
Well child	V20.2

Fractured mandible, closed   802.20

CDT-2 CODES

DENTAL SERVICE

DIAGNOSTIC

	CODE	FEE
Periodic exam	00120	
Limited exam	00140	
Comprehensive exam	00150	
Extensive exam	00160	

PREVENTIVE

	CODE	FEE
Intraoral–FMX	00210	
Intraoral–PA	00220	
BW	0027_	
Single posteroanterior	00290	
Panoramic X-ray	00330	
Prophylaxis adult	01110	
Prophylaxis child	01120	
Topical fluoride	012__	

DENTAL SERVICE

RESTORATIVE

	CODE	FEE
Amalgams (decid) Tooth #_____	021__	
Amalgams (perm) Tooth #_____	021__	

CROWNS AND BRIDGES

	CODE	FEE
PFG crown	02750	
FG cast crown	02790	
3/4 gold cast crown	02810	
FC bridge pontic	06210	
Porcelain bridge ( )	062__	

OTHER PROCEDURES

DOCTOR'S STATEMENT: I certify that I personally provided the above services and that fees shown represent my usual fees

Michael Lane, M.D.   3/15/--

Signature   Date

TOTAL	$	
AMOUNT PAID	$	0
BALANCE DUE	$	

Record #7 2 of 2

Medical & Dental Associates, P.C.

3733 Professional Drive #300   317/123-4567
Indianapolis, IN 46260   Tax ID# 99-9999999

CONFIDENTIAL PATIENT INFORMATION RECORD

(please print)

Patient Name	Robert R. Tillis	**Patient Employer**	Weber's Candy Co.
Address	1525 Mary Lane	Address	15 W. 8th St.
	Indpls, IN 47213		Indpls, IN 46233

Telephone	555-8911
Birthdate	11/21/-- 30 yrs old
Sex	M Marital Status M
Social Security No.	699-14-1398

Telephone	555-6111
Occupation	Accountant

Responsible Party (if other than patient)

Relationship to patient

Address

Primary insured date of birth	See aside
Secondary insured date of birth	3/9/-- (31)
Third insured date of birth	
Fourth insured date of birth	

(Please use the back of the form to write information about the third and fourth insured parties, if applicable.)

INSURANCE INFORMATION

Primary insured	Self	Secondary insured	Jane P. Tillis
Subscriber	"	Subscriber	Same
Address	Same	Address	Same
Telephone		Telephone	
Employer		Employer	IN Bell Tel Co.
Address		Address	5555 N. Mergan St.
			Indpls, IN 46222
Job/Union No.		Job/Union No.	
Subscriber's SS#	699-14-1398	Subscriber's SS#	511-00-1398
Relationship to patient		Relationship to patient	Wife
Insurance		Insurance	Goodman Ins. Co.
Address	Heart Ins. Co.	Address	15 W. Goode Hwy.
	120 N. High St., Col, OH 47555		NY, NY 10099
Policy No.		Policy No.	
Subscriber ID No.	HE 141398	Subscriber ID No.	511-00-1398
Group Name/No.	—	Group Name/No.	
Effective date	10/10/95	Effective date	1/1/96
Expiration date	10/10/2005	Expiration date	—

Record #8 1 of 2

194

Medical & Dental Associates, P.C.

3733 Professional Drive #300
Indianapolis, IN 46260

317/123-4567
Tax ID# 99-9999999

Patient name *Robt R. Tillis*

CPT-4 CODES

OFFICE SERVICES

	CODE	FEE
New patient, problem focused	99201	
New patient, expanded problem focused	99202	
New patient, detailed	99203	
New patient, comprehensive, mod.	99204	
New patient, comprehensive, high	99205	
Established patient, RN	99211	
Established patient, problem focused	99212	
Established patient, expanded problem	99213	
Established patient, detailed	99214	
Established patient, comprehensive	99215	
(Consultation)	*99245*	*200—*

LABORATORY

	CODE	FEE
X-ray, chest/ribs; single view, frontal	71010	
X-ray, chest/ribs; stereo, frontal	71015	
Therapeutic injections ( )	907__	
Drugs, trays, supplies	99070	
Educational supplies, books, tapes	99071	
Urinalysis, routine, dip stick	81000	
Urine pregnancy test, visual color	81025	
Blood count, hemoglobin	85018	
Pap smear	88150	

ICD-9-CM

DIAGNOSES

Anxiety reaction	300.00
Bleeding rectal	569.3
Benign prostatic hypertrophy	600
Bronchitis, acute	466.0
Bronchitis, chronic	491.9
Cardiac arrhythmia	427.9
Chest pain	786.50
Cirrhosis of liver	571.5
Conjunctivitis, acute	372.00
Depression	300.4
Flu	487.0
Fracture–nasal, closed	802.0
Fractured tibia	891.2
Headache, vascular	794.0
Herpes zoster	053.9
Irritable bowel syndrome	564.1
Menopause	627.2
Myocardial infarction, unspecified	410.90
Otitis, acute	381.01
Pharyngitis, acute	462
Pneumonia	486
Sinusitis, acute	461.9
Tendonitis	726.90
Tennis elbow	726.32
Pregnancy	V22.2
Sprained ankle	842.5
Tonsillitis	474.0
Vertigo	386.0
Well child	V20.2

Uncontrolled diabetes with diabetic retinopathy

CDT-2 CODES

DENTAL SERVICE

DIAGNOSTIC

	CODE	FEE
Periodic exam	00120	
Limited exam	00140	
Comprehensive exam	00150	
Extensive exam	00160	

PREVENTIVE

	CODE	FEE
Intraoral–FMX	00210	
Intraoral–PA	00220	
BW	0027_	
Single posteroanterior	00290	
Panoramic X-ray	00330	
Prophylaxis adult	01110	
Prophylaxis child	01120	
Topical fluoride	012__	

DENTAL SERVICE

RESTORATIVE

	CODE	FEE
Amalgams (decid) Tooth #_____	021__	
Amalgams (perm) Tooth #_____	021__	

CROWNS AND BRIDGES

	CODE	FEE
PFG crown	02750	
FG cast crown	02790	
3/4 gold cast crown	02810	
FC bridge pontic	06210	
Porcelain bridge ( )	062__	

OTHER PROCEDURES

DOCTOR'S STATEMENT: I certify that I personally provided the above services and that fees shown represent my usual fees

James P. Cartman, M.D.   *4/18/--*

Signature   Date

TOTAL	$	*200—*
AMOUNT PAID	$	*—*
BALANCE DUE	$	*200—*

Record #8 2 of 2

Medical & Dental Associates, P.C.

3733 Professional Drive #300   317/123-4567
Indianapolis, IN 46260   Tax ID# 99-9999999

CONFIDENTIAL PATIENT INFORMATION RECORD

(please print)

Patient Name	*Ai Vang*
Address	*9 Peace Lane*
	White Bear, IN 45110
Telephone	*(812) 555-8181*
Birthdate	*10/31/-- (38)*
Sex	*F* Marital Status *M*
Social Security No.	*301-98-4040*

Responsible Party (if other than patient)

Relationship to patient

Address

Patient Employer	*City of White Bear*
Address	*City Hall*
	W.B., IN 45119
Telephone	*(812) 555-1616*
Occupation	*City Manager*

Primary insured date of birth   *10/3/--*

Secondary insured date of birth   *4/11/-- (40)*

Third insured date of birth   —

Fourth insured date of birth   —

(Please use the back of the form to write information about the third and fourth insured parties, if applicable.)

INSURANCE INFORMATION

Primary insured	*Same*	Secondary insured	*Mao Vang*
Subscriber		Subscriber	*"*
Address		Address	*Same*
Telephone		Telephone	
Employer		Employer	*Ramsey Dodge*
Address		Address	*1510 Valley Creek Rd.*
			White Bear, IN 45110
Job/Union No.		Job/Union No.	
Subscriber's SS#	*301-98-4040*	Subscriber's SS#	*304-3308517*
Relationship to patient	*Same*	Relationship to patient	*Spouse*
Insurance	*Gen Ins.*	Insurance	*Blue Cross/Blue Shield*
Address	*1010 South Way*	Address	*P.O. Box 14888*
	Blgtn, IN 44313		*Gary, IN 47511*
Policy No.	*1515-9083W*	Policy No.	—
Subscriber ID No.	*301984040-1515*	Subscriber ID No.	*304338517RD*
Group Name/No.	*CH14*	Group Name/No.	—
Effective date	*1/1/96*	Effective date	*10/1/95*
Expiration date	—	Expiration date	

Record #9 1 of 3

Medical & Dental Associates, P.C.

3733 Professional Drive #300
Indianapolis, IN 46260

317/123-4567
Tax ID# 99-9999999

Patient name Mrs. Ai Vang

CPT-4 CODES

OFFICE SERVICES

	CODE	FEE
New patient, problem focused	99201	
New patient, expanded problem focused	99202	
New patient, detailed	99203	
New patient, comprehensive, mod.	99204	
New patient, comprehensive, high	99205	
Established patient, RN	99211	
Established patient, problem focused	99212	
Established patient, expanded problem	(99213)	?
Established patient, detailed	99214	
Established patient, comprehensive	99215	
Consultation		
Colposcopy c̄ biopsy of cervix		_320—_

LABORATORY

	CODE	FEE
X-ray, chest/ribs; single view, frontal	71010	
X-ray, chest/ribs; stereo, frontal	71015	
Therapeutic injections ( )	907__	
Drugs, trays, supplies	99070	
Educational supplies, books, tapes	99071	
Urinalysis, routine, dip stick	81000	
Urine pregnancy test, visual color	81025	
Blood count, hemoglobin	85018	
Pap smear	88150	

ICD-9-CM

DIAGNOSES

Anxiety reaction	300.00
Bleeding rectal	569.3
Benign prostatic hypertrophy	600
Bronchitis, acute	466.0
Bronchitis, chronic	491.9
Cardiac arrhythmia	427.9
Chest pain	786.50
Cirrhosis of liver	571.5
Conjunctivitis, acute	372.00
Depression	300.4
Flu	487.0
Fracture–nasal, closed	802.0
Fractured tibia	891.2
Headache, vascular	794.0
Herpes zoster	053.9
Irritable bowel syndrome	564.1
Menopause	627.2
Myocardial infarction, unspecified	410.90
Otitis, acute	381.01
Pharyngitis, acute	462
Pneumonia	486
Sinusitis, acute	461.9
Tendonitis	726.90
Tennis elbow	726.32
Pregnancy	V22.2
Sprained ankle	842.5
Tonsillitis	474.0
Vertigo	386.0
Well child	V20.2

Abnormal Pap test results

CDT-2 CODES

DENTAL SERVICE

DIAGNOSTIC

	CODE	FEE
Periodic exam	00120	
Limited exam	00140	
Comprehensive exam	00150	
Extensive exam	00160	

PREVENTIVE

	CODE	FEE
Intraoral–FMX	00210	
Intraoral–PA	00220	
BW	0027_	
Single posteroanterior	00290	
Panoramic X-ray	00330	
Prophylaxis adult	01110	
Prophylaxis child	01120	
Topical fluoride	012__	

DENTAL SERVICE

RESTORATIVE

	CODE	FEE
Amalgams (decid) Tooth #____	021__	
Amalgams (perm) Tooth #____	021__	

CROWNS AND BRIDGES

	CODE	FEE
PFG crown	02750	
FG cast crown	02790	
3/4 gold cast crown	02810	
FC bridge pontic	06210	
Porcelain bridge ( )	062__	

OTHER PROCEDURES

DOCTOR'S STATEMENT: I certify that I personally provided the above services and that fees shown represent my usual fees
Jane R. Portia, M.D.   6/3/--
Signature   Date

TOTAL	$	_320—_
AMOUNT PAID	$	_—_
BALANCE DUE	$	_320—_

Record #9 2 of 3

Medical & Dental Associates, P.C.

3733 Professional Drive #300
Indianapolis, IN 46260
317/123-4567
Tax ID# 99-9999999

STATEMENT OF ACCOUNT

VANG, Mrs. Ai
9 Peace Lane
White Bear, IN 45110

19--

DATE	CODE	CHARGE		CREDITS PAYMENT		ADJ		CURRENT BALANCE	
		BALANCE FORWARD ➡️						94	00
5/10	Ck. Pymt			94	00			0	
6/3	57454	320	00					320	00

PLEASE PAY LAST AMOUNT IN THIS COLUMN ↑

THIS IS A COPY OF YOUR ACCOUNT

Record #9 3 of 3

Medical & Dental Associates, P.C.

3733 Professional Drive #300   317/123-4567
Indianapolis, IN 46260   Tax ID# 99-9999999

CONFIDENTIAL PATIENT INFORMATION RECORD

(please print)

Patient Name	James X. Moyer, Jr.	**Patient Employer**	Student
Address	14 Crowe Dr.	Address	
	Beechline, IN 47888		

Telephone	555-8200	Telephone	
Birthdate	9/9/-- Age 10	Occupation	
Sex M	Marital Status S		
Social Security No.	488-16-3121		

Primary insured date of birth   4/10/-- Age 38

Secondary insured date of birth 10/11/-- 39

Responsible Party (if other than patient)

James Moyer Sr.

Third insured date of birth   —

Relationship to patient	Father
Address	Same

Fourth insured date of birth   —

(Please use the back of the form to write information about the
third and fourth insured parties, if applicable.)

INSURANCE INFORMATION

Primary insured	James X. Moyer, Sr.	Secondary insured	Charlotte Moyer
Subscriber	"	Subscriber	"s
Address	Same as Pt.	Address	Same

Telephone		Telephone	
Employer	North Bank	Employer	County Tyme Co.
Address	1700 Main St.	Address	Beechline Mall
	Beechline, IN 47888		Beechline, IN 47886
Job/Union No.		Job/Union No.	
Subscriber's SS#	484-91-1688	Subscriber's SS#	400-12-3344
Relationship to patient	FA	Relationship to patient	Mom
Insurance	Good Gold Ins. Co.	Insurance	Elreed Ins. Co.
Address	8900 W. Tree Lane	Address	2150 W. 67th St.
	Chicago, IL 60606		Indpls., IN 46280
Policy No.		Policy No.	
Subscriber ID No.	484-91-1688	Subscriber ID No.	400-12-3344
Group Name/No.	30668	Group Name/No.	
Effective date	4/7/94	Effective date	1/1/90
Expiration date		Expiration date	

Record #10 1 of 1

Medical & Dental Associates, P.C.

3733 Professional Drive #300 317/123-4567
Indianapolis, IN 46260 Tax ID# 99-9999999

CONFIDENTIAL PATIENT INFORMATION RECORD

(please print)

Patient Name Aleeshaa Mobutuu

Address 315 W. 91st St.
Indpls., IN 46240

Telephone 555-8433

Birthdate 10/6/-- Age 9

Sex M Marital Status S

Social Security No. 411-16-1488

Responsible Party (if other than patient)
Mr. Kareem Mobutuu

Relationship to patient Father

Address Same

Patient Employer Elementary School Student

Address

Telephone

Occupation

Primary insured date of birth 7/8/-- 33

Secondary insured date of birth 9/6/-- 33

Third insured date of birth —

Fourth insured date of birth —

(Please use the back of the form to write information about the third and fourth insured parties, if applicable.)

INSURANCE INFORMATION

Primary insured Father	Secondary insured Sherrae Mobutuu
Subscriber "	Subscriber "
Address Same	Address Same
Telephone	Telephone
Employer Hook's Drug Co.	Employer Northside Elem. School
Address 1400 W. Straight St. Carmel, IN 49411	Address 388 N. Rue Way Carmel, IN 49420
Job/Union No.	Job/Union No. #188
Subscriber's SS# 389-34-3668	Subscriber's SS# 325-06-4980
Relationship to patient FA	Relationship to patient Mother
Insurance Hook's Medical Ins.	Insurance
Address 845 W. 38th St. Indpls., IN 46222	Address Ridgeway Ins. Co. 311 W. 10th St., Ball, IN 47490
Policy No. —	Policy No.
Subscriber ID No. 61438QR9	Subscriber ID No. 325-064980
Group Name/No. Hook 241	Group Name/No. —
Effective date 10/1/90	Effective date 10/10/92
Expiration date —	Expiration date

Record #11 1 of 2

200

Medical & Dental Associates, P.C.

3733 Professional Drive #300
Indianapolis, IN 46260

317/123-4567
Tax ID# 99-9999999

Patient name *Aleeshaa Mobutuu*

CPT-4 CODES

OFFICE SERVICES

	CODE	FEE
New patient, problem focused	99201	
New patient, expanded problem focused	99202	
New patient, detailed	99203	
New patient, comprehensive, mod.	99204	
New patient, comprehensive, high	99205	
Established patient, RN	99211	
Established patient, problem focused	99212	
Established patient, expanded problem	(99213)	40—
Established patient, detailed	99214	
Established patient, comprehensive	99215	
Consultation		

LABORATORY

	CODE	FEE
X-ray, chest/ribs; single view, frontal	71010	
X-ray, chest/ribs; stereo, frontal	(71015)	45—
Therapeutic injections ( )	907_	
Drugs, trays, supplies	99070	
Educational supplies, books, tapes	99071	
Urinalysis, routine, dip stick	81000	
Urine pregnancy test, visual color	81025	
Blood count, hemoglobin	85018	
Pap smear	88150	

ICD-9-CM

DIAGNOSES

Anxiety reaction	300.00
Bleeding rectal	569.3
Benign prostatic hypertrophy	600
Bronchitis, acute	466.0
Bronchitis, chronic	491.9
Cardiac arrhythmia	427.9
Chest pain	786.50
Cirrhosis of liver	571.5
Conjunctivitis, acute	372.00
Depression	300.4
Flu	487.0
Fracture–nasal, closed	802.0
Fractured tibia	891.2
Headache, vascular	794.0
Herpes zoster	053.9
Irritable bowel syndrome	564.1
Menopause	627.2
Myocardial infarction, unspecified	410.90
Otitis, acute	381.01
Pharyngitis, acute	462
Pneumonia	486
Sinusitis, acute	461.9
Tendonitis	726.90
Tennis elbow	726.32
Pregnancy	V22.2
Sprained ankle	842.5
Tonsillitis	474.0
Vertigo	386.0
Well child	V20.2

Closed fractured ribs — 2

CDT-2 CODES

DENTAL SERVICE

DIAGNOSTIC

	CODE	FEE
Periodic exam	00120	
Limited exam	00140	
Comprehensive exam	00150	
Extensive exam	00160	

PREVENTIVE

	CODE	FEE
Intraoral–FMX	00210	
Intraoral–PA	00220	
BW	0027_	
Single posteroanterior	00290	
Panoramic X-ray	00330	
Prophylaxis adult	01110	
Prophylaxis child	01120	
Topical fluoride	012_	

DENTAL SERVICE

RESTORATIVE

	CODE	FEE
Amalgams (decid) Tooth #_____	021_	
Amalgams (perm) Tooth #_____	021_	

CROWNS AND BRIDGES

	CODE	FEE
PFG crown	02750	
FG cast crown	02790	
3/4 gold cast crown	02810	
FC bridge pontic	06210	
Porcelain bridge ( )	062_	

OTHER PROCEDURES

TOTAL	$	85—
AMOUNT PAID	$	—
BALANCE DUE	$	85—

DOCTOR'S STATEMENT: I certify that I personally provided the above services and that fees shown represent my usual fees

Harold S. Beckermann, M.D.   7/8/--

Signature   Date

Record #11 2 of 2

Medical & Dental Associates, P.C.

3733 Professional Drive #300   317/123-4567
Indianapolis, IN 46260   Tax ID# 99-9999999

CONFIDENTIAL PATIENT INFORMATION RECORD

(please print)

Patient Name	Timothy Small
Address	1400 E. 49th St.
	Indpls., IN 46244
Telephone	555-0155
Birthdate	2/27/-- Age 3
Sex M Marital Status S	
Social Security No.	411-14-6868

Responsible Party (if other than patient)

Marianne Thomas

Relationship to patient   Mother

Address   Same as Pt.

Patient Employer

Address

Telephone

Occupation

Primary insured date of birth   5/15/-- Age 28

Secondary insured date of birth 11/8/-- Age 25

Third insured date of birth   —

Fourth insured date of birth   —

(Please use the back of the form to write information about the third and fourth insured parties, if applicable.)

INSURANCE INFORMATION

Primary insured	Thomas Small	Secondary insured	Christopher Thomas
Subscriber	"	Subscriber	"
Address	5520 N. Meridian St.	Address	Same as Pt.
	Indpls., IN 46299		
Telephone	555-9138	Telephone	"
Employer	Baker Bros. Ins. Co.	Employer	Royal Electric
Address	740 N. Phea St.	Address	38 W. Spree St.
	Indpls., IN 46238		Indpls., IN 46250
Job/Union No.		Job/Union No.	—
Subscriber's SS#	425-21-8778	Subscriber's SS#	418-81-3266
Relationship to patient	Father	Relationship to patient	Stepfather
Insurance	Healthmen's Ins. Co.	Insurance	Blue Ribbon Ins.
Address	5800 S. Green St.	Address	14 N. Willis St.
	Harold, OH 34668		Chicago, IL 61661
Policy No.	—	Policy No.	4238-65
Subscriber ID No.	HE 42521-8778	Subscriber ID No.	418813266-41
Group Name/No.	—	Group Name/No.	6558
Effective date	2/1/--	Effective date	9/15/--
Expiration date		Expiration date	

Record #12 1 of 2

202

Medical & Dental Associates, P.C.

3733 Professional Drive #300
Indianapolis, IN 46260

317/123-4567
Tax ID# 99-9999999

Patient name   *Tim Small*

CPT-4 CODES

OFFICE SERVICES

	CODE	FEE
New patient, problem focused	99201	
New patient, expanded problem focused	99202	
New patient, detailed	99203	
New patient, comprehensive, mod.	99204	
New patient, comprehensive, high	99205	
Established patient, RN	99211	
Established patient, problem focused	99212	
Established patient, expanded problem	(99213)	40—
Established patient, detailed	99214	
Established patient, comprehensive	99215	
Consultation		

LABORATORY

	CODE	FEE
X-ray, chest/ribs; single view, frontal	71010	
X-ray, chest/ribs; stereo, frontal	71015	
Therapeutic injections ( )	907_	
Drugs, trays, supplies	(99070)	20—
Educational supplies, books, tapes	99071	
Urinalysis, routine, dip stick	81000	
Urine pregnancy test, visual color	81025	
Blood count, hemoglobin	85018	
Pap smear	88150	

ICD-9-CM

DIAGNOSES

Anxiety reaction	300.00
Bleeding rectal	569.3
Benign prostatic hypertrophy	600
Bronchitis, acute	466.0
Bronchitis, chronic	491.9
Cardiac arrhythmia	427.9
Chest pain	786.50
Cirrhosis of liver	571.5
Conjunctivitis, acute	372.00
Depression	300.4
Flu	487.0
Fracture–nasal, closed	802.0
Fractured tibia	891.2
Headache, vascular	794.0
Herpes zoster	053.9
Irritable bowel syndrome	564.1
Menopause	627.2
Myocardial infarction, unspecified	410.90
Otitis, acute	(381.01)
Pharyngitis, acute	462
Pneumonia	486
Sinusitis, acute	461.9
Tendonitis	726.90
Tennis elbow	726.32
Pregnancy	V22.2
Sprained ankle	842.5
Tonsillitis *1st*	(474.0)
Vertigo	386.0
Well child	V20.2

CDT-2 CODES

DENTAL SERVICE

DIAGNOSTIC

	CODE	FEE
Periodic exam	00120	
Limited exam	00140	
Comprehensive exam	00150	
Extensive exam	00160	

PREVENTIVE

	CODE	FEE
Intraoral–FMX	00210	
Intraoral–PA	00220	
BW	0027_	
Single posteroanterior	00290	
Panoramic X-ray	00330	
Prophylaxis adult	01110	
Prophylaxis child	01120	
Topical fluoride	012_	

DENTAL SERVICE

RESTORATIVE

	CODE	FEE
Amalgams (decid) Tooth #_____	021_	
Amalgams (perm) Tooth #_____	021_	

CROWNS AND BRIDGES

	CODE	FEE
PFG crown	02750	
FG cast crown	02790	
3/4 gold cast crown	02810	
FC bridge pontic	06210	
Porcelain bridge ( )	062_	

OTHER PROCEDURES

DOCTOR'S STATEMENT: I certify that I personally provided the above services and that fees shown represent my usual fees

Harold S. Beckermann, M.D.   7/20/--

Signature   Date

TOTAL	$	60—
AMOUNT PAID	$	—
BALANCE DUE	$	60—

Record #12 2 of 2

Medical & Dental Associates, P.C.

3733 Professional Drive #300   317/123-4567
Indianapolis, IN 46260   Tax ID# 99-9999999

CONFIDENTIAL PATIENT INFORMATION RECORD

(please print)

Patient Name	Ritchey Bacon	**Patient Employer**	
Address	1200 N. State St.	Address	
	Burl, IN 43400		

Telephone	(317) 555-1189	Telephone	
Birthdate	1/25/-- Age 12	Occupation	Student
Sex M	Marital Status S		
Social Security No.	400-91-6724		

Primary insured date of birth 12/1/-- (42)

Responsible Party (if other than patient)

Melanie Beeker

Secondary insured date of birth 8/14/-- (40)

Relationship to patient	Mother	Third insured date of birth	2/27/-- (38)
Address	7470 N. Woods Dr.	Fourth insured date of birth	
	Salton, IN 48411		

(Please use the back of the form to write information about the third and fourth insured parties, if applicable.)

Over ———→

INSURANCE INFORMATION

Primary insured	Melanie Beeker	Secondary insured	Charles Bacon
Subscriber	"	Subscriber	"
Address	See above	Address	Same as Pt.
Telephone	(317) 555-2314	Telephone	
Employer	James & Sons	Employer	4-Star Tire Co.
Address	15 N. Constance Dr.	Address	Burl, IN 43420
	Greenway, IN 43411		
Job/Union No.		Job/Union No.	
Subscriber's SS#	389-41-6707	Subscriber's SS#	391-61-3206
Relationship to patient	Mother	Relationship to patient	Father
Insurance	BC/BS	Insurance	Aetna Ins. Co.
Address	15 S. Wolfson	Address	Box 2119
	Springfield, IL 61228		Ft. Wayne, IN 47382
Policy No.		Policy No.	
Subscriber ID No.	389416707	Subscriber ID No.	391-61-3206
Group Name/No.		Group Name/No.	—
Effective date	8/15/94	Effective date	9/20/90
Expiration date		Expiration date	

Record #13 1 of 3

204

3rd Insured
    Cheryl Bacon
    Lives with patient
SS# 311-18-6240
Emp: Conway R.R.
     320 E. Main
     Greenway, IN 46288
Step-mother
Ins: Blue Cross/Blue Shield
    3366 Northside Way
    Chicago, IL 60611
ID# 311-18-6240
Effective: 11/14/92

Record #13 2 of 3

Medical & Dental Associates, P.C.

3733 Professional Drive #300
Indianapolis, IN 46260

317/123-4567
Tax ID# 99-9999999

Patient name *Ritchey Bacon*

CPT-4 CODES

OFFICE SERVICES	CODE	FEE
New patient, problem focused	99201	
New patient, expanded problem focused	99202	
New patient, detailed	99203	
New patient, comprehensive, mod.	99204	
New patient, comprehensive, high	99205	
Established patient, RN	99211	
Established patient, problem focused	99212	
Established patient, expanded problem	99213	
Established patient, detailed	(99214)	?48
Established patient, comprehensive	99215	
Consultation		

LABORATORY

	CODE	FEE
X-ray, chest/ribs; single view, frontal	71010	
X-ray, chest/ribs; stereo, frontal	71015	
Therapeutic injections ( )	907 *04*	*20—*
Drugs, trays, supplies	99070	
Educational supplies, books, tapes	99071	
Urinalysis, routine, dip stick	81000	
Urine pregnancy test, visual color	81025	
Blood count, hemoglobin	85018	
Pap smear	88150	

ICD-9-CM

DIAGNOSES	
Anxiety reaction	300.00
Bleeding rectal	569.3
Benign prostatic hypertrophy	600
Bronchitis, acute	466.0
Bronchitis, chronic	491.9
Cardiac arrhythmia	427.9
Chest pain	786.50
Cirrhosis of liver	571.5
Conjunctivitis, acute	372.00
Depression	300.4
Flu	487.0
Fracture–nasal, closed	802.0
Fractured tibia	891.2
Headache, vascular	794.0
Herpes zoster	053.9
Irritable bowel syndrome	564.1
Menopause	627.2
Myocardial infarction, unspecified	410.90
Otitis, acute	381.01
Pharyngitis, acute	462
Pneumonia	486
Sinusitis, acute	461.9
Tendonitis	726.90
Tennis elbow	726.32
Pregnancy	V22.2
Sprained ankle	842.5
Tonsillitis	474.0
Vertigo	386.0
Well child	(V20.2)

Annual check-up

CDT-2 CODES

DENTAL SERVICE

DIAGNOSTIC	CODE	FEE
Periodic exam	00120	
Limited exam	00140	
Comprehensive exam	00150	
Extensive exam	00160	
PREVENTIVE		
Intraoral–FMX	00210	
Intraoral–PA	00220	
BW	0027_	
Single posteroanterior	00290	
Panoramic X-ray	00330	
Prophylaxis adult	01110	
Prophylaxis child	01120	
Topical fluoride	012__	

DENTAL SERVICE

RESTORATIVE	CODE	FEE
Amalgams (decid) Tooth #_____	021__	
Amalgams (perm) Tooth #_____	021__	
CROWNS AND BRIDGES		
PFG crown	02750	
FG cast crown	02790	
3/4 gold cast crown	02810	
FC bridge pontic	06210	
Porcelain bridge ( )	062__	
OTHER PROCEDURES		

DOCTOR'S STATEMENT: I certify that I personally provided the above services and that fees shown represent my usual fees

Harold S. Beckermann, M.D.   *1/20/--*

Signature   Date

TOTAL	$	
AMOUNT PAID	$	*0*
BALANCE DUE	$	

Record #13 3 of 3

Medical & Dental Associates, P.C.

3733 Professional Drive #300   317/123-4567
Indianapolis, IN 46260   Tax ID# 99-9999999

CONFIDENTIAL PATIENT INFORMATION RECORD

(please print)

Patient Name Barbara M. O'Leary	**Patient Employer** Retired
Address 59986 10th St.	Address
Indpls., IN 46294	
Telephone 555-1111	Telephone
Birthdate 6/23/-- Age 66	Occupation
Sex F Marital Status M	
Social Security No. 482-40-1640	
	Primary insured date of birth
Responsible Party (if other than patient)	Secondary insured date of birth
	Third insured date of birth
Relationship to patient	Fourth insured date of birth
Address	(Please use the back of the form to write information about the
	third and fourth insured parties, if applicable.)

No referral — Dx: Rt. tennis elbow — Dr. Gregory

INSURANCE INFORMATION

Primary insured Same	Secondary insured None
Subscriber "	Subscriber
Address "	Address
Telephone	Telephone
Employer	Employer
Address	Address
Job/Union No.	Job/Union No.
Subscriber's SS# 482-40-1640	Subscriber's SS#
Relationship to patient Same	Relationship to patient
Insurance Medicare	Insurance
Address c/o Blue Cross/Blue Shield	Address
1500 E. 10th, Indpls. 46215	
Policy No.	Policy No. ,
Subscriber ID No. 482-40-1640AB	Subscriber ID No.
Group Name/No.	Group Name/No.
Effective date 6/23/--	Effective date
Expiration date	Expiration date

Record #14 1 of 2

Medical & Dental Associates, P.C.

3733 Professional Drive #300
Indianapolis, IN 46260
317/123-4567
Tax ID# 99-9999999

STATEMENT OF ACCOUNT

O'LEARY, Mrs. Barbara
59986 10th Street
Indianapolis, IN 46294

19--

DATE	CODE	CHARGE	CREDITS		CURRENT BALANCE
			PAYMENT	ADJ	
BALANCE FORWARD ➡					0
8/6	99212	32 00			32 00
8/6	73070	43 00			75 00
8/6	L3700	45 00			120 00
8/10	97010	20 00			140 00
8/12	97010	20 00			160 00
8/14	97010	20 00			180 00

PLEASE PAY LAST AMOUNT IN THIS COLUMN ↑

THIS IS A COPY OF YOUR ACCOUNT

Record #14 2 of 2

Medical & Dental Associates, P.C.

3733 Professional Drive #300   317/123-4567
Indianapolis, IN 46260   Tax ID# 99-9999999

CONFIDENTIAL PATIENT INFORMATION RECORD

(please print)

Patient Name	Willa F. Johnson
Address	4130 N. Ellen Dr.
	Indpls., IN 46230
Telephone	555-4791
Birthdate	5/12/-- Age 65
Sex	F Marital Status W
Social Security No.	243-16-8101

Responsible Party (if other than patient)

Relationship to patient

Address

Patient Employer

Address

Telephone

Occupation

Primary insured date of birth

Secondary insured date of birth

Third insured date of birth

Fourth insured date of birth

(Please use the back of the form to write information about the third and fourth insured parties, if applicable.)

INSURANCE INFORMATION

Primary insured	Pt.	Secondary insured	
Subscriber		Subscriber	
Address		Address	
Telephone		Telephone	
Employer		Employer	
Address		Address	
Job/Union No.		Job/Union No.	
Subscriber's SS#	243-16-8101	Subscriber's SS#	
Relationship to patient		Relationship to patient	
Insurance	Medicare	Insurance	
Address	c/o BC/BS	Address	
	1500 E. 10th St, Indpls 46215		
Policy No.		Policy No.	
Subscriber ID No.	243-16-8101AB	Subscriber ID No.	
Group Name/No.		Group Name/No.	
Effective date		Effective date	
Expiration date		Expiration date	

Record #15 1 of 3

Medical & Dental Associates, P.C.

3733 Professional Drive #300
Indianapolis, IN 46260

317/123-4567
Tax ID# 99-9999999

Patient name   *Willa F. Johnson*

CPT-4 CODES

OFFICE SERVICES

	CODE	FEE
New patient, problem focused	99201	
New patient, expanded problem focused	99202	
New patient, detailed	(99203)	*60—*
New patient, comprehensive, mod.	99204	
New patient, comprehensive, high	99205	
Established patient, RN	99211	
Established patient, problem focused	99212	
Established patient, expanded problem	99213	
Established patient, detailed	99214	
Established patient, comprehensive	99215	
Consultation		

LABORATORY

	CODE	FEE
X-ray, chest/ribs; single view, frontal	71010	
X-ray, chest/ribs; stereo, frontal	71015	
Therapeutic injections ( )	907__	
Drugs, trays, supplies	99070	
Educational supplies, books, tapes	99071	
Urinalysis, routine, dip stick	81000	
Urine pregnancy test, visual color	81025	
Blood count, hemoglobin	85018	
Pap smear	(88150)	*20—*

(our cost $18.00 from outside lab)

ICD-9-CM

DIAGNOSES

Anxiety reaction	(300.00)
Bleeding rectal	569.3
Benign prostatic hypertrophy	600
Bronchitis, acute	466.0
Bronchitis, chronic	491.9
Cardiac arrhythmia	427.9
Chest pain	786.50
Cirrhosis of liver	571.5
Conjunctivitis, acute	372.00
Depression	300.4
Flu	487.0
Fracture–nasal, closed	802.0
Fractured tibia	891.2
Headache, vascular	794.0
Herpes zoster	053.9
Irritable bowel syndrome	564.1
Menopause	627.2
Myocardial infarction, unspecified	410.90
Otitis, acute	381.01
Pharyngitis, acute	462
Pneumonia	486
Sinusitis, acute	461.9
Tendonitis	726.90
Tennis elbow	726.32
Pregnancy	V22.2
Sprained ankle	842.5
Tonsillitis	474.0
Vertigo	386.0
Well child	V20.2

1st Dx

Postmenopausal bleeding

CDT-2 CODES

DENTAL SERVICE

DIAGNOSTIC

	CODE	FEE
Periodic exam	00120	
Limited exam	00140	
Comprehensive exam	00150	
Extensive exam	00160	

PREVENTIVE

	CODE	FEE
Intraoral–FMX	00210	
Intraoral–PA	00220	
BW	0027_	
Single posteroanterior	00290	
Panoramic X-ray	00330	
Prophylaxis adult	01110	
Prophylaxis child	01120	
Topical fluoride	012__	

DENTAL SERVICE

RESTORATIVE

	CODE	FEE
Amalgams (decid) Tooth #_____	021__	
Amalgams (perm) Tooth #_____	021__	

CROWNS AND BRIDGES

	CODE	FEE
PFG crown	02750	
FG cast crown	02790	
3/4 gold cast crown	02810	
FC bridge pontic	06210	
Porcelain bridge ( )	062__	

OTHER PROCEDURES

DOCTOR'S STATEMENT: I certify that I personally provided the above services and that fees shown represent my usual fees

Jane R. Portia, M.D.   *6/15/--*

Signature   Date

TOTAL	$	*80—*
AMOUNT PAID	$	*—*
BALANCE DUE	$	*80—*

Medical & Dental Associates, P.C.

3733 Professional Drive #300
Indianapolis, IN 46260
317/123-4567
Tax ID# 99-9999999

STATEMENT OF ACCOUNT

JOHNSON, Mrs. Willa F.
4130 N. Ellen Drive
Indianapolis, IN 46230

19--

DATE	CODE	CHARGE		CREDITS PAYMENT	ADJ	CURRENT BALANCE	
			BALANCE FORWARD ➡			0	
6/15	99203	60	00			60	00
6/15	88150	20	00			80	00
6/25	99212	32	00			112	00
6/30	99212	32	00			144	00
7/3	99212	32	00			176	00

PLEASE PAY LAST AMOUNT IN THIS COLUMN ⬆

THIS IS A COPY OF YOUR ACCOUNT

Record #15 3 of 3

Medical & Dental Associates, P.C.

3733 Professional Drive #300   317/123-4567
Indianapolis, IN 46260   Tax ID# 99-9999999

CONFIDENTIAL PATIENT INFORMATION RECORD

(please print)

Patient Name	Mary Dawson
Address	4646 Pleasant Run
	Indpls., 46250
Telephone	555-7850
Birthdate	10/4/-- (66)
Sex	F Marital Status M
Social Security No.	366-21-7346

Responsible Party (if other than patient)

Relationship to patient

Address

Patient Employer	Retired
Address	
Telephone	
Occupation	

Primary insured date of birth   7/3/-- 60

Secondary insured date of birth   10/4/-- 65

Third insured date of birth

Fourth insured date of birth

(Please use the back of the form to write information about the third and fourth insured parties, if applicable.)

INSURANCE INFORMATION

Primary insured	Harlan Dawson	Secondary insured	Patient
Subscriber	"	Subscriber	"
Address	4646 Pleasant Run	Address	"
	Indpls., IN 46250		
Telephone		Telephone	
Employer	Golden Oats Co.	Employer	
Address	1480 W 82nd St.	Address	
	Indpls., 46260		
Job/Union No.		Job/Union No.	
Subscriber's SS#	289-09-6588	Subscriber's SS#	366-21-7346
Relationship to patient	Husband	Relationship to patient	Same
Insurance	Aetna Ins. Co.	Insurance	Medicare
Address	1411 N. Pearl St.	Address	c/o BC-BS
	Acton, IN 46239		1500 E. 10th St. City 46215
Policy No.		Policy No.	
Subscriber ID No.	289-09-6588-404	Subscriber ID No.	366-21-7346C4
Group Name/No.	—	Group Name/No.	
Effective date	10/1/90	Effective date	10/4/--
Expiration date		Expiration date	

Record #16 1 of 2

212

Medical & Dental Associates, P.C.

3733 Professional Drive #300
Indianapolis, IN 46260

317/123-4567
Tax ID# 99-9999999

Patient name *Mary Dawson*

CPT-4 CODES

OFFICE SERVICES	CODE	FEE
New patient, problem focused	99201	
New patient, expanded problem focused	99202	
New patient, detailed	99203	
New patient, comprehensive, mod.	99204	
New patient, comprehensive, high	99205	
Established patient, RN	99211	
Established patient, problem focused	(99212)	*32—*
Established patient, expanded problem	99213	
Established patient, detailed	99214	
Established patient, comprehensive	99215	
Consultation		

LABORATORY	CODE	FEE
X-ray, chest/ribs; single view, frontal	71010	
X-ray, chest/ribs; stereo, frontal	71015	
Therapeutic injections ( )	907__	
Drugs, trays, supplies	99070	
Educational supplies, books, tapes	(99071)	*8—*
Urinalysis, routine, dip stick	81000	
Urine pregnancy test, visual color	81025	
Blood count, hemoglobin	(85018)	*13—*
Pap smear	88150	

ICD-9-CM

DIAGNOSES

Anxiety reaction	300.00
Bleeding rectal	569.3
Benign prostatic hypertrophy	600
Bronchitis, acute	466.0
Bronchitis, chronic	491.9
Cardiac arrhythmia	427.9
Chest pain	786.50
Cirrhosis of liver	571.5
Conjunctivitis, acute	372.00
Depression	300.4
Flu	487.0
Fracture–nasal, closed	802.0
Fractured tibia	891.2
Headache, vascular	794.0
Herpes zoster	053.9
Irritable bowel syndrome	564.1
Menopause	627.2
Myocardial infarction, unspecified	410.90
Otitis, acute	381.01
Pharyngitis, acute	462
Pneumonia	486
Sinusitis, acute	461.9
Tendonitis	726.90
Tennis elbow	726.32
Pregnancy	V22.2
Sprained ankle	842.5
Tonsillitis	474.0
Vertigo	386.0
Well child	V20.2

Cervical CA c̄ metastasis

CDT-2 CODES

DENTAL SERVICE DIAGNOSTIC	CODE	FEE
Periodic exam	00120	
Limited exam	00140	
Comprehensive exam	00150	
Extensive exam	00160	
PREVENTIVE		
Intraoral–FMX	00210	
Intraoral–PA	00220	
BW	0027_	
Single posteroanterior	00290	
Panoramic X-ray	00330	
Prophylaxis adult	01110	
Prophylaxis child	01120	
Topical fluoride	012__	

DENTAL SERVICE RESTORATIVE	CODE	FEE
Amalgams (decid) Tooth #_____	021__	
Amalgams (perm) Tooth #_____	021__	
CROWNS AND BRIDGES		
PFG crown	02750	
FG cast crown	02790	
3/4 gold cast crown	02810	
FC bridge pontic	06210	
Porcelain bridge ( )	062__	
OTHER PROCEDURES		

DOCTOR'S STATEMENT: I certify that I personally provided the above services and that fees shown represent my usual fees

L.R. Gregory, M.D./sc   *8/4/--*

Signature   Date

TOTAL	$	*53—*
AMOUNT PAID	$	*—*
BALANCE DUE	$	*53—*

Record #16 2 of 2

Medical & Dental Associates, P.C.

3733 Professional Drive #300   317/123-4567
Indianapolis, IN 46260   Tax ID# 99-9999999

CONFIDENTIAL PATIENT INFORMATION RECORD

(please print)

Patient Name Gerald Steinbert	**Patient Employer**
Address 110 S. State St.	Address
City 46203	
Telephone 555-6311	Telephone
Birthdate 2/2/-- Age 70	Occupation
Sex M Marital Status D	
Social Security No. 211-88-5244	
	Primary insured date of birth
Responsible Party (if other than patient)	Secondary insured date of birth
	Third insured date of birth
Relationship to patient	Fourth insured date of birth
Address	(Please use the back of the form to write information about the
	third and fourth insured parties, if applicable.)

INSURANCE INFORMATION

Primary insured Gerald	Secondary insured Gerald
Subscriber	Subscriber
Address	Address
Telephone	Telephone
Employer	Employer
Address	Address
Job/Union No.	Job/Union No.
Subscriber's SS# 211-88-5244	Subscriber's SS#
Relationship to patient	Relationship to patient
Insurance Medicare	Insurance Metro Medigap
Address	Address 10 Market St.
	City 46201
Policy No. 211-88-5244-B3	Policy No.
Subscriber ID No. 211-88-5244-B3	Subscriber ID No. 5244AB
Group Name/No.	Group Name/No. #7707
Effective date 2/2/--	Effective date 2/2/--
Expiration date	Expiration date

Record #17 1 of 2

214

Medical & Dental Associates, P.C.

3733 Professional Drive #300
Indianapolis, IN 46260

317/123-4567
Tax ID# 99-9999999

Patient name *Gerald Steinbert*

CPT-4 CODES

OFFICE SERVICES

	CODE	FEE
New patient, problem focused	99201	
New patient, expanded problem focused	99202	
New patient, detailed	99203	
New patient, comprehensive, mod.	99204	
New patient, comprehensive, high	99205	
Established patient, RN	99211	
Established patient, problem focused	99212	
Established patient, expanded problem	99213	
Established patient, detailed	(99214)	?
Established patient, comprehensive	99215	
Consultation		

LABORATORY

	CODE	FEE
X-ray, chest/ribs; single view, frontal	71010	
X-ray, chest/ribs; stereo, frontal	(71015)	?
Therapeutic injections ( )	907__	
Drugs, trays, supplies	99070	
Educational supplies, books, tapes	99071	
Urinalysis, routine, dip stick	81000	
Urine pregnancy test, visual color	81025	
Blood count, hemoglobin	85018	
Pap smear	88150	

ICD-9-CM

DIAGNOSES

Anxiety reaction	300.00
Bleeding rectal	569.3
Benign prostatic hypertrophy	(600)
Bronchitis, acute	466.0
Bronchitis, chronic	491.9
Cardiac arrhythmia	427.9
Chest pain *Primary*	(786.50)
Cirrhosis of liver	571.5
Conjunctivitis, acute	372.00
Depression	300.4
Flu	487.0
Fracture–nasal, closed	802.0
Fractured tibia	891.2
Headache, vascular	794.0
Herpes zoster	053.9
Irritable bowel syndrome	564.1
Menopause	627.2
Myocardial infarction, unspecified	410.90
Otitis, acute	381.01
Pharyngitis, acute	462
Pneumonia	486
Sinusitis, acute	461.9
Tendonitis	726.90
Tennis elbow	726.32
Pregnancy	V22.2
Sprained ankle	842.5
Tonsillitis	474.0
Vertigo	386.0
Well child	V20.2

CDT-2 CODES

DENTAL SERVICE

DIAGNOSTIC

	CODE	FEE
Periodic exam	00120	
Limited exam	00140	
Comprehensive exam	00150	
Extensive exam	00160	

PREVENTIVE

	CODE	FEE
Intraoral–FMX	00210	
Intraoral–PA	00220	
BW	0027_	
Single posteroanterior	00290	
Panoramic X-ray	00330	
Prophylaxis adult	01110	
Prophylaxis child	01120	
Topical fluoride	012__	

DENTAL SERVICE

RESTORATIVE

	CODE	FEE
Amalgams (decid) Tooth #_____	021__	
Amalgams (perm) Tooth #_____	021__	

CROWNS AND BRIDGES

	CODE	FEE
PFG crown	02750	
FG cast crown	02790	
3/4 gold cast crown	02810	
FC bridge pontic	06210	
Porcelain bridge ( )	062__	

OTHER PROCEDURES

DOCTOR'S STATEMENT: I certify that I personally provided the above services and that fees shown represent my usual fees

L.R. Gregory, M.D./sc   9/4/--

Signature   Date

TOTAL	$	?
AMOUNT PAID	$	0
BALANCE DUE	$	

Record #17 2 of 2

Medical & Dental Associates, P.C.

3733 Professional Drive #300   317/123-4567
Indianapolis, IN 46260   Tax ID# 99-9999999

CONFIDENTIAL PATIENT INFORMATION RECORD

(please print)

Patient Name	Hoyt Styvesant	**Patient Employer** —
Address	1511 N. Illinois St.	Address
	Amber, IN 46231	
Telephone	(317) 555-6181	Telephone
Birthdate	12/15/-- Age 67	Occupation
Sex M Marital Status Div		
Social Security No. 334-90-2121		Primary insured date of birth
Responsible Party (if other than patient)		Secondary insured date of birth
		Third insured date of birth
Relationship to patient		Fourth insured date of birth
Address		(Please use the back of the form to write information about the third and fourth insured parties, if applicable.)

INSURANCE INFORMATION

Primary insured		Secondary insured	
Subscriber		Subscriber	
Address		Address	
Telephone		Telephone	
Employer		Employer	
Address		Address	
Job/Union No.		Job/Union No.	
Subscriber's SS#		Subscriber's SS#	
Relationship to patient		Relationship to patient	
Insurance	Medicare	Insurance	Medicaid
Address		Address	
Policy No.		Policy No.	
Subscriber ID No.	334092121C4	Subscriber ID No.	43-116449800-1
Group Name/No.		Group Name/No.	
Effective date	12/15/--	Effective date	7/1/--
Expiration date		Expiration date	

Record #18 1 of 2

216

Medical & Dental Associates, P.C.

3733 Professional Drive #300
Indianapolis, IN 46260

317/123-4567
Tax ID# 99-9999999

Patient name   *Hoyt Styvesant*

CPT-4 CODES

OFFICE SERVICES

	CODE	FEE
New patient, problem focused	99201	
New patient, expanded problem focused	99202	
New patient, detailed	99203	
New patient, comprehensive, mod.	99204	
New patient, comprehensive, high	99205	
Established patient, RN	(99211)	25—
Established patient, problem focused	99212	
Established patient, expanded problem	99213	
Established patient, detailed	99214	
Established patient, comprehensive	99215	
Consultation		

LABORATORY

	CODE	FEE
X-ray, chest/ribs; single view, frontal	71010	
X-ray, chest/ribs; stereo, frontal	71015	
Therapeutic injections ( )	907__	
Drugs, trays, supplies	99070	
Educational supplies, books, tapes	99071	
Urinalysis, routine, dip stick	81000	
Urine pregnancy test, visual color	81025	
Blood count, hemoglobin	85018	
Pap smear	88150	
	J1631	*38—*

ICD-9-CM

DIAGNOSES

Anxiety reaction	300.00
Bleeding rectal	569.3
Benign prostatic hypertrophy	600
Bronchitis, acute	466.0
Bronchitis, chronic	491.9
Cardiac arrhythmia	427.9
Chest pain	786.50
Cirrhosis of liver	571.5
Conjunctivitis, acute	372.00
Depression	300.4
Flu	487.0
Fracture–nasal, closed	802.0
Fractured tibia	891.2
Headache, vascular	794.0
Herpes zoster	053.9
Irritable bowel syndrome	564.1
Menopause	627.2
Myocardial infarction, unspecified	410.90
Otitis, acute	381.01
Pharyngitis, acute	462
Pneumonia	486
Sinusitis, acute	461.9
Tendonitis	726.90
Tennis elbow	726.32
Pregnancy	V22.2
Sprained ankle	842.5
Tonsillitis	474.0
Vertigo	386.0
Well child	V20.2

Schizo-affective psychosis

CDT-2 CODES

DENTAL SERVICE

DIAGNOSTIC	CODE	FEE
Periodic exam	00120	
Limited exam	00140	
Comprehensive exam	00150	
Extensive exam	00160	
PREVENTIVE		
Intraoral–FMX	00210	
Intraoral–PA	00220	
BW	0027_	
Single posteroanterior	00290	
Panoramic X-ray	00330	
Prophylaxis adult	01110	
Prophylaxis child	01120	
Topical fluoride	012__	

DENTAL SERVICE

RESTORATIVE	CODE	FEE
Amalgams (decid) Tooth #_____	021__	
Amalgams (perm) Tooth #_____	021__	
CROWNS AND BRIDGES		
PFG crown	02750	
FG cast crown	02790	
3/4 gold cast crown	02810	
FC bridge pontic	06210	
Porcelain bridge ( )	062__	
OTHER PROCEDURES		

DOCTOR'S STATEMENT: I certify that I personally provided the above services and that fees shown represent my usual fees

James P. Cartman, M.D.   *7/15/--*

Signature   Date

TOTAL	$	63—
AMOUNT PAID	$	—
BALANCE DUE	$	63—

Record #18 2 of 2

Medical & Dental Associates, P.C.

3733 Professional Drive #300   317/123-4567
Indianapolis, IN 46260   Tax ID# 99-9999999

CONFIDENTIAL PATIENT INFORMATION RECORD

(please print)

Patient Name	Diana Higson	**Patient Employer**	Unemployed
Address	31 Glenna Lane	Address	
	Indpls. 46239		

Telephone	555-1688
Birthdate	9/15/-- Age 42
Sex	F Marital Status S
Social Security No.	472-31-9842

Responsible Party (if other than patient)

Relationship to patient

Address

Telephone

Occupation

Primary insured date of birth

Secondary insured date of birth

Third insured date of birth

Fourth insured date of birth

(Please use the back of the form to write information about the third and fourth insured parties, if applicable.)

INSURANCE INFORMATION

Primary insured		Secondary insured	
Subscriber		Subscriber	
Address		Address	
Telephone		Telephone	
Employer		Employer	
Address		Address	
Job/Union No.		Job/Union No.	
Subscriber's SS#		Subscriber's SS#	
Relationship to patient		Relationship to patient	
Insurance	Medicaid	Insurance	
Address	P.O. Box 688888	Address	
	Indpls., IN 46288		
Policy No.		Policy No.	
Subscriber ID No.	42-394166571-5	Subscriber ID No.	
Group Name/No.		Group Name/No.	
Effective date	12/1/--	Effective date	
Expiration date	12/31/--	Expiration date	

Record #19 1 of 2

218

Medical & Dental Associates, P.C.

3733 Professional Drive #300
Indianapolis, IN 46260

317/123-4567
Tax ID# 99-9999999

Patient name *Diana Higson*

CPT-4 CODES

OFFICE SERVICES	CODE	FEE
New patient, problem focused	99201	
New patient, expanded problem focused	99202	
New patient, detailed	(99203)	60—
New patient, comprehensive, mod.	99204	
New patient, comprehensive, high	99205	
Established patient, RN	99211	
Established patient, problem focused	99212	
Established patient, expanded problem	99213	
Established patient, detailed	99214	
Established patient, comprehensive	99215	
Consultation		

LABORATORY

	CODE	FEE
X-ray, chest/ribs; single view, frontal	71010	
X-ray, chest/ribs; stereo, frontal	71015	
Therapeutic injections ( )	907__	
Drugs, trays, supplies	99070	
Educational supplies, books, tapes	99071	
Urinalysis, routine, dip stick	81000	
Urine pregnancy test, visual color	81025	
Blood count, hemoglobin	85018	
Pap smear	88150	

ICD-9-CM

DIAGNOSES	
Anxiety reaction	300.00
Bleeding rectal	569.3
Benign prostatic hypertrophy	600
Bronchitis, acute	466.0
Bronchitis, chronic	491.9
Cardiac arrhythmia	427.9
Chest pain	786.50
Cirrhosis of liver	(571.5)
Conjunctivitis, acute	372.00
Depression	300.4
Flu	487.0
Fracture–nasal, closed	802.0
Fractured tibia	891.2
Headache, vascular	794.0
Herpes zoster	053.9
Irritable bowel syndrome	564.1
Menopause	627.2
Myocardial infarction, unspecified	410.90
Otitis, acute	381.01
Pharyngitis, acute	462
Pneumonia	486
Sinusitis, acute	461.9
Tendonitis	726.90
Tennis elbow	726.32
Pregnancy	V22.2
Sprained ankle	842.5
Tonsillitis	474.0
Vertigo	386.0
Well child	V20.2

CDT-2 CODES

DENTAL SERVICE

DIAGNOSTIC	CODE	FEE
Periodic exam	00120	
Limited exam	00140	
Comprehensive exam	00150	
Extensive exam	00160	

PREVENTIVE		
Intraoral–FMX	00210	
Intraoral–PA	00220	
BW	0027_	
Single posteroanterior	00290	
Panoramic X-ray	00330	
Prophylaxis adult	01110	
Prophylaxis child	01120	
Topical fluoride	012__	

DENTAL SERVICE

RESTORATIVE	CODE	FEE
Amalgams (decid) Tooth #_____	021__	
Amalgams (perm) Tooth #_____	021__	

CROWNS AND BRIDGES		
PFG crown	02750	
FG cast crown	02790	
3/4 gold cast crown	02810	
FC bridge pontic	06210	
Porcelain bridge ( )	062__	

OTHER PROCEDURES

DOCTOR'S STATEMENT: I certify that I personally provided the above services and that fees shown represent my usual fees

James P. Cartman, M.D.   12/10/--

Signature   Date

TOTAL	$	60—
AMOUNT PAID	$	—
BALANCE DUE	$	60—

Medical & Dental Associates, P.C.

3733 Professional Drive #300   317/123-4567
Indianapolis, IN 46260   Tax ID# 99-9999999

CONFIDENTIAL PATIENT INFORMATION RECORD

(please print)

Patient Name Everett B. White	**Patient Employer** —
Address 43 Harding Way	Address
Indpls., IN 46901	
Telephone None	Telephone
Birthdate 6/11/-- Age 38	Occupation
Sex M Marital Status D	
Social Security No. 336-97-2345	
	Primary insured date of birth
Responsible Party (if other than patient) —	Secondary insured date of birth
	Third insured date of birth
Relationship to patient	Fourth insured date of birth
Address	(Please use the back of the form to write information about the
	third and fourth insured parties, if applicable.)

INSURANCE INFORMATION

Primary insured	Secondary insured —
Subscriber	Subscriber
Address	Address
Telephone	Telephone
Employer	Employer
Address	Address
Job/Union No.	Job/Union No.
Subscriber's SS#	Subscriber's SS#
Relationship to patient	Relationship to patient
Insurance Medicaid	Insurance
Address P.O. Box 688-888	Address
Indpls., IN 46288	
Policy No.	Policy No.
Subscriber ID No. 49-333449380-2	Subscriber ID No.
Group Name/No.	Group Name/No.
Effective date 2/1/--	Effective date
Expiration date 2/28/--	Expiration date

Record #20 1 of 2

Medical & Dental Associates, P.C.

3733 Professional Drive #300
Indianapolis, IN 46260

317/123-4567
Tax ID# 99-9999999

Patient name *E.B. White*

CPT-4 CODES

OFFICE SERVICES

	CODE	FEE
New patient, problem focused	99201	_____
New patient, expanded problem focused	99202	_____
New patient, detailed	99203	_____
New patient, comprehensive, mod.	99204	_____
New patient, comprehensive, high	99205	_____
Established patient, RN	99211	_____
Established patient, problem focused	(99212)	_____
Established patient, expanded problem	99213	_____
Established patient, detailed	99214	_____
Established patient, comprehensive	99215	_____
Consultation		

LABORATORY

	CODE	FEE
X-ray, chest/ribs; single view, frontal	71010	_____
X-ray, chest/ribs; stereo, frontal	71015	_____
Therapeutic injections ( )	907__	_____
Drugs, trays, supplies	99070	_____
Educational supplies, books, tapes	99071	_____
Urinalysis, routine, dip stick	81000	_____
Urine pregnancy test, visual color	81025	_____
Blood count, hemoglobin	85018	_____
Pap smear	88150	_____
	J0540	*12.50*

ICD-9-CM

DIAGNOSES

Anxiety reaction	300.00
Bleeding rectal	569.3
Benign prostatic hypertrophy	600
Bronchitis, acute	466.0
Bronchitis, chronic	491.9
Cardiac arrhythmia	427.9
Chest pain	786.50
Cirrhosis of liver	571.5
Conjunctivitis, acute	372.00
Depression	300.4
Flu	487.0
Fracture–nasal, closed	802.0
Fractured tibia	891.2
Headache, vascular	794.0
Herpes zoster	053.9
Irritable bowel syndrome	564.1
Menopause	627.2
Myocardial infarction, unspecified	410.90
Otitis, acute	381.01
Pharyngitis, acute	462
Pneumonia	486
Sinusitis, acute	461.9
Tendonitis	726.90
Tennis elbow	726.32
Pregnancy	V22.2
Sprained ankle	842.5
Tonsillitis	474.0
Vertigo	386.0
Well child	V20.2

Acc. hypertension

CDT-2 CODES

DENTAL SERVICE

DIAGNOSTIC

	CODE	FEE
Periodic exam	00120	_____
Limited exam	00140	_____
Comprehensive exam	00150	_____
Extensive exam	00160	_____

PREVENTIVE

	CODE	FEE
Intraoral–FMX	00210	_____
Intraoral–PA	00220	_____
BW	0027_	_____
Single posteroanterior	00290	_____
Panoramic X-ray	00330	_____
Prophylaxis adult	01110	_____
Prophylaxis child	01120	_____
Topical fluoride	012__	_____

DENTAL SERVICE

RESTORATIVE

	CODE	FEE
Amalgams (decid) Tooth #_____	021__	_____
Amalgams (perm) Tooth #_____	021__	_____

CROWNS AND BRIDGES

	CODE	FEE
PFG crown	02750	_____
FG cast crown	02790	_____
3/4 gold cast crown	02810	_____
FC bridge pontic	06210	_____
Porcelain bridge ( )	062__	_____

OTHER PROCEDURES

DOCTOR'S STATEMENT: I certify that I personally provided the above services and that fees shown represent my usual fees

James P. Cartman, M.D.   *2/10/--*

Signature   Date

TOTAL	$	
AMOUNT PAID	$	
BALANCE DUE	$	_____

Record #20 2 of 2

Medical & Dental Associates, P.C.

3733 Professional Drive #300   317/123-4567
Indianapolis, IN 46260   Tax ID# 99-9999999

CONFIDENTIAL PATIENT INFORMATION RECORD

(please print)

Patient Name	Philip P. Woods
Address	8623 Cooks Lane
	Melrose, IN 46230
Telephone	(317) 555-7891
Birthdate	11/13/-- Age 60
Sex	M Marital Status M
Social Security No.	204-14-1702

Responsible Party (if other than patient)

Relationship to patient

Address

Patient Employer —

Address

Telephone

Occupation   Carpenter

Primary insured date of birth

Secondary insured date of birth

Third insured date of birth

Fourth insured date of birth

(Please use the back of the form to write information about the third and fourth insured parties, if applicable.)

INSURANCE INFORMATION

Primary insured	Secondary insured
Subscriber	Subscriber
Address	Address
Telephone	Telephone
Employer	Employer
Address	Address
Job/Union No.	Job/Union No.
Subscriber's SS#	Subscriber's SS#
Relationship to patient	Relationship to patient
Insurance Medicaid	Insurance
Address	Address
Policy No.	Policy No.
Subscriber ID No. 62-8000-28620-2	Subscriber ID No.
Group Name/No.	Group Name/No.
Effective date 3/1/--	Effective date
Expiration date 3/31/--	Expiration date

Record #21 1 of 2

222

Medical & Dental Associates, P.C.

3733 Professional Drive #300
Indianapolis, IN 46260

317/123-4567
Tax ID# 99-9999999

Patient name *Philip P. Woods*

Referred by Dr. Lukoskie
Medicaid Prov. #218603419

CPT-4 CODES

OFFICE SERVICES	CODE	FEE
New patient, problem focused	99201	
New patient, expanded problem focused	99202	
New patient, detailed	99203	
New patient, comprehensive, mod.	99204	
New patient, comprehensive, high	99205	
Established patient, RN	99211	
Established patient, problem focused	99212	
Established patient, expanded problem	99213	
Established patient, detailed	99214	
Established patient, comprehensive	99215	
(Consultation)	*99243*	*$125—*

LABORATORY

	CODE	FEE
X-ray, chest/ribs; single view, frontal	71010	
X-ray, chest/ribs; stereo, frontal	71015	
Therapeutic injections ( )	907_	
Drugs, trays, supplies	99070	
Educational supplies, books, tapes	99071	
Urinalysis, routine, dip stick	81000	
Urine pregnancy test, visual color	81025	
Blood count, hemoglobin	85018	
Pap smear	88150	

80059–$12, 80050–$45, 80058–$12,
86593–$12 — in house

ICD-9-CM

DIAGNOSES	
Anxiety reaction	300.00
Bleeding rectal	569.3
Benign prostatic hypertrophy	600
Bronchitis, acute	466.0
Bronchitis, chronic	491.9
Cardiac arrhythmia	427.9
Chest pain	786.50
Cirrhosis of liver *Primary*	(571.5)
Conjunctivitis, acute	372.00
Depression	300.4
Flu	487.0
Fracture–nasal, closed	802.0
Fractured tibia	891.2
Headache, vascular	794.0
Herpes zoster	053.9
Irritable bowel syndrome	564.1
Menopause	627.2
Myocardial infarction, unspecified	410.90
Otitis, acute	381.01
Pharyngitis, acute	462
Pneumonia	486
Sinusitis, acute	461.9
Tendonitis	726.90
Tennis elbow	726.32
Pregnancy	V22.2
Sprained ankle	842.5
Tonsillitis	474.0
Vertigo	386.0
Well child	V20.2

Hematuria

CDT-2 CODES

DENTAL SERVICE

DIAGNOSTIC	CODE	FEE
Periodic exam	00120	
Limited exam	00140	
Comprehensive exam	00150	
Extensive exam	00160	

PREVENTIVE	CODE	FEE
Intraoral–FMX	00210	
Intraoral–PA	00220	
BW	0027_	
Single posteroanterior	00290	
Panoramic X-ray	00330	
Prophylaxis adult	01110	
Prophylaxis child	01120	
Topical fluoride	012_	

DENTAL SERVICE

RESTORATIVE	CODE	FEE
Amalgams (decid) Tooth #_____	021_	
Amalgams (perm) Tooth #_____	021_	

CROWNS AND BRIDGES	CODE	FEE
PFG crown	02750	
FG cast crown	02790	
3/4 gold cast crown	02810	
FC bridge pontic	06210	
Porcelain bridge ( )	062_	

OTHER PROCEDURES

DOCTOR'S STATEMENT: I certify that I personally provided the above services and that fees shown represent my usual fees

Linda R. Gregory, M.D.   *3/18/--*

Signature   Date

TOTAL	$	*206—*
AMOUNT PAID	$	*—*
BALANCE DUE	$	*206—*

Record #21 2 of 2

Medical & Dental Associates, P.C.

3733 Professional Drive #300   317/123-4567
Indianapolis, IN 46260   Tax ID# 99-9999999

CONFIDENTIAL PATIENT INFORMATION RECORD

(please print)

Patient Name Daniel O'Shea	**Patient Employer** 33M
Address 1510 Sunfish Lake Rd.	Address 33M Center
Forest, IN 46711	Indpls., IN 46277
Telephone (812) 555-1212	Telephone 555-1110
Birthdate 1/1/-- Age 33	Occupation Engineer
Sex M Marital Status D	
Social Security No. 350-27-7780	

Primary insured date of birth

Responsible Party (if other than patient)

Secondary insured date of birth

Third insured date of birth

Relationship to patient

Fourth insured date of birth

Address

(Please use the back of the form to write information about the third and fourth insured parties, if applicable.)

INSURANCE INFORMATION

Primary insured	Self	Secondary insured	
Subscriber		Subscriber	
Address		Address	
Telephone		Telephone	*called work:*
Employer		Employer	*W.C. Claim #4288*
Address		Address	*send claim to employer*
Job/Union No.		Job/Union No.	
Subscriber's SS#		Subscriber's SS#	
Relationship to patient		Relationship to patient	
Insurance	Engineers Ins.	Insurance	
Address	395 West Ave.	Address	
	Gary, IN 47790		
Policy No.	A9875021-43	Policy No.	
Subscriber ID No.	350277780-328	Subscriber ID No.	
Group Name/No.		Group Name/No.	
Effective date	6/25/91	Effective date	
Expiration date		Expiration date	

Record #22 1 of 5

Medical & Dental Associates, P.C.

3733 Professional Drive #300
Indianapolis, IN 46260

317/123-4567
Tax ID# 99-9999999

MEDICAL HISTORY

Patient Name _Danial O'Shea_	Today's Date _5/20/--_

Are you currently in good health? _Yes_

Are you under a physician's regular care at this time? | If so, state reason(s) for regular treatment:

_No_

Are you currently taking prescribed medication? | If so, state brand name and dosage schedule:

_No_

Circle the names of the following diseases for which you have been treated:

Alcoholism	Allergies	Amenorrhea	Anemia	Arthritis
Asthma	Cancer	Colitis	Depression	Diabetes
Gingivitis	Heart Disease	Hemorrhoids	Hepatitis	Hernia _ulcer,_
Hypertension	Hypoglycemia	Kidney Disease	Lumbago	Migraine _tension_
Mononucleosis	Periodontal Dis.	Rheumatic fever	Rubella	(Other) _headaches_

Have you ever had prolonged bleeding? If yes, explain: _Yes. Stomach ulcer — surgery in '93_

Have you ever had an unusual reaction to a drug, antibiotic or anesthetic, such as novocaine or penicillin?

If yes, explain: _No_

Is there any other information we should know about you or your health? _Had a blood transfusion in '93_

Is there any other information we should know about previous treatments you have had?

Have you ever been exposed to the HIV/AIDS virus? _Maybe — I'd like an AIDS test today_

Purpose of the first visit _Job injury_

Family physician _—_ | Who referred you to this practice? _Work_

Authorization for Release of Medical Information to the Insurance Carrier and Assignment of Benefits to Medical & Dental Associates, P.C.

Commercial Insurance

I hereby authorize release of medical information necessary to file a claim with my insurance company and assign benefits otherwise payable to me to Medical & Dental Associates, P.C. I understand I am financially responsible for any balance due not covered by my insurance carrier or denied by my insurance carrier for lack of coverage. A copy of this signature is as valid as the original.

Signature of Patient or Legal Guardian _Daniel O'Shea_

Medicare Insurance

Beneficiary _____ Medicare Number _____

I request that payment of authorized Medicare benefits be made either to me or on my behalf to Medical & Dental Associates, P.C. for any services furnished to me by that association. I authorize any holder of medical information about me to release to the Health Care Financing Administration and its agents any information needed to determine these benefits payable for related services.

Beneficiary Signature _____

Medicare Supplemental Insurance

Beneficiary _____ Medicare Number _____

Medigap ID Number _____

I request that payment of authorized Medigap benefits be made either to me or on my behalf to Medical & Dental Associates, P.C. for any services furnished to me by that physician. I authorize any holder of Medicare information about me to release to Medical & Dental Associates, P.C. any information needed to determine these benefits payable for related services.

Beneficiary Signature _____

Record #22 2 of 5

Medical & Dental Associates, P.C.

3733 Professional Drive #300
Indianapolis, IN 46260

317/123-4567
Tax ID# 99-9999999

MEDICAL TREATMENT RECORD

Patient _Daniel O'Shea_	Date _5/20/--_
Occupation	DOB _____ Age _33_
Insurance Carrier	Social Security No.
Admitted _____ Discharged	Consults
Hospital _____ Other	Referred by: ~~Dr.~~ _Urgicenter_

CC: _Pain in (L) ankle after fall at work_
(tripped over rug)

Previous symptom: Yes / (No)

First Symptom: _3:30 PM_

Physical Examination _BP 105/70; Pulse 88 & Reg — T 37.8° C orally_

General _Resp. 14_

Appearance _Healthy, alert cauc. male, appearing stated age_

HEENT ⎫
Lungs ⎬ _WNL_

Cardiac _Clear to P&A — NSR, No M_

ABD _WNL_

Extremities _Edema (L) lateral malledus—ROM limited to 30° due to pain_

Dx (Primary): _Muscoluligamentous sprain, (L) ankle (X-ray showed no FX)_

Dx (Secondary): —

Dx (Postoperative): —

Procedures: _DX exam — 3" elastic bandage to ankle X-rays interpreted by me_

Complications: —

Dx testing (place of service): _X-rays taken at Urgicenter — not read there — (L) ankle,_
complete (AP & Oblique) neg for injury, FX
AIDS test

Plan:
RTW 2 days (5/23)
See me PRN
Will contact him for test results

Linda R. Gregory, M.D.
Attending physician

Record #22 3 of 5

226

Medical & Dental Associates, P.C.

3733 Professional Drive #300
Indianapolis, IN 46260
317/123-4567
Tax ID# 99-9999999

STATEMENT OF ACCOUNT

O'SHEA, Daniel
1510 Sunfish Lake Rd.
Forest, IN 46711

19--   WORKER'S COMP

DATE	CODE	CHARGE		CREDITS PAYMENT	ADJ		CURRENT BALANCE	
		BALANCE FORWARD ➡					0	
5/20	99203	60	00				60	00
5/20	76140	40	00				100	00
5/20	A4460	8	00				108	00

PLEASE PAY LAST AMOUNT IN THIS COLUMN ↑

THIS IS A COPY OF YOUR ACCOUNT

Record #22 4 of 5

Medical & Dental Associates, P.C.

3733 Professional Drive #300
Indianapolis, IN 46260
317/123-4567
Tax ID# 99-9999999

STATEMENT OF ACCOUNT

O'SHEA, Daniel
1510 Sunfish Lake Rd.
Forest, IN 46711

19--

| DATE | CODE | CHARGE | CREDITS | | CURRENT BALANCE |
			PAYMENT	ADJ	
		BALANCE FORWARD ⟶			0
5/20	Lab HTLV 86687	30 00			30 00

PLEASE PAY LAST AMOUNT IN THIS COLUMN ↑

THIS IS A COPY OF YOUR ACCOUNT

Record #22 5 of 5

Medical & Dental Associates, P.C.

3733 Professional Drive #300   317/123-4567
Indianapolis, IN 46260   Tax ID# 99-9999999

CONFIDENTIAL PATIENT INFORMATION RECORD

(please print)

Patient Name Donald Ebner	**Patient Employer** Self
Address 6018 Orchard Lane	Address Ebner Gallery
Blgtn, IN 47437-1237	Sunset Lane
	Blgtn, IN 47437-1237
Telephone (812) 555-1844	Telephone (812) 555-5067
Birthdate 12/15/-- Age 52	Occupation Artist
Sex M Marital Status W	
Social Security No. 132-60-8001	
	Primary insured date of birth 12/15/--
Responsible Party (if other than patient)	Secondary insured date of birth
	Third insured date of birth
Relationship to patient	Fourth insured date of birth
Address	(Please use the back of the form to write information about the
	third and fourth insured parties, if applicable.)

INSURANCE INFORMATION

Primary insured	Secondary insured
Subscriber	Subscriber
Address	Address
Telephone	Telephone
Employer U.S. Navy Retired	Employer
Address VA Station #558	Address
Job/Union No.	Job/Union No.
Subscriber's SS# 132-60-8000	Subscriber's SS#
Relationship to patient Self	Relationship to patient
Insurance CHAMPUS	Insurance
Address BC/BS of R.I.	Address
P.O. B. 33	
Policy No. Providence, RI 02901	Policy No.
Subscriber ID No. 132-60-8000	Subscriber ID No.
Group Name/No. USN (GR9) Ret	Group Name/No.
Effective date 10/10/94	Effective date
Expiration date	Expiration date

Record #23 1 of 3

Medical & Dental Associates, P.C.

3733 Professional Drive #300
Indianapolis, IN 46260

317/123-4567
Tax ID# 99-9999999

MEDICAL TREATMENT RECORD

Patient *Donald Ebner*	Date *3/11/--*
Occupation	DOB Age *52*
Insurance Carrier	Social Security No.
Admitted Discharged	Consults
Hospital Other	Referred by: Dr.

CC: *Complete urinary retention*

Previous symptom: Yes / (No)

First Symptom: *Gradual onset*

Physical Examination	*BP 140/90 – P 94 & Reg – Temp 37.2° 0 – Resp 26/min & somewhat*
General	*labored*
Appearance	*Some distention of jugular in supine position; pupils equal; extraocular*
HEENT	*movements WNL*
Lungs	*↑AP dimensions – breath sounds ↓ – lut. wheezing & narrowing*
Cardiac	*grade II systolic ejection murmur at apex*
ABD	*distended urinary bladder*
Extremities	*distol pulses WNL – femoral pulse ↓ lut. Rectal – enlarged prostate*

Dx (Primary): *BPH c̄ urinary retention*

Dx (Secondary): *Pulmonary emphysema; arteriosclerosis onset*

Dx (Postoperative): —

Procedures: *Today – cystourethroscopy*
Schedule TURP ASAP at Good Sam

Complications: *none expected*

Dx testing (place of service): *IVP*
chest X-ray
serum electrolytes   *BUN*
EKG
arterial blood gases   } *in hospital*

Plan:

Return Post-Op as directed

Linda Gregory, M.D.

Attending physician

Record #23 2 of 3

230

Medical & Dental Associates, P.C.

3733 Professional Drive #300
Indianapolis, IN 46260
317/123-4567
Tax ID# 99-9999999

STATEMENT OF ACCOUNT

EBNER, Donald
6018 Orchard Lane
Bloomington, IN 47437-1237

19--

DATE	CODE	CHARGE	CREDITS PAYMENT	ADJ	CURRENT BALANCE
BALANCE FORWARD ➡					
3/11	52000	200 00			200 00
3/18	52601	1800 00			2000 00

PLEASE PAY LAST AMOUNT IN THIS COLUMN ⬆

THIS IS A COPY OF YOUR ACCOUNT

Record #23 3 of 3

Medical & Dental Associates, P.C.

3733 Professional Drive #300
Indianapolis, IN 46260

317/123-4567
Tax ID# 99-9999999

CONFIDENTIAL PATIENT INFORMATION RECORD

(please print)

Patient Name	Nancy J. Hawkins	**Patient Employer**	Homemaker
Address	2301 Bushe	Address	
	Indpls., IN 46298		
Telephone	555-8955	Telephone	
Birthdate	8/9/-- Age 25	Occupation	
Sex F Marital Status M			
Social Security No.	364-36-5761		
		Primary insured date of birth	11/10/-- (25)
Responsible Party (if other than patient)		Secondary insured date of birth	
	Greg P. Hawkins	Third insured date of birth	
Relationship to patient	Husband	Fourth insured date of birth	
Address	Same	(Please use the back of the form to write information about the third and fourth insured parties, if applicable.)	

INSURANCE INFORMATION

Primary insured	Husb.	Secondary insured	
Subscriber	"	Subscriber	
Address	Same	Address	
Telephone		Telephone	
Employer	InTemp Services	Employer	
Address	1400 N. Main Pkwy	Address	
	Indpls., IN 46265		
Job/Union No.		Job/Union No.	
Subscriber's SS#	431-67-7980	Subscriber's SS#	
Relationship to patient	Husb.	Relationship to patient	
Insurance	Minnesota Dental Assoc.	Insurance	
Address	873 2nd St.	Address	
	Minn, MN 55014		
Policy No.		Policy No.	
Subscriber ID No.	431-67-7980	Subscriber ID No.	
Group Name/No.	37145	Group Name/No.	
Effective date	7/25/95	Effective date	
Expiration date		Expiration date	

Record #24 1 of 4

232

Medical & Dental Associates, P.C.

3733 Professional Drive #300
Indianapolis, IN 46260

317/123-4567
Tax ID# 99-9999999

MEDICAL HISTORY

Patient Name *Nancy J. Hawkins*   Today's Date *1/21/--*

Are you currently in good health? *Yes*

Are you under a physician's regular care at this time? *No*   If so, state reason(s) for regular treatment:

Are you currently taking prescribed medication? *No*   If so, state brand name and dosage schedule:

Circle the names of the following diseases for which you have been treated:

Alcoholism	Allergies	Amenorrhea	Anemia	Arthritis
Asthma	Cancer	Colitis	Depression	Diabetes
Gingivitis	Heart Disease	Hemorrhoids	Hepatitis	Hernia
Hypertension	Hypoglycemia	Kidney Disease	Lumbago	(Migraine)
Mononucleosis	Periodontal Dis.	Rheumatic fever	Rubella	Other _____

Have you ever had prolonged bleeding? If yes, explain: *No*

Have you ever had an unusual reaction to a drug, antibiotic or anesthetic, such as novocaine or penicillin?

If yes, explain: *No*

Is there any other information we should know about you or your health? *No*

Is there any other information we should know about previous treatments you have had? *No*

Have you ever been exposed to the HIV/AIDS virus? *No*

Purpose of the first visit *Cleaning, gen. exam*

Family physician   Who referred you to this practice? *Pt.*

Authorization for Release of Medical Information to the Insurance Carrier and Assignment of Benefits to Medical & Dental Associates, P.C.

Commercial Insurance

I hereby authorize release of medical information necessary to file a claim with my insurance company and assign benefits otherwise payable to me to Medical & Dental Associates, P.C. I understand I am financially responsible for any balance due not covered by my insurance carrier or denied by my insurance carrier for lack of coverage. A copy of this signature is as valid as the original.

Signature of Patient or Legal Guardian *Nancy J. Hawkins*

Medicare Insurance

Beneficiary _____ Medicare Number _____

I request that payment of authorized Medicare benefits be made either to me or on my behalf to Medical & Dental Associates, P.C. for any services furnished to me by that association. I authorize any holder of medical information about me to release to the Health Care Financing Administration and its agents any information needed to determine these benefits payable for related services.

Beneficiary Signature _____

Medicare Supplemental Insurance

Beneficiary _____ Medicare Number _____

Medigap ID Number _____

I request that payment of authorized Medigap benefits be made either to me or on my behalf to Medical & Dental Associates, P.C. for any services furnished to me by that physician. I authorize any holder of Medicare information about me to release to Medical & Dental Associates, P.C. any information needed to determine these benefits payable for related services.

Beneficiary Signature _____

Record #24 2 of 4

DENTAL TREATMENT RECORD
Medical & Dental Associates, P.C.

Name Nancy J. Hawkins

Parent or Guardian —

Occupation Homemaker

Dentist Dr. Lane

Date of Exam 01/21/--

Recommended by Self

ORAL FINDINGS

Chief Complaint

General Physical Condition   Excellent

Condition of Teeth and Gums   Good

Occlusion

Abnormalities

Blood Pressure
130/90

Hygiene	① 2 3 4
Deposits	1 ② 3 4
Periodontal Condition	① 2 3 4

SERVICES RENDERED

Date	Tooth	Service Rendered	Fee		Paid	Balance
01/21		Periodic Eval.	20	00		
"		Prophylaxis	25	00		
"		Bitewings—4	20	00		

DENTAL HISTORY

Date, Last Dental Visit   04/03/--

History of Bleeding?   No

Reaction to Anesthetic   No

Allergies?   No

Anemia?   No

Chronic Disorders-Heart?   No

Diabetes?   No

Infectious Hepatitis?   No

Nervousness?   No

Rheumatic Fever?   No

Date, Last X-rays: FMX

BW   04/03/--

Date of Models

Record #24 3 of 4

Medical & Dental Associates, P.C.

3733 Professional Drive #300
Indianapolis, IN 46260
317/123-4567
Tax ID# 99-9999999

STATEMENT OF ACCOUNT

HAWKINS, Nancy J.
c/o HAWKINS, Gregory
2301 Bushe
Indianapolis, IN 46298

19--

DATE	CODE	CHARGE	CREDITS		CURRENT BALANCE
			PAYMENT	ADJ	
BALANCE FORWARD ➡					0
1/21	00120	20 00			20 00
1/21	00274	20 00			40 00
1/21	01110	37 00			77 00

PLEASE PAY LAST AMOUNT IN THIS COLUMN ↑

THIS IS A COPY OF YOUR ACCOUNT

Record #24 4 of 4

Medical & Dental Associates, P.C.

3733 Professional Drive #300
Indianapolis, IN 46260

317/123-4567
Tax ID# 99-9999999

CONFIDENTIAL PATIENT INFORMATION RECORD

(please print)

Patient Name Stacy J. Bogan

Address 2150 Kristy Lane

Indpls., IN 46203

Telephone 555-8144

Birthdate 12/1/-- Age 29

Sex F   Marital Status S

Social Security No. 311-48-6120

Responsible Party (if other than patient)

Relationship to patient

Address

Patient Employer Bogan Studios

Address 2500 Cliff St.

Indpls., IN 46230

Telephone 555-2130

Occupation Pres./CEO

Primary insured date of birth

Secondary insured date of birth

Third insured date of birth

Fourth insured date of birth

(Please use the back of the form to write information about the

third and fourth insured parties, if applicable.)

INSURANCE INFORMATION

Primary insured

Subscriber

Address

Telephone

Employer

Address

Job/Union No.

Subscriber's SS#

Relationship to patient

Insurance Prudential Dental Plan

Address P.O. Box 210

Westbrook, IL 61630

Policy No.

Subscriber ID No. 311-48-6120

Group Name/No.

Effective date 10/1/94

Expiration date

Secondary insured

Subscriber

Address

Telephone

Employer

Address

Job/Union No.

Subscriber's SS#

Relationship to patient

Insurance

Address

Policy No.

Subscriber ID No.

Group Name/No.

Effective date

Expiration date

Record #25 1 of 2

Medical & Dental Associates, P.C.

3733 Professional Drive #300
Indianapolis, IN 46260

317/123-4567
Tax ID# 99-9999999

Patient name *Stacy J. Bogan*

CPT-4 CODES

OFFICE SERVICES

OFFICE SERVICES	CODE	FEE
New patient, problem focused	99201	
New patient, expanded problem focused	99202	
New patient, detailed	99203	
New patient, comprehensive, mod.	99204	
New patient, comprehensive, high	99205	
Established patient, RN	99211	
Established patient, problem focused	99212	
Established patient, expanded problem	99213	
Established patient, detailed	99214	
Established patient, comprehensive	99215	
Consultation		

LABORATORY

LABORATORY	CODE	FEE
X-ray, chest/ribs; single view, frontal	71010	
X-ray, chest/ribs; stereo, frontal	71015	
Therapeutic injections ( )	907__	
Drugs, trays, supplies	99070	
Educational supplies, books, tapes	99071	
Urinalysis, routine, dip stick	81000	
Urine pregnancy test, visual color	81025	
Blood count, hemoglobin	85018	
Pap smear	88150	

ICD-9-CM

DIAGNOSES

DIAGNOSES	
Anxiety reaction	300.00
Bleeding rectal	569.3
Benign prostatic hypertrophy	600
Bronchitis, acute	466.0
Bronchitis, chronic	491.9
Cardiac arrhythmia	427.9
Chest pain	786.50
Cirrhosis of liver	571.5
Conjunctivitis, acute	372.00
Depression	300.4
Flu	487.0
Fracture–nasal, closed	802.0
Fractured tibia	891.2
Headache, vascular	794.0
Herpes zoster	053.9
Irritable bowel syndrome	564.1
Menopause	627.2
Myocardial infarction, unspecified	410.90
Otitis, acute	381.01
Pharyngitis, acute	462
Pneumonia	486
Sinusitis, acute	461.9
Tendonitis	726.90
Tennis elbow	726.32
Pregnancy	V22.2
Sprained ankle	842.5
Tonsillitis	474.0
Vertigo	386.0
Well child	V20.2

CDT-2 CODES

DENTAL SERVICE

DIAGNOSTIC

DIAGNOSTIC	CODE	FEE
Periodic exam	(00120)	20—
Limited exam	00140	
Comprehensive exam	00150	
Extensive exam	00160	

PREVENTIVE

PREVENTIVE	CODE	FEE
Intraoral–FMX	00210	
Intraoral–PA	00220	
BW *— 2 films*	0027*2*	12—
Single posteroanterior	00290	
Panoramic X-ray	00330	37—
Prophylaxis adult	(01110)	
Prophylaxis child	01120	
Topical fluoride	012__	

DENTAL SERVICE

RESTORATIVE

RESTORATIVE	CODE	FEE
Amalgams (decid) Tooth #_____	021__	
Amalgams (perm) Tooth #_____	021__	

CROWNS AND BRIDGES

CROWNS AND BRIDGES	CODE	FEE
PFG crown	02750	
FG cast crown	02790	
3/4 gold cast crown	02810	
FC bridge pontic	06210	
Porcelain bridge ( )	062__	

OTHER PROCEDURES

	TOTAL	$	69—
	AMOUNT PAID	$	10—
	BALANCE DUE	$	59—

DOCTOR'S STATEMENT: I certify that I personally provided the above services and that fees shown represent my usual fees

Patrick Zunkel, DDS   4/3/--
Signature   Date

Medical & Dental Associates, P.C.

3733 Professional Drive #300   317/123-4567
Indianapolis, IN 46260   Tax ID# 99-9999999

CONFIDENTIAL PATIENT INFORMATION RECORD

(please print)

Patient Name Stephanie McCullough, Ph.D.	**Patient Employer** Northside Clinic
Address 1500 W. Toohey Ln.	Address 14000 N. Meridian St.
Indpls., IN 46233	Indpls., IN 46388
Telephone 555-6280	Telephone 555-8840
Birthdate 2/27/-- Age 35	Occupation Psychologist
Sex F Marital Status S	
Social Security No. 389-41-6000	
	Primary insured date of birth
Responsible Party (if other than patient)	Secondary insured date of birth
	Third insured date of birth
Relationship to patient	Fourth insured date of birth
Address	(Please use the back of the form to write information about the
	third and fourth insured parties, if applicable.)

INSURANCE INFORMATION

Primary insured	Secondary insured
Subscriber	Subscriber
Address	Address
Telephone	Telephone
Employer	Employer
Address	Address
Job/Union No.	Job/Union No.
Subscriber's SS# 389-41-6000	Subscriber's SS#
Relationship to patient	Relationship to patient
Insurance Gateway Dental	Insurance
Address 311 N. Michigan Ave	Address
Chicago, IL 60611	
Policy No.	Policy No.
Subscriber ID No. 389-41-6000	Subscriber ID No.
Group Name/No.	Group Name/No.
Effective date 10/8/96	Effective date
Expiration date	Expiration date

Record #26 1 of 2

238

Medical & Dental Associates, P.C.

3733 Professional Drive #300
Indianapolis, IN 46260

317/123-4567
Tax ID# 99-9999999

Patient name   _Dr. McCullough_

CPT-4 CODES

OFFICE SERVICES	CODE	FEE
New patient, problem focused	99201	
New patient, expanded problem focused	99202	
New patient, detailed	99203	
New patient, comprehensive, mod.	99204	
New patient, comprehensive, high	99205	
Established patient, RN	99211	
Established patient, problem focused	99212	
Established patient, expanded problem	99213	
Established patient, detailed	99214	
Established patient, comprehensive	99215	
Consultation		

LABORATORY		
X-ray, chest/ribs; single view, frontal	71010	
X-ray, chest/ribs; stereo, frontal	71015	
Therapeutic injections ( )	907__	
Drugs, trays, supplies	99070	
Educational supplies, books, tapes	99071	
Urinalysis, routine, dip stick	81000	
Urine pregnancy test, visual color	81025	
Blood count, hemoglobin	85018	
Pap smear	88150	

ICD-9-CM

DIAGNOSES	
Anxiety reaction	300.00
Bleeding rectal	569.3
Benign prostatic hypertrophy	600
Bronchitis, acute	466.0
Bronchitis, chronic	491.9
Cardiac arrhythmia	427.9
Chest pain	786.50
Cirrhosis of liver	571.5
Conjunctivitis, acute	372.00
Depression	300.4
Flu	487.0
Fracture–nasal, closed	802.0
Fractured tibia	891.2
Headache, vascular	794.0
Herpes zoster	053.9
Irritable bowel syndrome	564.1
Menopause	627.2
Myocardial infarction, unspecified	410.90
Otitis, acute	381.01
Pharyngitis, acute	462
Pneumonia	486
Sinusitis, acute	461.9
Tendonitis	726.90
Tennis elbow	726.32
Pregnancy	V22.2
Sprained ankle	842.5
Tonsillitis	474.0
Vertigo	386.0
Well child	V20.2

New Pt

CDT-2 CODES

DENTAL SERVICE

DIAGNOSTIC	CODE	FEE
Periodic exam	(00120)	20—
Limited exam	00140	
Comprehensive exam	00150	
Extensive exam	00160	

PREVENTIVE		
Intraoral–FMX	00210	
Intraoral–PA	00220	
BW	0027_	
Single posteroanterior	00290	
Panoramic X-ray	(00330)	40—
Prophylaxis adult	(01110)	37—
Prophylaxis child	01120	
Topical fluoride	012__	

DENTAL SERVICE

RESTORATIVE	CODE	FEE
Amalgams (decid) Tooth #_____	021__	
Amalgams (perm) Tooth #_____	021__	
CROWNS AND BRIDGES		
PFG crown	02750	
FG cast crown	02790	
3/4 gold cast crown	02810	
FC bridge pontic	06210	
Porcelain bridge ( )	062__	
OTHER PROCEDURES		

DOCTOR'S STATEMENT: I certify that I personally provided the above services and that fees shown represent my usual fees

Michael Lane, DDS   7/11/--
Signature   Date

TOTAL	$	97—
AMOUNT PAID	$	97—
BALANCE DUE	$	0

Medical & Dental Associates, P.C.

3733 Professional Drive #300   317/123-4567
Indianapolis, IN 46260   Tax ID# 99-9999999

CONFIDENTIAL PATIENT INFORMATION RECORD

(please print)

Patient Name	Keith Konklin	**Patient Employer**	Ind. Univ.
Address	1010 Sunview Dr.	Address	Box 3200
	Bloomington, IN 48211		Bloomington, IN 48200

Telephone	(812) 555-3113
Birthdate	10/20/-- Age 40
Sex	M Marital Status M
Social Security No.	471-20-0800

Telephone   (812) 555-2060

Occupation

Responsible Party (if other than patient)

Relationship to patient

Address

Primary insured date of birth

Secondary insured date of birth

Third insured date of birth

Fourth insured date of birth

(Please use the back of the form to write information about the third and fourth insured parties, if applicable.)

INSURANCE INFORMATION

Primary insured	Self	Secondary insured	
Subscriber	"	Subscriber	
Address		Address	
Telephone		Telephone	
Employer		Employer	
Address		Address	
Job/Union No.		Job/Union No.	
Subscriber's SS#		Subscriber's SS#	
Relationship to patient		Relationship to patient	
Insurance	Dental Ins. of IN	Insurance	
Address	2229 S. Hillway	Address	
	Fishers, IN 48411		
Policy No.		Policy No.	
Subscriber ID No.	471-20-0800-90	Subscriber ID No.	
Group Name/No.	—	Group Name/No.	
Effective date	1/1/90	Effective date	
Expiration date	—	Expiration date	

Record #27 1 of 3

240

Medical & Dental Associates, P.C.

3733 Professional Drive #300
Indianapolis, IN 46260

317/123-4567
Tax ID# 99-9999999

Patient name *Keith Konklin*

CPT-4 CODES

OFFICE SERVICES

	CODE	FEE
New patient, problem focused	99201	
New patient, expanded problem focused	99202	
New patient, detailed	99203	
New patient, comprehensive, mod.	99204	
New patient, comprehensive, high	99205	
Established patient, RN	99211	
Established patient, problem focused	99212	
Established patient, expanded problem	99213	
Established patient, detailed	99214	
Established patient, comprehensive	99215	
Consultation		

LABORATORY

X-ray, chest/ribs; single view, frontal	71010	
X-ray, chest/ribs; stereo, frontal	71015	
Therapeutic injections ( )	907__	
Drugs, trays, supplies	99070	
Educational supplies, books, tapes	99071	
Urinalysis, routine, dip stick	81000	
Urine pregnancy test, visual color	81025	
Blood count, hemoglobin	85018	
Pap smear	88150	

ICD-9-CM

DIAGNOSES

Anxiety reaction	300.00
Bleeding rectal	569.3
Benign prostatic hypertrophy	600
Bronchitis, acute	466.0
Bronchitis, chronic	491.9
Cardiac arrhythmia	427.9
Chest pain	786.50
Cirrhosis of liver	571.5
Conjunctivitis, acute	372.00
Depression	300.4
Flu	487.0
Fracture–nasal, closed	802.0
Fractured tibia	891.2
Headache, vascular	794.0
Herpes zoster	053.9
Irritable bowel syndrome	564.1
Menopause	627.2
Myocardial infarction, unspecified	410.90
Otitis, acute	381.01
Pharyngitis, acute	462
Pneumonia	486
Sinusitis, acute	461.9
Tendonitis	726.90
Tennis elbow	726.32
Pregnancy	V22.2
Sprained ankle	842.5
Tonsillitis	474.0
Vertigo	386.0
Well child	V20.2

CDT-2 CODES

DENTAL SERVICE

DIAGNOSTIC

	CODE	FEE
Periodic exam	(00120)	20—
Limited exam	00140	
Comprehensive exam	00150	
Extensive exam	00160	

PREVENTIVE

Intraoral–FMX	00210	
Intraoral–PA	(00220)	10—
BW	0027_	
Single posteroanterior	00290	
Panoramic X-ray	00330	
Prophylaxis adult	(01110)	37—
Prophylaxis child	01120	
Topical fluoride	012__	

DENTAL SERVICE

RESTORATIVE

	CODE	FEE
Amalgams (decid) Tooth #_____	021__	
Amalgams (perm) Tooth #_____	021__	

CROWNS AND BRIDGES

PFG crown	02750	
FG cast crown	02790	
3/4 gold cast crown	02810	
FC bridge pontic	06210	
Porcelain bridge ( )	062__	

OTHER PROCEDURES

Resin restoration #14	*02330*	*$37*

DOCTOR'S STATEMENT: I certify that I personally provided the above services and that fees shown represent my usual fees

M.P. Lane, DDS   *2/15/--*

Signature   Date

TOTAL	$	104—
AMOUNT PAID	$	25—
BALANCE DUE	$	79—

Record #27 2 of 3

Medical & Dental Associates, P.C.

3733 Professional Drive #300
Indianapolis, IN 46260

317/123-4567
Tax ID# 99-9999999

Patient name *Keith Konklin*

CPT-4 CODES

OFFICE SERVICES

	CODE	FEE
New patient, problem focused	99201	_____
New patient, expanded problem focused	99202	_____
New patient, detailed	99203	_____
New patient, comprehensive, mod.	99204	_____
New patient, comprehensive, high	99205	_____
Established patient, RN	99211	_____
Established patient, problem focused	99212	_____
Established patient, expanded problem	99213	_____
Established patient, detailed	99214	_____
Established patient, comprehensive	99215	_____
Consultation		

LABORATORY

	CODE	FEE
X-ray, chest/ribs; single view, frontal	71010	_____
X-ray, chest/ribs; stereo, frontal	71015	_____
Therapeutic injections ( )	907__	_____
Drugs, trays, supplies	99070	_____
Educational supplies, books, tapes	99071	_____
Urinalysis, routine, dip stick	81000	_____
Urine pregnancy test, visual color	81025	_____
Blood count, hemoglobin	85018	_____
Pap smear	88150	_____

ICD-9-CM

DIAGNOSES

Anxiety reaction	300.00
Bleeding rectal	569.3
Benign prostatic hypertrophy	600
Bronchitis, acute	466.0
Bronchitis, chronic	491.9
Cardiac arrhythmia	427.9
Chest pain	786.50
Cirrhosis of liver	571.5
Conjunctivitis, acute	372.00
Depression	300.4
Flu	487.0
Fracture–nasal, closed	802.0
Fractured tibia	891.2
Headache, vascular	794.0
Herpes zoster	053.9
Irritable bowel syndrome	564.1
Menopause	627.2
Myocardial infarction, unspecified	410.90
Otitis, acute	381.01
Pharyngitis, acute	462
Pneumonia	486
Sinusitis, acute	461.9
Tendonitis	726.90
Tennis elbow	726.32
Pregnancy	V22.2
Sprained ankle	842.5
Tonsillitis	474.0
Vertigo	386.0
Well child	V20.2

CDT-2 CODES

DENTAL SERVICE

DIAGNOSTIC

	CODE	FEE
Periodic exam	00120	_____
Limited exam	00140	_____
Comprehensive exam	00150	_____
Extensive exam	00160	_____

PREVENTIVE

	CODE	FEE
Intraoral–FMX	00210	_____
Intraoral–PA	00220	_____
BW	0027_	_____
Single posteroanterior	00290	_____
Panoramic X-ray	00330	_____
Prophylaxis adult	01110	_____
Prophylaxis child	01120	_____
Topical fluoride	012__	_____

DENTAL SERVICE

RESTORATIVE

	CODE	FEE
Amalgams (decid) Tooth #_____	021__	_____
Amalgams (perm) Tooth #_____	021__	_____

CROWNS AND BRIDGES

	CODE	FEE
PFG crown	02750	_____
FG cast crown	02790	_____
3/4 gold cast crown *#14*	(02810)	*475—*
FC bridge pontic	06210	_____
Porcelain bridge ( )	062__	_____

OTHER PROCEDURES

DOCTOR'S STATEMENT: I certify that I personally provided the above services and that fees shown represent my usual fees

M.P. Lane, DDS   *3/1/--*

Signature   Date

TOTAL	$	*475—*
AMOUNT PAID	$	*—*
BALANCE DUE	$	*475—*

Record #27 3 of 3

242

Good Samaritan Hospital

1212 West 88th Street • Indianapolis, IN 46260 • 317/555-1212

EMERGENCY ROOM PATIENT INFORMATION

Date 9/14/--   Time 0750   Account

Patient Name Aaron Marshall   Address 2140 Westside Canal Dr.

City Indpls.   State IN   Zip 46288

Telephone No. 555-8799   Date of Birth Age 67 10/20/-- (M) F

Responsible party name and address, if different than above

Insurance company name and address Medicare – 1500 E. 10th St – Indpls. 46215

No other

ID number 347-89-0322AB   Group number —

Insured name Aaron Marshall   SS# 347-89-0322

Nature of complaints Passenger in auto accident — sustained injury to the mouth, lips, gums

DX: 802.37, 802.8, 804.61

I do hereby agree to be responsible for any charges resulting from this visit in the event my insurance company denies payment of benefits. I agree to authorize payment for any insurance benefits directly to Good Samaritan Hospital, 1212 West 88th Street, Indianapolis, IN, 46260.

Signature of patient or guardian Aaron Marshall

Name

Date 9/14/--

Record #28 1 of 2

Medical & Dental Associates, P.C.

3733 Professional Drive #300
Indianapolis, IN 46260
317/123-4567
Tax ID# 99-9999999

STATEMENT OF ACCOUNT

MARSHALL, Aaron
2140 Westside Canal Drive
Indianapolis, IN 46288

19--

DATE	CODE	CHARGE		CREDITS		CURRENT BALANCE	
				PAYMENT	ADJ		
BALANCE FORWARD ➡							
9/14	99252	175	00			175	00
914	D4355	100	00			275	00

PLEASE PAY LAST AMOUNT IN THIS COLUMN ↑

THIS IS A COPY OF YOUR ACCOUNT

Record #28 2 of 2

Medical & Dental Associates, P.C.

3733 Professional Drive #300   317/123-4567
Indianapolis, IN 46260   Tax ID# 99-9999999

CONFIDENTIAL PATIENT INFORMATION RECORD

(please print)

Patient Name Terrence James	**Patient Employer** Disabled
Address 210 N. Mount St.	Address
Hope, IN 47233	
Telephone (789) 555-3128	Telephone
Birthdate 4/18/-- Age 55	Occupation
Sex M Marital Status D	
Social Security No.	
	Primary insured date of birth
Responsible Party (if other than patient)	Secondary insured date of birth
	Third insured date of birth
Relationship to patient	Fourth insured date of birth
Address	(Please use the back of the form to write information about the
	third and fourth insured parties, if applicable.)

INSURANCE INFORMATION

Primary insured	Secondary insured
Subscriber	Subscriber
Address	Address
Telephone	Telephone
Employer	Employer
Address	Address
Job/Union No.	Job/Union No.
Subscriber's SS#	Subscriber's SS#
Relationship to patient	Relationship to patient
Insurance Medicaid Dental	Insurance
Address	Address
Policy No.	Policy No.
Subscriber ID No. 62-404039731-1	Subscriber ID No.
Group Name/No.	Group Name/No.
Effective date 1/1/--	Effective date
Expiration date 1/31/--	Expiration date

Record #29 1 of 2

Medical & Dental Associates, P.C.

3733 Professional Drive #300
Indianapolis, IN 46260

317/123-4567
Tax ID# 99-9999999

Patient name *Terrence James*

CPT-4 CODES

OFFICE SERVICES	CODE	FEE
New patient, problem focused	99201	_____
New patient, expanded problem focused	99202	_____
New patient, detailed	99203	_____
New patient, comprehensive, mod.	99204	_____
New patient, comprehensive, high	99205	_____
Established patient, RN	99211	_____
Established patient, problem focused	99212	_____
Established patient, expanded problem	99213	_____
Established patient, detailed	99214	_____
Established patient, comprehensive	99215	_____
Consultation		

LABORATORY

	CODE	FEE
X-ray, chest/ribs; single view, frontal	71010	_____
X-ray, chest/ribs; stereo, frontal	71015	_____
Therapeutic injections ( )	907__	_____
Drugs, trays, supplies	99070	_____
Educational supplies, books, tapes	99071	_____
Urinalysis, routine, dip stick	81000	_____
Urine pregnancy test, visual color	81025	_____
Blood count, hemoglobin	85018	_____
Pap smear	88150	_____

ICD-9-CM

DIAGNOSES	
Anxiety reaction	300.00
Bleeding rectal	569.3
Benign prostatic hypertrophy	600
Bronchitis, acute	466.0
Bronchitis, chronic	491.9
Cardiac arrhythmia	427.9
Chest pain	786.50
Cirrhosis of liver	571.5
Conjunctivitis, acute	372.00
Depression	300.4
Flu	487.0
Fracture–nasal, closed	802.0
Fractured tibia	891.2
Headache, vascular	794.0
Herpes zoster	053.9
Irritable bowel syndrome	564.1
Menopause	627.2
Myocardial infarction, unspecified	410.90
Otitis, acute	381.01
Pharyngitis, acute	462
Pneumonia	486
Sinusitis, acute	461.9
Tendonitis	726.90
Tennis elbow	726.32
Pregnancy	V22.2
Sprained ankle	842.5
Tonsillitis	474.0
Vertigo	386.0
Well child	V20.2

CDT-2 CODES

DENTAL SERVICE

DIAGNOSTIC	CODE	FEE
Periodic exam	(00120)	20—
Limited exam	00140	_____
Comprehensive exam	00150	_____
Extensive exam	00160	_____
PREVENTIVE		
Intraoral–FMX	00210	_____
Intraoral–PA	00220	_____
BW	0027_	_____
Single posteroanterior	00290	_____
Panoramic X-ray	00330	_____
Prophylaxis adult	(01110)	37—
Prophylaxis child	01120	_____
Topical fluoride	012__	_____

DENTAL SERVICE

RESTORATIVE	CODE	FEE
Amalgams (decid) Tooth #_____	021__	_____
Amalgams (perm) Tooth #_____	021__	_____
CROWNS AND BRIDGES		
PFG crown	02750	_____
FG cast crown	02790	_____
3/4 gold cast crown	02810	_____
FC bridge pontic	06210	_____
Porcelain bridge ( )	062__	_____
OTHER PROCEDURES		

DOCTOR'S STATEMENT: I certify that I personally provided the above services and that fees shown represent my usual fees

M. Lane, DDS   *1/20/--*

Signature   Date

TOTAL	$	57—
AMOUNT PAID	$	—
BALANCE DUE	$	57—

Record #29 2 of 2

Medical & Dental Associates, P.C.

3733 Professional Drive #300   317/123-4567
Indianapolis, IN 46260   Tax ID# 99-9999999

CONFIDENTIAL PATIENT INFORMATION RECORD

(please print)

Patient Name	Bill Williams, Ph.D.	**Patient Employer**	Ecological Planning
Address	342 N. Waverly	Address	820 W. Mars Ave
	Indpls., IN 46299		Indpls., IN 46232

Telephone	555-8089	Telephone	555-8089
Birthdate	10/14/-- Age 32	Occupation	Pres. of Co.
Sex M Marital Status M			
Social Security No.	312-30-6032		

Primary insured date of birth

Responsible Party (if other than patient)

Secondary insured date of birth

Third insured date of birth

Relationship to patient

Fourth insured date of birth

Address

(Please use the back of the form to write information about the

third and fourth insured parties, if applicable.)

INSURANCE INFORMATION

Primary insured		Secondary insured	
Subscriber		Subscriber	
Address		Address	
Telephone		Telephone	
Employer		Employer	
Address		Address	
Job/Union No.		Job/Union No.	
Subscriber's SS#		Subscriber's SS#	
Relationship to patient		Relationship to patient	
Insurance	Day Bright Dental Co.	Insurance	
Address	110 W. State St.	Address	
	Pittsburgh, PA 32190		
Policy No.	2166802	Policy No.	
Subscriber ID No.	312306032-2	Subscriber ID No.	
Group Name/No.		Group Name/No.	
Effective date	10/10/93	Effective date	
Expiration date		Expiration date	

Record #30 1 of 2

Medical & Dental Associates, P.C.

3733 Professional Drive #300
Indianapolis, IN 46260

317/123-4567
Tax ID# 99-9999999

Patient name _Dr. Bill Williams_

CPT-4 CODES

OFFICE SERVICES

	CODE	FEE
New patient, problem focused	99201	_____
New patient, expanded problem focused	99202	_____
New patient, detailed	99203	_____
New patient, comprehensive, mod.	99204	_____
New patient, comprehensive, high	99205	_____
Established patient, RN	99211	_____
Established patient, problem focused	99212	_____
Established patient, expanded problem	99213	_____
Established patient, detailed	99214	_____
Established patient, comprehensive	99215	_____
Consultation		

LABORATORY

	CODE	FEE
X-ray, chest/ribs; single view, frontal	71010	_____
X-ray, chest/ribs; stereo, frontal	71015	_____
Therapeutic injections ( )	907__	_____
Drugs, trays, supplies	99070	_____
Educational supplies, books, tapes	99071	_____
Urinalysis, routine, dip stick	81000	_____
Urine pregnancy test, visual color	81025	_____
Blood count, hemoglobin	85018	_____
Pap smear	88150	_____

ICD-9-CM

DIAGNOSES

Anxiety reaction	300.00
Bleeding rectal	569.3
Benign prostatic hypertrophy	600
Bronchitis, acute	466.0
Bronchitis, chronic	491.9
Cardiac arrhythmia	427.9
Chest pain	786.50
Cirrhosis of liver	571.5
Conjunctivitis, acute	372.00
Depression	300.4
Flu	487.0
Fracture–nasal, closed	802.0
Fractured tibia	891.2
Headache, vascular	794.0
Herpes zoster	053.9
Irritable bowel syndrome	564.1
Menopause	627.2
Myocardial infarction, unspecified	410.90
Otitis, acute	381.01
Pharyngitis, acute	462
Pneumonia	486
Sinusitis, acute	461.9
Tendonitis	726.90
Tennis elbow	726.32
Pregnancy	V22.2
Sprained ankle	842.5
Tonsillitis	474.0
Vertigo	386.0
Well child	V20.2

CDT-2 CODES

DENTAL SERVICE

DIAGNOSTIC

	CODE	FEE
Periodic exam	00120	_____
Limited exam	00140	_____
Comprehensive exam	00150	_____
Extensive exam	00160	_____

PREVENTIVE

	CODE	FEE
Intraoral–FMX	00210	_____
Intraoral–PA	(00220)	_10—_
BW	0027_	_____
Single posteroanterior	00290	_____
Panoramic X-ray	00330	_____
Prophylaxis adult	01110	_____
Prophylaxis child	01120	_____
Topical fluoride	012__	_____

(marked ① next to Intraoral–PA)

DENTAL SERVICE

RESTORATIVE

	CODE	FEE
Amalgams (decid) Tooth #_____	021__	_____
Amalgams (perm) Tooth #_____	021__	_____

CROWNS AND BRIDGES

	CODE	FEE
PFG crown _Tooth #12_	(02750)	_450—_
FG cast crown	02790	_____
3/4 gold cast crown	02810	_____
FC bridge pontic	06210	_____
Porcelain bridge ( )	062__	_____

OTHER PROCEDURES

_03320 $320_

_02954 150_   (_Tx started 10-1_)

TOTAL	$	_930—_
AMOUNT PAID	$	_—_
BALANCE DUE	$	_930—_

DOCTOR'S STATEMENT: I certify that I personally provided the above services and that fees shown represent my usual fees

Patrick M. Zunkel, DDS   _11/15/--_

Signature   Date

Part Five

NUMBERED FORMS
AND WORKSHEETS

JOB DESCRIPTION

TITLE: Insurance Billing Specialist

IMMEDIATE SUPERVISOR: Office Manager

JOB DUTIES: Part I. To gather sufficient patient information to complete and file health insurance claims for reimbursement for services rendered by the physicians and dentists of this office. Actual patient records will be examined

Part II. To complete the insurance forms correctly in accordance with the general requirements of most fee-for-service third-party payers. Patient records of this office will be accessed for clarification.

Part III. To adapt the insurance form completion process, as determined by specific patient records, to the general requirements of the major insurers, such as Medicare, Medicaid, Workers' Compensation, CHAMPUS, and certain other managed care insurance plans.

Part IV. To provide the references and resources necessary to complete the insurance billing process.

Part V. To furnish the forms and worksheets needed to complete all required tasks.

APPROVED OMB-0938-0008

General Ins Co
1010 Southway
Gavy 48431 blvd

CARRIER

☐☐ PICA

HEALTH INSURANCE CLAIM FORM

PICA ☐☐

1. MEDICARE	MEDICAID	CHAMPUS	CHAMPVA	GROUP HEALTH PLAN	FECA BLK LUNG	OTHER	1a. INSURED'S I.D. NUMBER	(FOR PROGRAM IN ITEM 1)
☒ (Medicare #)	☐ (Medicaid #)	☐ (Sponsor's SSN)	☐ (VA File #)	☐ (SSN or ID)	☐ (SSN)	☐ (ID)	334 04 2121 C A	

2. PATIENT'S NAME (Last Name, First Name, Middle Initial)
Stuyvesant Hoyt

3. PATIENT'S BIRTH DATE
MM 12 DD 25 YY   SEX M ☒   F ☐

4. INSURED'S NAME (Last Name, First Name, Middle Initial)

5. PATIENT'S ADDRESS (No. Street)
1511 N Illionis St

6. PATIENT RELATIONSHIP TO INSURED
Self ☐ Spouse ☐ Child ☐ Other ☐

7. INSURED'S ADDRESS (No. Street)

CITY
Amber

STATE
IN

8. PATIENT STATUS
Single ☒   Married ☐   Other ☐

CITY

STATE

ZIP CODE
46231

TELEPHONE (Include Area Code)
(   )

Employed ☐   Full-Time Student ☐   Part-Time Student ☐

ZIP CODE

TELEPHONE (INCLUDE AREA CODE)
(   )

9. OTHER INSURED'S NAME (Last Name, First Name, Middle Initial)

10. IS PATIENT'S CONDITION RELATED TO:

11. INSURED'S POLICY GROUP OR FECA NUMBER

a. OTHER INSURED'S POLICY OR GROUP NUMBER

a. EMPLOYMENT? (CURRENT OR PREVIOUS)
☐ YES   ☐ NO

a. INSURED'S DATE OF BIRTH
MM DD YY   SEX M ☐ F ☐

b. OTHER INSURED'S DATE OF BIRTH
MM DD YY   SEX M ☐ F ☐

b. AUTO ACCIDENT?   PLACE (State)
☐ YES   ☒ NO

b. EMPLOYER'S NAME OR SCHOOL NAME

c. EMPLOYER'S NAME OR SCHOOL NAME

c. OTHER ACCIDENT?
☐ YES   ☒ NO

c. INSURANCE PLAN NAME OR PROGRAM NAME

d. INSURANCE PLAN NAME OR PROGRAM NAME

10d. RESERVED FOR LOCAL USE

d. IS THERE ANOTHER HEALTH BENEFIT PLAN?
☐ YES   ☐ NO   If yes, return to and complete item 9 a – d.

READ BACK OF FORM BEFORE COMPLETING & SIGNING THIS FORM.
12. PATIENT'S OR AUTHORIZED PERSON'S SIGNATURE I authorize the release of any medical or other information necessary to process this claim. I also request payment of government benefits either to myself or to the party who accepts assignment below.

SIGNED Signature on file   DATE Today

13. INSURED'S OR AUTHORIZED PERSON'S SIGNATURE I authorize payment of medical benefits to the undersigned physician or supplier for services described below.

SIGNED Signature on file

14. DATE OF CURRENT: MM DD YY   ◄ ILLNESS (First symptom) OR INJURY (Accident) OR PREGNANCY (LMP)

15. IF PATIENT HAS HAD SAME OR SIMILAR ILLNESS, GIVE FIRST DATE MM DD YY

16. DATES PATIENT UNABLE TO WORK IN CURRENT OCCUPATION
FROM MM DD YY   TO MM DD YY

17. NAME OF REFERRING PHYSICIAN OR OTHER SOURCE

17a. I.D. NUMBER OF REFERRING PHYSICIAN

18. HOSPITALIZATION DATES RELATED TO CURRENT SERVICES
FROM MM DD YY   TO MM DD YY

19. RESERVED FOR LOCAL USE

20. OUTSIDE LAB? $ CHARGES
☐ YES   ☐ NO

21. DIAGNOSIS OR NATURE OF ILLNESS OR INJURY. (RELATE ITEMS 1, 2, 3, OR 4 TO ITEM 24E BY LINE)

1. |___|___.___|
2. |___|___.___|
3. |___|___.___|
4. |___|___.___|

22. MEDICAID RESUBMISSION CODE   ORIGINAL REF. NO.

23. PRIOR AUTHORIZATION NUMBER

24. A DATE(S) OF SERVICE		B	C	D	E	F	G	H	I	J	K
From MM DD YY	To MM DD YY	Place of Service	Type of Service	PROCEDURES, SERVICES, OR SUPPLIES (Explain Unusual Circumstances) CPT/HCPCS MODIFIER	DIAGNOSIS CODE	$ CHARGES	DAYS OR UNITS	EPSDT Family Plan	EMG	COB	RESERVED FOR LOCAL USE

25. FEDERAL TAX I.D. NUMBER   SSN ☐ EIN ☐

26. PATIENT'S ACCOUNT NO.

27. ACCEPT ASSIGNMENT? (For govt. claims, see back)
☐ YES   ☐ NO

28. TOTAL CHARGE
$

29. AMOUNT PAID
$

30. BALANCE DUE
$

31. SIGNATURE OF PHYSICIAN OR SUPPLIER INCLUDING DEGREES OR CREDENTIALS (I certify that the statements on the reverse apply to this bill and are made a part thereof.)

SIGNED   DATE

32. NAME AND ADDRESS OF FACILITY WHERE SERVICES WERE RENDERED (If other than home or office)

33. PHYSICIAN'S SUPPLIER'S BILLING NAME, ADDRESS, ZIP CODE & PHONE #

PIN#   GRP#

(APPROVED BY AMA COUNCIL ON MEDICAL SERVICE 8/88)   PLEASE PRINT OR TYPE

FORM HCFA-1500 (12-90)
FORM OWCP-1500   FORM RRB-1500
FORM AMA OP050192

PATIENT AND INSURED INFORMATION

PHYSICIAN OR SUPPLIER INFORMATION

FORM 1

NOT THE INSURED

PLEASE
DO NOT
STAPLE
IN THIS
AREA

CARRIER

☐☐ PICA

HEALTH INSURANCE CLAIM FORM

PICA ☐☐☐

| 1. MEDICARE ☐ (Medicare #) | MEDICAID ☐ (Medicaid #) | CHAMPUS ☐ (Sponsor's SSN) | CHAMPVA ☐ (VA File #) | GROUP HEALTH PLAN ☐ (SSN or ID) | FECA BLK LUNG ☐ (SSN) | OTHER ☐ (ID) | 1a. INSURED'S I.D. NUMBER (FOR PROGRAM IN ITEM 1) 451-03-4672 |

2. PATIENT'S NAME (Last Name, First Name, Middle Initial)
JR, ROBERTS RICHARD O

3. PATIENT'S BIRTH DATE
MM 11 | DD 01 | YY   SEX M ☒ F ☐

4. INSURED'S NAME (Last Name, First Name, Middle Initial)
Sr. ROBERTS RICHARDS O

5. PATIENT'S ADDRESS (No. Street)
312 HILL ST

6. PATIENT RELATIONSHIP TO INSURED
Self ☐ Spouse ☐ Child ☒ Other ☐

7. INSURED'S ADDRESS (No. Street)
SAME

CITY
DOLOTH   STATE IN

8. PATIENT STATUS
Single ☐ Married ☐ Other ☐

CITY   STATE

ZIP CODE
46233
TELEPHONE (Include Area Code)
(   )

Employed ☐ Full-Time Student ☐ Part-Time Student ☐

ZIP CODE   TELEPHONE (INCLUDE AREA CODE)
(   )

9. OTHER INSURED'S NAME (Last Name, First Name, Middle Initial)

10. IS PATIENT'S CONDITION RELATED TO:

11. INSURED'S POLICY GROUP OR FECA NUMBER

a. OTHER INSURED'S POLICY OR GROUP NUMBER

a. EMPLOYMENT? (CURRENT OR PREVIOUS)
☐ YES ☐ NO

a. INSURED'S DATE OF BIRTH
MM 06 | DD 05 | YY   SEX M ☒ F ☐

b. OTHER INSURED'S DATE OF BIRTH
MM | DD | YY   SEX M ☐ F ☐

b. AUTO ACCIDENT?   PLACE (State)
☐ YES ☐ NO

b. EMPLOYER'S NAME OR SCHOOL NAME
WALL DEPOT. STORE

c. EMPLOYER'S NAME OR SCHOOL NAME

c. OTHER ACCIDENT?
☐ YES ☐ NO

c. INSURANCE PLAN NAME OR PROGRAM NAME

d. INSURANCE PLAN NAME OR PROGRAM NAME

10d. RESERVED FOR LOCAL USE

d. IS THERE ANOTHER HEALTH BENEFIT PLAN?
☐ YES ☐ NO   If yes, return to and complete item 9 a – d.

READ BACK OF FORM BEFORE COMPLETING & SIGNING THIS FORM.
12. PATIENT'S OR AUTHORIZED PERSON'S SIGNATURE I authorize the release of any medical or other information necessary to process this claim. I also request payment of government benefits either to myself or to the party who accepts assignment below.

SIGNED _____   DATE _____

13. INSURED'S OR AUTHORIZED PERSON'S SIGNATURE I authorize payment of medical benefits to the undersigned physician or supplier for services described below.

SIGNED _____

14. DATE OF CURRENT: ◄ ILLNESS (First symptom) OR
MM | DD | YY   INJURY (Accident) OR
PREGNANCY (LMP)

15. IF PATIENT HAS HAD SAME OR SIMILAR ILLNESS, GIVE FIRST DATE   MM | DD | YY

16. DATES PATIENT UNABLE TO WORK IN CURRENT OCCUPATION
MM | DD | YY   MM | DD | YY
FROM   TO

17. NAME OF REFERRING PHYSICIAN OR OTHER SOURCE

17a. I.D. NUMBER OF REFERRING PHYSICIAN

18. HOSPITALIZATION DATES RELATED TO CURRENT SERVICES
MM | DD | YY   MM | DD | YY
FROM   TO

19. RESERVED FOR LOCAL USE

20. OUTSIDE LAB? $ CHARGES
☐ YES ☐ NO

21. DIAGNOSIS OR NATURE OF ILLNESS OR INJURY. (RELATE ITEMS 1, 2, 3, OR 4 TO ITEM 24E BY LINE)

1. _____   3. _____

2. _____   4. _____

22. MEDICAID RESUBMISSION
CODE   ORIGINAL REF. NO.

23. PRIOR AUTHORIZATION NUMBER

24. A DATE(S) OF SERVICE						B Place of Service	C Type of Service	D PROCEDURES, SERVICES, OR SUPPLIES (Explain Unusual Circumstances)		E DIAGNOSIS CODE	F $ CHARGES	G DAYS OR UNITS	H EPSDT Family Plan	I EMG	J COB	K RESERVED FOR LOCAL USE
From MM	DD	YY	To MM	DD	YY			CPT/HCPCS	MODIFIER							
1																
2																
3																
4																
5																
6																

25. FEDERAL TAX I.D. NUMBER   SSN ☐ EIN ☐

26. PATIENT'S ACCOUNT NO.

27. ACCEPT ASSIGNMENT? (For govt. claims, see back)
☐ YES ☐ NO

28. TOTAL CHARGE
$

29. AMOUNT PAID
$

30. BALANCE DUE
$

31. SIGNATURE OF PHYSICIAN OR SUPPLIER INCLUDING DEGREES OR CREDENTIALS (I certify that the statements on the reverse apply to this bill and are made a part thereof.)

SIGNED _____ DATE _____

32. NAME AND ADDRESS OF FACILITY WHERE SERVICES WERE RENDERED (If other than home or office)

33. PHYSICIAN'S SUPPLIER'S BILLING NAME, ADDRESS, ZIP CODE & PHONE #

PIN#   GRP#

PHYSICIAN OR SUPPLIER INFORMATION

PATIENT AND INSURED INFORMATION

(APPROVED BY AMA COUNCIL ON MEDICAL SERVICE 8/88)

PLEASE PRINT OR TYPE

FORM HCFA-1500 (12-90)
FORM OWCP-1500   FORM RRB-1500
FORM AMA OP050192

FORM 2

APPROVED OMB-0938-0008

CARRIER

| | PICA

HEALTH INSURANCE CLAIM FORM

PICA | |

1. MEDICARE MEDICAID CHAMPUS CHAMPVA GROUP HEALTH PLAN FECA BLK LUNG OTHER	1a. INSURED'S I.D. NUMBER (FOR PROGRAM IN ITEM 1)
☐ (Medicare #) ☐ (Medicaid #) ☐ (Sponsor's SSN) ☐ (VA File #) ☐ (SSN or ID) ☐ (SSN) ☐ (ID)	

2. PATIENT'S NAME (Last Name, First Name, Middle Initial)	3. PATIENT'S BIRTH DATE MM DD YY SEX M ☐ F ☐	4. INSURED'S NAME (Last Name, First Name, Middle Initial)

5. PATIENT'S ADDRESS (No. Street)	6. PATIENT RELATIONSHIP TO INSURED Self ☐ Spouse ☐ Child ☐ Other ☐	7. INSURED'S ADDRESS (No. Street)
CITY STATE	8. PATIENT STATUS Single ☐ Married ☐ Other ☐	CITY STATE
ZIP CODE TELEPHONE (Include Area Code) ( )	Employed ☐ Full-Time Student ☐ Part-Time Student ☐	ZIP CODE TELEPHONE (INCLUDE AREA CODE) ( )

9. OTHER INSURED'S NAME (Last Name, First Name, Middle Initial)	10. IS PATIENT'S CONDITION RELATED TO:	11. INSURED'S POLICY GROUP OR FECA NUMBER
a. OTHER INSURED'S POLICY OR GROUP NUMBER	a. EMPLOYMENT? (CURRENT OR PREVIOUS) ☐ YES ☐ NO	a. INSURED'S DATE OF BIRTH MM DD YY SEX M ☐ F ☐
b. OTHER INSURED'S DATE OF BIRTH MM DD YY SEX M ☐ F ☐	b. AUTO ACCIDENT? PLACE (State) ☐ YES ☐ NO	b. EMPLOYER'S NAME OR SCHOOL NAME
c. EMPLOYER'S NAME OR SCHOOL NAME	c. OTHER ACCIDENT? ☐ YES ☐ NO	c. INSURANCE PLAN NAME OR PROGRAM NAME
d. INSURANCE PLAN NAME OR PROGRAM NAME	10d. RESERVED FOR LOCAL USE	d. IS THERE ANOTHER HEALTH BENEFIT PLAN? ☐ YES ☐ NO If yes, return to and complete item 9 a – d.

READ BACK OF FORM BEFORE COMPLETING & SIGNING THIS FORM.
12. PATIENT'S OR AUTHORIZED PERSON'S SIGNATURE I authorize the release of any medical or other information necessary to process this claim. I also request payment of government benefits either to myself or to the party who accepts assignment below.

SIGNED _____ DATE _____

13. INSURED'S OR AUTHORIZED PERSON'S SIGNATURE I authorize payment of medical benefits to the undersigned physician or supplier for services described below.

SIGNED _____

PATIENT AND INSURED INFORMATION

14. DATE OF CURRENT: ILLNESS (First symptom) OR MM DD YY INJURY (Accident) OR PREGNANCY (LMP)	15. IF PATIENT HAS HAD SAME OR SIMILAR ILLNESS, GIVE FIRST DATE MM DD YY	16. DATES PATIENT UNABLE TO WORK IN CURRENT OCCUPATION MM DD YY MM DD YY FROM TO
17. NAME OF REFERRING PHYSICIAN OR OTHER SOURCE	17a. I.D. NUMBER OF REFERRING PHYSICIAN	18. HOSPITALIZATION DATES RELATED TO CURRENT SERVICES MM DD YY MM DD YY FROM TO
19. RESERVED FOR LOCAL USE		20. OUTSIDE LAB? $ CHARGES ☐ YES ☐ NO

21. DIAGNOSIS OR NATURE OF ILLNESS OR INJURY. (RELATE ITEMS 1, 2, 3, OR 4 TO ITEM 24E BY LINE)

1. |___|.|___| 3. |___|.|___|

2. |___|.|___| 4. |___|.|___|

22. MEDICAID RESUBMISSION CODE ORIGINAL REF. NO.
23. PRIOR AUTHORIZATION NUMBER

24. A DATE(S) OF SERVICE		B Place of Service	C Type of Service	D PROCEDURES, SERVICES, OR SUPPLIES (Explain Unusual Circumstances)		E DIAGNOSIS CODE	F $ CHARGES	G DAYS OR UNITS	H EPSDT Family Plan	I EMG	J COB	K RESERVED FOR LOCAL USE
From MM DD YY	To MM DD YY			CPT/HCPCS	MODIFIER							
1												
2												
3												
4												
5												
6												

25. FEDERAL TAX I.D. NUMBER SSN EIN ☐ ☐	26. PATIENT'S ACCOUNT NO.	27. ACCEPT ASSIGNMENT? (For govt. claims, see back) ☐ YES ☐ NO	28. TOTAL CHARGE $	29. AMOUNT PAID $	30. BALANCE DUE $

31. SIGNATURE OF PHYSICIAN OR SUPPLIER INCLUDING DEGREES OR CREDENTIALS (I certify that the statements on the reverse apply to this bill and are made a part thereof.) SIGNED DATE	32. NAME AND ADDRESS OF FACILITY WHERE SERVICES WERE RENDERED (If other than home or office)	33. PHYSICIAN'S SUPPLIER'S BILLING NAME, ADDRESS, ZIP CODE & PHONE # PIN# GRP#

PHYSICIAN OR SUPPLIER INFORMATION

(APPROVED BY AMA COUNCIL ON MEDICAL SERVICE 8/88)

PLEASE PRINT OR TYPE

FORM HCFA-1500 (12-90)
FORM OWCP-1500   FORM RRB-1500
FORM AMA OP050192

FORM 3

HEALTH INSURANCE CLAIM FORM

| | PICA | | | | | | PICA | |

1. MEDICARE	MEDICAID	CHAMPUS	CHAMPVA	GROUP HEALTH PLAN	FECA BLK LUNG	OTHER	1a. INSURED'S I.D. NUMBER	(FOR PROGRAM IN ITEM 1)
☐ (Medicare #)	☒ (Medicaid #)	☒ (Sponsor's SSN)	☐ (VA File #)	☐ (SSN or ID)	☐ (SSN)	☐ (ID)		

2. PATIENT'S NAME (Last Name, First Name, Middle Initial)
stuuesant Hoyt

3. PATIENT'S BIRTH DATE MM DD YY
12 13

SEX M ☒ F ☐

4. INSURED'S NAME (Last Name, First Name, Middle Initial)

5. PATIENT'S ADDRESS (No. Street)
11511 N. Illians St

6. PATIENT RELATIONSHIP TO INSURED
Self ☐ Spouse ☐ Child ☐ Other ☐

7. INSURED'S ADDRESS (No. Street)

CITY Amber **STATE** FN

8. PATIENT STATUS
Single ☐ Married ☐ Other ☒
Employed ☐ Full-Time Student ☐ Part-Time Student ☐

CITY **STATE**

ZIP CODE 46231 **TELEPHONE (Include Area Code)** ( )

ZIP CODE **TELEPHONE (INCLUDE AREA CODE)** ( )

9. OTHER INSURED'S NAME (Last Name, First Name, Middle Initial)

10. IS PATIENT'S CONDITION RELATED TO:

11. INSURED'S POLICY GROUP OR FECA NUMBER

a. OTHER INSURED'S POLICY OR GROUP NUMBER

a. EMPLOYMENT? (CURRENT OR PREVIOUS) ☐ YES ☐ NO

a. INSURED'S DATE OF BIRTH MM DD YY **SEX** M ☐ F ☐

b. OTHER INSURED'S DATE OF BIRTH MM DD YY **SEX** M ☐ F ☐

b. AUTO ACCIDENT? **PLACE (State)** ☐ YES ☐ NO

b. EMPLOYER'S NAME OR SCHOOL NAME

c. EMPLOYER'S NAME OR SCHOOL NAME

c. OTHER ACCIDENT? ☐ YES ☐ NO

c. INSURANCE PLAN NAME OR PROGRAM NAME

d. INSURANCE PLAN NAME OR PROGRAM NAME
medicare

10d. RESERVED FOR LOCAL USE

d. IS THERE ANOTHER HEALTH BENEFIT PLAN?
☐ YES ☐ NO If yes, return to and complete item 9 a – d.

READ BACK OF FORM BEFORE COMPLETING & SIGNING THIS FORM.

12. PATIENT'S OR AUTHORIZED PERSON'S SIGNATURE I authorize the release of any medical or other information necessary to process this claim. I also request payment of government benefits either to myself or to the party who accepts assignment below.

SIGNED _____ DATE _____

13. INSURED'S OR AUTHORIZED PERSON'S SIGNATURE I authorize payment of medical benefits to the undersigned physician or supplier for services described below.

SIGNED _____

14. DATE OF CURRENT: ILLNESS (First symptom) OR INJURY (Accident) OR PREGNANCY (LMP) MM DD YY

15. IF PATIENT HAS HAD SAME OR SIMILAR ILLNESS, GIVE FIRST DATE MM DD YY

16. DATES PATIENT UNABLE TO WORK IN CURRENT OCCUPATION MM DD YY FROM TO MM DD YY

17. NAME OF REFERRING PHYSICIAN OR OTHER SOURCE

17a. I.D. NUMBER OF REFERRING PHYSICIAN

18. HOSPITALIZATION DATES RELATED TO CURRENT SERVICES MM DD YY FROM TO MM DD YY

19. RESERVED FOR LOCAL USE

20. OUTSIDE LAB? ☐ YES ☐ NO **$ CHARGES**

21. DIAGNOSIS OR NATURE OF ILLNESS OR INJURY. (RELATE ITEMS 1, 2, 3, OR 4 TO ITEM 24E BY LINE)

1. ____.____
2. ____.____
3. ____.____
4. ____.____

22. MEDICAID RESUBMISSION CODE **ORIGINAL REF. NO.**

23. PRIOR AUTHORIZATION NUMBER

24. A DATE(S) OF SERVICE						B Place of Service	C Type of Service	D PROCEDURES, SERVICES, OR SUPPLIES (Explain Unusual Circumstances) CPT/HCPCS MODIFIER	E DIAGNOSIS CODE	F $ CHARGES	G DAYS OR UNITS	H EPSDT Family Plan	I EMG	J COB	K RESERVED FOR LOCAL USE
From MM	DD	YY	To MM	DD	YY										
1															
2															
3															
4															
5															
6															

25. FEDERAL TAX I.D. NUMBER SSN ☐ EIN ☐

26. PATIENT'S ACCOUNT NO.

27. ACCEPT ASSIGNMENT? (For govt. claims see back) ☐ YES ☐ NO

28. TOTAL CHARGE $

29. AMOUNT PAID $

30. BALANCE DUE $

31. SIGNATURE OF PHYSICIAN OR SUPPLIER INCLUDING DEGREES OR CREDENTIALS (I certify that the statements on the reverse apply to this bill and are made a part thereof.)

SIGNED _____ DATE _____

32. NAME AND ADDRESS OF FACILITY WHERE SERVICES WERE RENDERED (If other than home or office)

33. PHYSICIAN'S SUPPLIER'S BILLING NAME, ADDRESS, ZIP CODE & PHONE #

PIN# _____ GRP# _____

(APPROVED BY AMA COUNCIL ON MEDICAL SERVICE 8/88)

PLEASE PRINT OR TYPE

FORM HCFA-1500 (12-90)
FORM OWCP-1500 FORM RRB-1500
FORM AMA OP050192

FORM 4

APPROVED OMB-0938-0008

CARRIER

☐☐ PICA

HEALTH INSURANCE CLAIM FORM

PICA ☐☐

1.	MEDICARE	MEDICAID	CHAMPUS	CHAMPVA	GROUP HEALTH PLAN	FECA BLK LUNG	OTHER	1a. INSURED'S I.D. NUMBER	(FOR PROGRAM IN ITEM 1)
	☐ (Medicare #)	☐ (Medicaid #)	☐ (Sponsor's SSN)	☐ (VA File #)	☐ (SSN or ID)	☐ (SSN)	☐ (ID)		

2. PATIENT'S NAME (Last Name, First Name, Middle Initial)

3. PATIENT'S BIRTH DATE MM ☐ DD ☐ YY   SEX M ☐ F ☐

4. INSURED'S NAME (Last Name, First Name, Middle Initial)

5. PATIENT'S ADDRESS (No. Street)

6. PATIENT RELATIONSHIP TO INSURED   Self ☐ Spouse ☐ Child ☐ Other ☐

7. INSURED'S ADDRESS (No. Street)

CITY   STATE

8. PATIENT STATUS   Single ☐ Married ☐ Other ☐

CITY   STATE

ZIP CODE   TELEPHONE (Include Area Code) (   )

Employed ☐ Full-Time Student ☐ Part-Time Student ☐

ZIP CODE   TELEPHONE (INCLUDE AREA CODE) (   )

9. OTHER INSURED'S NAME (Last Name, First Name, Middle Initial)

10. IS PATIENT'S CONDITION RELATED TO:

11. INSURED'S POLICY GROUP OR FECA NUMBER

a. OTHER INSURED'S POLICY OR GROUP NUMBER

a. EMPLOYMENT? (CURRENT OR PREVIOUS) ☐ YES ☐ NO

a. INSURED'S DATE OF BIRTH MM ☐ DD ☐ YY   SEX M ☐ F ☐

b. OTHER INSURED'S DATE OF BIRTH MM ☐ DD ☐ YY   SEX M ☐ F ☐

b. AUTO ACCIDENT?   PLACE (State) ☐ YES ☐ NO

b. EMPLOYER'S NAME OR SCHOOL NAME

c. EMPLOYER'S NAME OR SCHOOL NAME

c. OTHER ACCIDENT? ☐ YES ☐ NO

c. INSURANCE PLAN NAME OR PROGRAM NAME

d. INSURANCE PLAN NAME OR PROGRAM NAME

10d. RESERVED FOR LOCAL USE

d. IS THERE ANOTHER HEALTH BENEFIT PLAN? ☐ YES ☐ NO   If yes, return to and complete item 9 a – d.

READ BACK OF FORM BEFORE COMPLETING & SIGNING THIS FORM.
12. PATIENT'S OR AUTHORIZED PERSON'S SIGNATURE I authorize the release of any medical or other information necessary to process this claim. I also request payment of government benefits either to myself or to the party who accepts assignment below.

SIGNED _____ DATE _____

13. INSURED'S OR AUTHORIZED PERSON'S SIGNATURE I authorize payment of medical benefits to the undersigned physician or supplier for services described below.

SIGNED _____

14. DATE OF CURRENT: MM ☐ DD ☐ YY ◄ ILLNESS (First symptom) OR INJURY (Accident) OR PREGNANCY (LMP)

15. IF PATIENT HAS HAD SAME OR SIMILAR ILLNESS, GIVE FIRST DATE MM ☐ DD ☐ YY

16. DATES PATIENT UNABLE TO WORK IN CURRENT OCCUPATION MM ☐ DD ☐ YY FROM   TO MM ☐ DD ☐ YY

17. NAME OF REFERRING PHYSICIAN OR OTHER SOURCE

17a. I.D. NUMBER OF REFERRING PHYSICIAN

18. HOSPITALIZATION DATES RELATED TO CURRENT SERVICES MM ☐ DD ☐ YY FROM   TO MM ☐ DD ☐ YY

19. RESERVED FOR LOCAL USE

20. OUTSIDE LAB? ☐ YES ☐ NO $ CHARGES

21. DIAGNOSIS OR NATURE OF ILLNESS OR INJURY. (RELATE ITEMS 1, 2, 3, OR 4 TO ITEM 24E BY LINE)

1. L___ . ___   3. L___ . ___

2. L___ . ___   4. L___ . ___

22. MEDICAID RESUBMISSION CODE   ORIGINAL REF. NO.

23. PRIOR AUTHORIZATION NUMBER

24. A DATE(S) OF SERVICE						B Place of Service	C Type of Service	D PROCEDURES, SERVICES, OR SUPPLIES (Explain Unusual Circumstances) CPT/HCPCS | MODIFIER	E DIAGNOSIS CODE	F $ CHARGES	G DAYS OR UNITS	H EPSDT Family Plan	I EMG	J COB	K RESERVED FOR LOCAL USE
From MM	DD	YY	To MM	DD	YY										
1															
2															
3															
4															
5															
6															

25. FEDERAL TAX I.D. NUMBER   SSN ☐ EIN ☐

26. PATIENT'S ACCOUNT NO.

27. ACCEPT ASSIGNMENT? (For govt. claims, see back) ☐ YES ☐ NO

28. TOTAL CHARGE $

29. AMOUNT PAID $

30. BALANCE DUE $

31. SIGNATURE OF PHYSICIAN OR SUPPLIER INCLUDING DEGREES OR CREDENTIALS (I certify that the statements on the reverse apply to this bill and are made a part thereof.)

SIGNED _____ DATE _____

32. NAME AND ADDRESS OF FACILITY WHERE SERVICES WERE RENDERED (If other than home or office)

33. PHYSICIAN'S SUPPLIER'S BILLING NAME, ADDRESS, ZIP CODE & PHONE #

PIN#   GRP#

PATIENT AND INSURED INFORMATION

PHYSICIAN OR SUPPLIER INFORMATION

(APPROVED BY AMA COUNCIL ON MEDICAL SERVICE 8/88)

PLEASE PRINT OR TYPE

FORM HCFA-1500 (12-90)
FORM OWCP-1500   FORM RRB-1500
FORM AMA OP050192

FORM 5

APPROVED OMB-0938-0008

CARRIER

HEALTH INSURANCE CLAIM FORM

PICA			PICA

1. MEDICARE MEDICAID CHAMPUS CHAMPVA GROUP HEALTH PLAN FECA BLK LUNG OTHER	1a. INSURED'S I.D. NUMBER (FOR PROGRAM IN ITEM 1)
☐ (Medicare #) ☐ (Medicaid #) ☐ (Sponsor's SSN) ☐ (VA File #) ☐ (SSN or ID) ☐ (SSN) ☐ (ID)	

2. PATIENT'S NAME (Last Name, First Name, Middle Initial)	3. PATIENT'S BIRTH DATE MM DD YY SEX M ☐ F ☐	4. INSURED'S NAME (Last Name, First Name, Middle Initial)

5. PATIENT'S ADDRESS (No. Street)	6. PATIENT RELATIONSHIP TO INSURED Self ☐ Spouse ☐ Child ☐ Other ☐	7. INSURED'S ADDRESS (No. Street)

CITY STATE	8. PATIENT STATUS Single ☐ Married ☐ Other ☐	CITY STATE

ZIP CODE TELEPHONE (Include Area Code) ( )	Employed ☐ Full-Time Student ☐ Part-Time Student ☐	ZIP CODE TELEPHONE (INCLUDE AREA CODE) ( )

9. OTHER INSURED'S NAME (Last Name, First Name, Middle Initial)	10. IS PATIENT'S CONDITION RELATED TO:	11. INSURED'S POLICY GROUP OR FECA NUMBER

a. OTHER INSURED'S POLICY OR GROUP NUMBER	a. EMPLOYMENT? (CURRENT OR PREVIOUS) ☐ YES ☐ NO	a. INSURED'S DATE OF BIRTH MM DD YY SEX M ☐ F ☐

b. OTHER INSURED'S DATE OF BIRTH MM DD YY SEX M ☐ F ☐	b. AUTO ACCIDENT? PLACE (State) ☐ YES ☐ NO	b. EMPLOYER'S NAME OR SCHOOL NAME

c. EMPLOYER'S NAME OR SCHOOL NAME	c. OTHER ACCIDENT? ☐ YES ☐ NO	c. INSURANCE PLAN NAME OR PROGRAM NAME

d. INSURANCE PLAN NAME OR PROGRAM NAME	10d. RESERVED FOR LOCAL USE	d. IS THERE ANOTHER HEALTH BENEFIT PLAN? ☐ YES ☐ NO If yes, return to and complete item 9 a – d.

READ BACK OF FORM BEFORE COMPLETING & SIGNING THIS FORM.

12. PATIENT'S OR AUTHORIZED PERSON'S SIGNATURE I authorize the release of any medical or other information necessary to process this claim. I also request payment of government benefits either to myself or to the party who accepts assignment below. SIGNED _____ DATE _____	13. INSURED'S OR AUTHORIZED PERSON'S SIGNATURE I authorize payment of medical benefits to the undersigned physician or supplier for services described below. SIGNED _____

14. DATE OF CURRENT: ILLNESS (First symptom) OR MM DD YY INJURY (Accident) OR PREGNANCY (LMP)	15. IF PATIENT HAS HAD SAME OR SIMILAR ILLNESS, GIVE FIRST DATE MM DD YY	16. DATES PATIENT UNABLE TO WORK IN CURRENT OCCUPATION MM DD YY MM DD YY FROM TO

17. NAME OF REFERRING PHYSICIAN OR OTHER SOURCE	17a. I.D. NUMBER OF REFERRING PHYSICIAN	18. HOSPITALIZATION DATES RELATED TO CURRENT SERVICES MM DD YY MM DD YY FROM TO

19. RESERVED FOR LOCAL USE	20. OUTSIDE LAB? $ CHARGES ☐ YES ☐ NO

21. DIAGNOSIS OR NATURE OF ILLNESS OR INJURY. (RELATE ITEMS 1, 2, 3, OR 4 TO ITEM 24E BY LINE) 1. ⌐ 3. ⌐ 2. ⌐ 4. ⌐	22. MEDICAID RESUBMISSION CODE ORIGINAL REF. NO.
	23. PRIOR AUTHORIZATION NUMBER

24. A DATE(S) OF SERVICE		B Place of Service	C Type of Service	D PROCEDURES, SERVICES, OR SUPPLIES (Explain Unusual Circumstances)		E DIAGNOSIS CODE	F $ CHARGES	G DAYS OR UNITS	H EPSDT Family Plan	I EMG	J COB	K RESERVED FOR LOCAL USE
From MM DD YY	To MM DD YY			CPT/HCPCS	MODIFIER							

25. FEDERAL TAX I.D. NUMBER SSN EIN ☐ ☐	26. PATIENT'S ACCOUNT NO.	27. ACCEPT ASSIGNMENT? (For govt. claims, see back) ☐ YES ☐ NO	28. TOTAL CHARGE $	29. AMOUNT PAID $	30. BALANCE DUE $

31. SIGNATURE OF PHYSICIAN OR SUPPLIER INCLUDING DEGREES OR CREDENTIALS (I certify that the statements on the reverse apply to this bill and are made a part thereof.) SIGNED _____ DATE _____	32. NAME AND ADDRESS OF FACILITY WHERE SERVICES WERE RENDERED (If other than home or office)	33. PHYSICIAN'S SUPPLIER'S BILLING NAME, ADDRESS, ZIP CODE & PHONE # PIN# GRP#

PATIENT AND INSURED INFORMATION

PHYSICIAN OR SUPPLIER INFORMATION

(APPROVED BY AMA COUNCIL ON MEDICAL SERVICE 8/88)

PLEASE PRINT OR TYPE

FORM HCFA-1500 (12-90)
FORM OWCP-1500 FORM RRB-1500
FORM AMA OP050192

FORM 6

APPROVED OMB-0938-0008

CARRIER

| | PICA | **HEALTH INSURANCE CLAIM FORM** | PICA | |

1. MEDICARE MEDICAID CHAMPUS CHAMPVA GROUP HEALTH PLAN FECA BLK LUNG OTHER
☐ (Medicare #) ☐ (Medicaid #) ☐ (Sponsor's SSN) ☐ (VA File #) ☐ (SSN or ID) ☐ (SSN) ☐ (ID)

1a. INSURED'S I.D. NUMBER (FOR PROGRAM IN ITEM 1)

2. PATIENT'S NAME (Last Name, First Name, Middle Initial)

3. PATIENT'S BIRTH DATE MM DD YY SEX M ☐ F ☐

4. INSURED'S NAME (Last Name, First Name, Middle Initial)

5. PATIENT'S ADDRESS (No. Street)

6. PATIENT RELATIONSHIP TO INSURED
Self ☐ Spouse ☐ Child ☐ Other ☐

7. INSURED'S ADDRESS (No. Street)

CITY STATE

8. PATIENT STATUS
Single ☐ Married ☐ Other ☐
Employed ☐ Full-Time Student ☐ Part-Time Student ☐

CITY STATE

ZIP CODE TELEPHONE (Include Area Code) ( )

ZIP CODE TELEPHONE (INCLUDE AREA CODE) ( )

9. OTHER INSURED'S NAME (Last Name, First Name, Middle Initial)

10. IS PATIENT'S CONDITION RELATED TO:

11. INSURED'S POLICY GROUP OR FECA NUMBER

a. OTHER INSURED'S POLICY OR GROUP NUMBER

a. EMPLOYMENT? (CURRENT OR PREVIOUS) ☐ YES ☐ NO

a. INSURED'S DATE OF BIRTH MM DD YY SEX M ☐ F ☐

b. OTHER INSURED'S DATE OF BIRTH MM DD YY SEX M ☐ F ☐

b. AUTO ACCIDENT? PLACE (State) ☐ YES ☐ NO

b. EMPLOYER'S NAME OR SCHOOL NAME

c. EMPLOYER'S NAME OR SCHOOL NAME

c. OTHER ACCIDENT? ☐ YES ☐ NO

c. INSURANCE PLAN NAME OR PROGRAM NAME

d. INSURANCE PLAN NAME OR PROGRAM NAME

10d. RESERVED FOR LOCAL USE

d. IS THERE ANOTHER HEALTH BENEFIT PLAN? ☐ YES ☐ NO If yes, return to and complete item 9 a – d.

READ BACK OF FORM BEFORE COMPLETING & SIGNING THIS FORM.
12. PATIENT'S OR AUTHORIZED PERSON'S SIGNATURE I authorize the release of any medical or other information necessary to process this claim. I also request payment of government benefits either to myself or to the party who accepts assignment below.

SIGNED _____ DATE _____

13. INSURED'S OR AUTHORIZED PERSON'S SIGNATURE I authorize payment of medical benefits to the undersigned physician or supplier for services described below.

SIGNED _____

PATIENT AND INSURED INFORMATION

14. DATE OF CURRENT: MM DD YY ◄ ILLNESS (First symptom) OR INJURY (Accident) OR PREGNANCY (LMP)

15. IF PATIENT HAS HAD SAME OR SIMILAR ILLNESS, GIVE FIRST DATE MM DD YY

16. DATES PATIENT UNABLE TO WORK IN CURRENT OCCUPATION MM DD YY MM DD YY FROM TO

17. NAME OF REFERRING PHYSICIAN OR OTHER SOURCE

17a. I.D. NUMBER OF REFERRING PHYSICIAN

18. HOSPITALIZATION DATES RELATED TO CURRENT SERVICES MM DD YY MM DD YY FROM TO

19. RESERVED FOR LOCAL USE

20. OUTSIDE LAB? ☐ YES ☐ NO $ CHARGES

21. DIAGNOSIS OR NATURE OF ILLNESS OR INJURY. (RELATE ITEMS 1, 2, 3, OR 4 TO ITEM 24E BY LINE)
1. L___ . ___ 3. L___ . ___
2. L___ . ___ 4. L___ . ___

22. MEDICAID RESUBMISSION CODE ORIGINAL REF. NO.

23. PRIOR AUTHORIZATION NUMBER

24.

A DATE(S) OF SERVICE						B Place of Service	C Type of Service	D PROCEDURES, SERVICES, OR SUPPLIES (Explain Unusual Circumstances)		E DIAGNOSIS CODE	F $ CHARGES	G DAYS OR UNITS	H EPSDT Family Plan	I EMG	J COB	K RESERVED FOR LOCAL USE
From MM	DD	YY	To MM	DD	YY			CPT/HCPCS	MODIFIER							
1																
2																
3																
4																
5																
6																

25. FEDERAL TAX I.D. NUMBER SSN ☐ EIN ☐

26. PATIENT'S ACCOUNT NO.

27. ACCEPT ASSIGNMENT? (For govt. claims, see back) ☐ YES ☐ NO

28. TOTAL CHARGE $

29. AMOUNT PAID $

30. BALANCE DUE $

31. SIGNATURE OF PHYSICIAN OR SUPPLIER INCLUDING DEGREES OR CREDENTIALS (I certify that the statements on the reverse apply to this bill and are made a part thereof.)

SIGNED _____ DATE _____

32. NAME AND ADDRESS OF FACILITY WHERE SERVICES WERE RENDERED (If other than home or office)

33. PHYSICIAN'S SUPPLIER'S BILLING NAME, ADDRESS, ZIP CODE & PHONE #

PIN# GRP#

PHYSICIAN OR SUPPLIER INFORMATION

(APPROVED BY AMA COUNCIL ON MEDICAL SERVICE 8/88) *PLEASE PRINT OR TYPE*

FORM HCFA-1500 (12-90)
FORM OWCP-1500 FORM RRB-1500
FORM AMA OP050192

FORM 7

SPOUSAL COVERAGE

PLEASE
DO NOT
STAPLE
IN THIS
AREA

CARRIER

HEALTH INSURANCE CLAIM FORM

| | PICA | | | | | | | | PICA | | |

1. MEDICARE	MEDICAID	CHAMPUS	CHAMPVA	GROUP HEALTH PLAN	FECA BLK LUNG	OTHER	1a. INSURED'S I.D. NUMBER	(FOR PROGRAM IN ITEM 1)
(Medicare #)	(Medicaid #)	(Sponsor's SSN)	(VA File #)	(SSN or ID)	(SSN)	(ID)		

2. PATIENT'S NAME (Last Name, First Name, Middle Initial)

3. PATIENT'S BIRTH DATE MM | DD | YY   SEX   M [ ]   F [ ]

4. INSURED'S NAME (Last Name, First Name, Middle Initial)

5. PATIENT'S ADDRESS (No. Street)

6. PATIENT RELATIONSHIP TO INSURED
Self [ ]   Spouse [ ]   Child [ ]   Other [ ]

7. INSURED'S ADDRESS (No. Street)

CITY   STATE

8. PATIENT STATUS
Single [ ]   Married [ ]   Other [ ]

CITY   STATE

ZIP CODE   TELEPHONE (Include Area Code)
(   )

Employed [ ]   Full-Time Student [ ]   Part-Time Student [ ]

ZIP CODE   TELEPHONE (INCLUDE AREA CODE)
(   )

9. OTHER INSURED'S NAME (Last Name, First Name, Middle Initial)
TJLLIS JANE P

10. IS PATIENT'S CONDITION RELATED TO:

11. INSURED'S POLICY GROUP OR FECA NUMBER

a. OTHER INSURED'S POLICY OR GROUP NUMBER
511-00-1398

a. EMPLOYMENT? (CURRENT OR PREVIOUS)
[ ] YES   [ ] NO

a. INSURED'S DATE OF BIRTH MM | DD | YY   SEX   M [ ]   F [ ]

b. OTHER INSURED'S DATE OF BIRTH
MM | DD | YY   03 | 09 | 10   M [ ]   F [X]

b. AUTO ACCIDENT?   PLACE (State)
[ ] YES   [ ] NO

b. EMPLOYER'S NAME OR SCHOOL NAME

c. EMPLOYER'S NAME OR SCHOOL NAME
IN BELL TEL. CO

c. OTHER ACCIDENT?
[ ] YES   [ ] NO

c. INSURANCE PLAN NAME OR PROGRAM NAME

d. INSURANCE PLAN NAME OR PROGRAM NAME
Goodman Ins Co.

10d. RESERVED FOR LOCAL USE

d. IS THERE ANOTHER HEALTH BENEFIT PLAN?
[X] YES   [ ] NO   If yes, return to and complete item 9 a – d.

READ BACK OF FORM BEFORE COMPLETING & SIGNING THIS FORM.
12. PATIENT'S OR AUTHORIZED PERSON'S SIGNATURE I authorize the release of any medical or other information necessary to process this claim. I also request payment of government benefits either to myself or to the party who accepts assignment below.

SIGNED _____   DATE _____

13. INSURED'S OR AUTHORIZED PERSON'S SIGNATURE I authorize payment of medical benefits to the undersigned physician or supplier for services described below.

SIGNED _____

PATIENT AND INSURED INFORMATION

FORM 8

APPROVED OMB-0938-0008

CARRIER

| | PICA | | |

HEALTH INSURANCE CLAIM FORM

PICA | | |

1. MEDICARE	MEDICAID	CHAMPUS	CHAMPVA	GROUP HEALTH PLAN	FECA BLK LUNG	OTHER	1a. INSURED'S I.D. NUMBER	(FOR PROGRAM IN ITEM 1)
☐ (Medicare #)	☐ (Medicaid #)	☐ (Sponsor's SSN)	☐ (VA File #)	☐ (SSN or ID)	☐ (SSN)	☐ (ID)		

2. PATIENT'S NAME (Last Name, First Name, Middle Initial)

3. PATIENT'S BIRTH DATE MM | DD | YY   SEX M ☐   F ☐

4. INSURED'S NAME (Last Name, First Name, Middle Initial)

5. PATIENT'S ADDRESS (No. Street)

6. PATIENT RELATIONSHIP TO INSURED Self ☐ Spouse ☐ Child ☐ Other ☐

7. INSURED'S ADDRESS (No. Street)

CITY   STATE

8. PATIENT STATUS Single ☐   Married ☐   Other ☐ Employed ☐   Full-Time Student ☐   Part-Time Student ☐

CITY   STATE

ZIP CODE   TELEPHONE (Include Area Code) (   )

ZIP CODE   TELEPHONE (INCLUDE AREA CODE) (   )

9. OTHER INSURED'S NAME (Last Name, First Name, Middle Initial)

10. IS PATIENT'S CONDITION RELATED TO:

11. INSURED'S POLICY GROUP OR FECA NUMBER

a. OTHER INSURED'S POLICY OR GROUP NUMBER

a. EMPLOYMENT? (CURRENT OR PREVIOUS) ☐ YES ☐ NO

a. INSURED'S DATE OF BIRTH MM | DD | YY   SEX M ☐   F ☐

b. OTHER INSURED'S DATE OF BIRTH MM | DD | YY   SEX M ☐   F ☐

b. AUTO ACCIDENT?   PLACE (State) ☐ YES ☐ NO

b. EMPLOYER'S NAME OR SCHOOL NAME

c. EMPLOYER'S NAME OR SCHOOL NAME

c. OTHER ACCIDENT? ☐ YES ☐ NO

c. INSURANCE PLAN NAME OR PROGRAM NAME

d. INSURANCE PLAN NAME OR PROGRAM NAME

10d. RESERVED FOR LOCAL USE

d. IS THERE ANOTHER HEALTH BENEFIT PLAN? ☐ YES ☐ NO   If yes, return to and complete item 9 a – d.

READ BACK OF FORM BEFORE COMPLETING & SIGNING THIS FORM.
12. PATIENT'S OR AUTHORIZED PERSON'S SIGNATURE I authorize the release of any medical or other information necessary to process this claim. I also request payment of government benefits either to myself or to the party who accepts assignment below.

SIGNED _____ DATE _____

13. INSURED'S OR AUTHORIZED PERSON'S SIGNATURE I authorize payment of medical benefits to the undersigned physician or supplier for services described below.

SIGNED _____

PATIENT AND INSURED INFORMATION

14. DATE OF CURRENT: ILLNESS (First symptom) OR INJURY (Accident) OR PREGNANCY (LMP) MM | DD | YY

15. IF PATIENT HAS HAD SAME OR SIMILAR ILLNESS, GIVE FIRST DATE MM | DD | YY

16. DATES PATIENT UNABLE TO WORK IN CURRENT OCCUPATION MM | DD | YY   FROM   TO MM | DD | YY

17. NAME OF REFERRING PHYSICIAN OR OTHER SOURCE

17a. I.D. NUMBER OF REFERRING PHYSICIAN

18. HOSPITALIZATION DATES RELATED TO CURRENT SERVICES MM | DD | YY FROM   TO MM | DD | YY

19. RESERVED FOR LOCAL USE

20. OUTSIDE LAB? ☐ YES ☐ NO $ CHARGES

21. DIAGNOSIS OR NATURE OF ILLNESS OR INJURY. (RELATE ITEMS 1, 2, 3, OR 4 TO ITEM 24E BY LINE)

1. └___ . ___
2. └___ . ___
3. └___ . ___
4. └___ . ___

22. MEDICAID RESUBMISSION CODE   ORIGINAL REF. NO.

23. PRIOR AUTHORIZATION NUMBER

24. A DATE(S) OF SERVICE						B Place of Service	C Type of Service	D PROCEDURES, SERVICES, OR SUPPLIES (Explain Unusual Circumstances) CPT/HCPCS MODIFIER	E DIAGNOSIS CODE	F $ CHARGES	G DAYS OR UNITS	H EPSDT Family Plan	I EMG	J COB	K RESERVED FOR LOCAL USE
From MM	DD	YY	To MM	DD	YY										
1															
2															
3															
4															
5															
6															

25. FEDERAL TAX I.D. NUMBER   SSN ☐ EIN ☐

26. PATIENT'S ACCOUNT NO.

27. ACCEPT ASSIGNMENT? (For govt. claims, see back) ☐ YES ☐ NO

28. TOTAL CHARGE $

29. AMOUNT PAID $

30. BALANCE DUE $

31. SIGNATURE OF PHYSICIAN OR SUPPLIER INCLUDING DEGREES OR CREDENTIALS (I certify that the statements on the reverse apply to this bill and are made a part thereof.)

SIGNED _____ DATE _____

32. NAME AND ADDRESS OF FACILITY WHERE SERVICES WERE RENDERED (If other than home or office)

33. PHYSICIAN'S SUPPLIER'S BILLING NAME, ADDRESS, ZIP CODE & PHONE #

PIN#   GRP#

PHYSICIAN OR SUPPLIER INFORMATION

(APPROVED BY AMA COUNCIL ON MEDICAL SERVICE 8/88)

PLEASE PRINT OR TYPE

FORM HCFA-1500 (12-90)
FORM OWCP-1500   FORM RRB-1500
FORM AMA OP050192

FORM 9

APPROVED OMB-0938-0008

□□□ PICA

HEALTH INSURANCE CLAIM FORM

PICA □□□

1.	MEDICARE	MEDICAID	CHAMPUS	CHAMPVA	GROUP HEALTH PLAN	FECA BLK LUNG	OTHER	1a. INSURED'S I.D. NUMBER (FOR PROGRAM IN ITEM 1)
	□ (Medicare #)	□ (Medicaid #)	□ (Sponsor's SSN)	□ (VA File #)	□ (SSN or ID)	□ (SSN)	□ (ID)	311-00-1398

2. PATIENT'S NAME (Last Name, First Name, Middle Initial)
TILLS JANE P

3. PATIENT'S BIRTH DATE   SEX
MM 11 | DD 2 | YY   M □ F □

4. INSURED'S NAME (Last Name, First Name, Middle Initial)
JANE P TILLS

5. PATIENT'S ADDRESS (No. Street)
1325 Mary Lane

6. PATIENT RELATIONSHIP TO INSURED
Self □ Spouse ☒ Child □ Other □

7. INSURED'S ADDRESS (No. Street)
SAME

CITY
Indpls
STATE
IN

8. PATIENT STATUS
Single □ Married ☒ Other □

Employed ☒ Full-Time Student □ Part-Time Student □

CITY
STATE

ZIP CODE
49213

TELEPHONE (Include Area Code)
(   )

ZIP CODE

TELEPHONE (INCLUDE AREA CODE)
(   )

9. OTHER INSURED'S NAME (Last Name, First Name, Middle Initial)
TILLS ROBERT R

10. IS PATIENT'S CONDITION RELATED TO:

11. INSURED'S POLICY GROUP OR FECA NUMBER

a. OTHER INSURED'S POLICY OR GROUP NUMBER

a. EMPLOYMENT? (CURRENT OR PREVIOUS)
□ YES ☒ NO

a. INSURED'S DATE OF BIRTH
MM | DD | YY
03 | 09 |
SEX
M □ F ☒

b. OTHER INSURED'S DATE OF BIRTH
MM 11 | DD 21 | YY   SEX M ☒ F □

b. AUTO ACCIDENT?   PLACE (State)
□ YES ☒ NO

b. EMPLOYER'S NAME OR SCHOOL NAME
IN BELL TEL. CO

c. EMPLOYER'S NAME OR SCHOOL NAME
KIEBER'S CANDY CO

c. OTHER ACCIDENT?
□ YES ☒ NO

c. INSURANCE PLAN NAME OR PROGRAM NAME

d. INSURANCE PLAN NAME OR PROGRAM NAME
HEART INS. CO.

10d. RESERVED FOR LOCAL USE
SEE ATTACHED EOB

d. IS THERE ANOTHER HEALTH BENEFIT PLAN?
☒ YES □ NO   If yes, return to and complete item 9 a – d.

READ BACK OF FORM BEFORE COMPLETING & SIGNING THIS FORM.
12. PATIENT'S OR AUTHORIZED PERSON'S SIGNATURE I authorize the release of any medical or other information necessary to process this claim. I also request payment of government benefits either to myself or to the party who accepts assignment below.

SIGNED JANE P TILLS   DATE 01-12-09

13. INSURED'S OR AUTHORIZED PERSON'S SIGNATURE I authorize payment of medical benefits to the undersigned physician or supplier for services described below.

SIGNED SIGNATURE ON FILE

14. DATE OF CURRENT:
MM | DD | YY
◄ ILLNESS (First symptom) OR INJURY (Accident) OR PREGNANCY (LMP)

15. IF PATIENT HAS HAD SAME OR SIMILAR ILLNESS, GIVE FIRST DATE MM | DD | YY

16. DATES PATIENT UNABLE TO WORK IN CURRENT OCCUPATION
MM | DD | YY   MM | DD | YY
FROM   TO

17. NAME OF REFERRING PHYSICIAN OR OTHER SOURCE
JAMES P. CARTMAN, M.D

17a. I.D. NUMBER OF REFERRING PHYSICIAN
99-9999999

18. HOSPITALIZATION DATES RELATED TO CURRENT SERVICES
MM | DD | YY   MM | DD | YY
FROM   TO

19. RESERVED FOR LOCAL USE

20. OUTSIDE LAB? $ CHARGES
□ YES □ NO

21. DIAGNOSIS OR NATURE OF ILLNESS OR INJURY. (RELATE ITEMS 1, 2, 3, OR 4 TO ITEM 24E BY LINE)

1. 99245

3. └___.___

2. └___.___

4. └___.___

22. MEDICAID RESUBMISSION
CODE   ORIGINAL REF. NO.

23. PRIOR AUTHORIZATION NUMBER

24. A DATE(S) OF SERVICE						B Place of Service	C Type of Service	D PROCEDURES, SERVICES, OR SUPPLIES (Explain Unusual Circumstances) CPT/HCPCS	MODIFIER	E DIAGNOSIS CODE	F $ CHARGES	G DAYS OR UNITS	H EPSDT Family Plan	I EMG	J COB	K RESERVED FOR LOCAL USE
	From MM	DD	YY	To MM	DD	YY											
1	04	18	10				11		99245		1,2	200 00	1				
2																
3																
4																
5																
6																

25. FEDERAL TAX I.D. NUMBER   SSN □ EIN ☒
99-9999999

26. PATIENT'S ACCOUNT NO.

27. ACCEPT ASSIGNMENT? (For govt. claims, see back)
□ YES □ NO

28. TOTAL CHARGE
$ 200.00

29. AMOUNT PAID
$ 128.00

30. BALANCE DUE
$ 72.00

31. SIGNATURE OF PHYSICIAN OR SUPPLIER INCLUDING DEGREES OR CREDENTIALS
(I certify that the statements on the reverse apply to this bill and are made a part thereof.)

SIGNED JAMES D CARTMAN, MD   DATE 01/12/0

32. NAME AND ADDRESS OF FACILITY WHERE SERVICES WERE RENDERED (If other than home or office)

33. PHYSICIAN'S SUPPLIER'S BILLING NAME, ADDRESS, ZIP CODE & PHONE #
James P Cartman
3733 Professional Dr
Indpls, IN 46260

PIN#   GRP#

(APPROVED BY AMA COUNCIL ON MEDICAL SERVICE 8/88)

PLEASE PRINT OR TYPE

FORM HCFA-1500 (12-90)
FORM OWCP-1500   FORM RRB-1500
FORM AMA OP050192

FORM 10

Genral Insurance Co.
1010 South Way
Bloomington, IN 44313-9010

EXPLANATION OF BENEFITS

Service	Dates	Charge	Covered Expense @ 70%	Not Covered
Colposcopy with Biopsy	06/03/--	$320.00	$224.00	

Totals:	$320.00
Copay and/or Deductible:	0.00
Balance:	0.00
Payable @	70%
Benefit:	$224.00

Provider:

Medical and Dental Associates, P.C.
3733 Professional Drive, #300
Indianapolis, IN 46260

Employee:

Mrs. Ai Vang
9 Peace Lane
White Bear, IN 45110

ID#:

301984040-1515

Claim No.:

06687

Policy No.:

1515-9083W

FORM 11

APPROVED OMB-0938-0008

CARRIER

HEALTH INSURANCE CLAIM FORM

| PICA | | PICA |

1. MEDICARE ☐ (Medicare #)   MEDICAID ☐ (Medicaid #)   CHAMPUS ☐ (Sponsor's SSN)   CHAMPVA ☐ (VA File #)   GROUP HEALTH PLAN ☐ (SSN or ID)   FECA BLK LUNG ☐ (SSN)   OTHER ☐ (ID)

1a. INSURED'S I.D. NUMBER   (FOR PROGRAM IN ITEM 1)

2. PATIENT'S NAME (Last Name, First Name, Middle Initial)

3. PATIENT'S BIRTH DATE   MM ☐ DD ☐ YY   SEX   M ☐ F ☐

4. INSURED'S NAME (Last Name, First Name, Middle Initial)

5. PATIENT'S ADDRESS (No. Street)

6. PATIENT RELATIONSHIP TO INSURED   Self ☐   Spouse ☐   Child ☐   Other ☐

7. INSURED'S ADDRESS (No. Street)

CITY   STATE

8. PATIENT STATUS   Single ☐   Married ☐   Other ☐

CITY   STATE

ZIP CODE   TELEPHONE (Include Area Code) ( )

Employed ☐   Full-Time Student ☐   Part-Time Student ☐

ZIP CODE   TELEPHONE (INCLUDE AREA CODE) ( )

9. OTHER INSURED'S NAME (Last Name, First Name, Middle Initial)

10. IS PATIENT'S CONDITION RELATED TO:

11. INSURED'S POLICY GROUP OR FECA NUMBER

a. OTHER INSURED'S POLICY OR GROUP NUMBER

a. EMPLOYMENT? (CURRENT OR PREVIOUS) ☐ YES ☐ NO

a. INSURED'S DATE OF BIRTH   MM ☐ DD ☐ YY   SEX   M ☐ F ☐

b. OTHER INSURED'S DATE OF BIRTH   MM ☐ DD ☐ YY   SEX   M ☐ F ☐

b. AUTO ACCIDENT?   PLACE (State) ☐ YES ☐ NO

b. EMPLOYER'S NAME OR SCHOOL NAME

c. EMPLOYER'S NAME OR SCHOOL NAME

c. OTHER ACCIDENT? ☐ YES ☐ NO

c. INSURANCE PLAN NAME OR PROGRAM NAME

d. INSURANCE PLAN NAME OR PROGRAM NAME

10d. RESERVED FOR LOCAL USE

d. IS THERE ANOTHER HEALTH BENEFIT PLAN? ☐ YES ☐ NO   If yes, return to and complete item 9 a – d.

READ BACK OF FORM BEFORE COMPLETING & SIGNING THIS FORM.
12. PATIENT'S OR AUTHORIZED PERSON'S SIGNATURE. I authorize the release of any medical or other information necessary to process this claim. I also request payment of government benefits either to myself or to the party who accepts assignment below.

SIGNED _____ DATE _____

13. INSURED'S OR AUTHORIZED PERSON'S SIGNATURE. I authorize payment of medical benefits to the undersigned physician or supplier for services described below.

SIGNED _____

PATIENT AND INSURED INFORMATION

14. DATE OF CURRENT: MM ☐ DD ☐ YY   ◄ ILLNESS (First symptom) OR INJURY (Accident) OR PREGNANCY (LMP)

15. IF PATIENT HAS HAD SAME OR SIMILAR ILLNESS, GIVE FIRST DATE   MM ☐ DD ☐ YY

16. DATES PATIENT UNABLE TO WORK IN CURRENT OCCUPATION   MM ☐ DD ☐ YY   FROM   TO   MM ☐ DD ☐ YY

17. NAME OF REFERRING PHYSICIAN OR OTHER SOURCE

17a. I.D. NUMBER OF REFERRING PHYSICIAN

18. HOSPITALIZATION DATES RELATED TO CURRENT SERVICES   MM ☐ DD ☐ YY   FROM   TO   MM ☐ DD ☐ YY

19. RESERVED FOR LOCAL USE

20. OUTSIDE LAB? ☐ YES ☐ NO $ CHARGES

21. DIAGNOSIS OR NATURE OF ILLNESS OR INJURY. (RELATE ITEMS 1, 2, 3, OR 4 TO ITEM 24E BY LINE)

1. ☐____.__   3. ☐____.__

2. ☐____.__   4. ☐____.__

22. MEDICAID RESUBMISSION CODE   ORIGINAL REF. NO.

23. PRIOR AUTHORIZATION NUMBER

24. A DATE(S) OF SERVICE						B Place of Service	C Type of Service	D PROCEDURES, SERVICES, OR SUPPLIES (Explain Unusual Circumstances) CPT/HCPCS MODIFIER	E DIAGNOSIS CODE	F $ CHARGES	G DAYS OR UNITS	H EPSDT Family Plan	I EMG	J COB	K RESERVED FOR LOCAL USE
From MM	DD	YY	To MM	DD	YY										
1															
2															
3															
4															
5															
6															

25. FEDERAL TAX I.D. NUMBER   SSN ☐ EIN ☐

26. PATIENT'S ACCOUNT NO.

27. ACCEPT ASSIGNMENT? (For govt. claims, see back) ☐ YES ☐ NO

28. TOTAL CHARGE $

29. AMOUNT PAID $

30. BALANCE DUE $

31. SIGNATURE OF PHYSICIAN OR SUPPLIER INCLUDING DEGREES OR CREDENTIALS (I certify that the statements on the reverse apply to this bill and are made a part thereof.)

SIGNED _____ DATE _____

32. NAME AND ADDRESS OF FACILITY WHERE SERVICES WERE RENDERED (If other than home or office)

33. PHYSICIAN'S SUPPLIER'S BILLING NAME, ADDRESS, ZIP CODE & PHONE #

PIN#   GRP#

PHYSICIAN OR SUPPLIER INFORMATION

(APPROVED BY AMA COUNCIL ON MEDICAL SERVICE 8/88)

PLEASE PRINT OR TYPE

FORM HCFA-1500 (12-90)
FORM OWCP-1500   FORM RRB-1500
FORM AMA OP050192

FORM 12

Part Five   Numbered Forms and Worksheets

APPROVED OMB-0938-0008

Good Golds Inc.Co
8900 W tree Lane
Chicago, IL
60606

CARRIER

| | PICA | | **HEALTH INSURANCE CLAIM FORM** | PICA | | |

1. MEDICARE MEDICAID CHAMPUS CHAMPVA	GROUP HEALTH PLAN	FECA BLK LUNG	OTHER	1a. INSURED'S I.D. NUMBER (FOR PROGRAM IN ITEM 1)
☐ (Medicare #) ☐ (Medicaid #) ☐ (Sponsor's SSN) ☐ (VA File #)	☐ (SSN or ID)	☐ (SSN)	☐ (ID)	484-91-1688

2. PATIENT'S NAME (Last Name, First Name, Middle Initial)	3. PATIENT'S BIRTH DATE	SEX	4. INSURED'S NAME (Last Name, First Name, Middle Initial)
Jr. Moyer James X	MM 09 DD 59 YY	M ☒ F ☐	Sr, moyer James

5. PATIENT'S ADDRESS (No. Street)	6. PATIENT RELATIONSHIP TO INSURED	7. INSURED'S ADDRESS (No. Street)
14 Crowe Dr	Self ☐ Spouse ☐ Child ☒ Other ☐	same

CITY	STATE	8. PATIENT STATUS	CITY	STATE
Beechline	TN	Single ☒ Married ☐ Other ☐		

ZIP CODE	TELEPHONE (Include Area Code)		ZIP CODE	TELEPHONE (INCLUDE AREA CODE)
47888	( )	Employed ☐ Full-Time Student ☒ Part-Time Student ☐		( )

9. OTHER INSURED'S NAME (Last Name, First Name, Middle Initial)	10. IS PATIENT'S CONDITION RELATED TO:	11. INSURED'S POLICY GROUP OR FECA NUMBER
moyer Charolette		30668

a. OTHER INSURED'S POLICY OR GROUP NUMBER	a. EMPLOYMENT? (CURRENT OR PREVIOUS)	a. INSURED'S DATE OF BIRTH SEX
400-12-1344	☐ YES ☒ NO	MM 4 DD 10 YY M ☒ F ☐

b. OTHER INSURED'S DATE OF BIRTH SEX	b. AUTO ACCIDENT? PLACE (State)	b. EMPLOYER'S NAME OR SCHOOL NAME
MM 10 DD 11 YY M ☐ F ☒	☐ YES ☒ NO	North Bank

c. EMPLOYER'S NAME OR SCHOOL NAME	c. OTHER ACCIDENT?	c. INSURANCE PLAN NAME OR PROGRAM NAME
County Tyme	☐ YES ☒ NO	Good Gold Inc.

d. INSURANCE PLAN NAME OR PROGRAM NAME	10d. RESERVED FOR LOCAL USE	d. IS THERE ANOTHER HEALTH BENEFIT PLAN?
Elreed Inc. Co		☒ YES ☐ NO If yes, return to and complete item 9 a – d.

READ BACK OF FORM BEFORE COMPLETING & SIGNING THIS FORM.

12. PATIENT'S OR AUTHORIZED PERSON'S SIGNATURE I authorize the release of any medical or other information necessary to process this claim. I also request payment of government benefits either to myself or to the party who accepts assignment below.	13. INSURED'S OR AUTHORIZED PERSON'S SIGNATURE I authorize payment of medical benefits to the undersigned physician or supplier for services described below.
SIGNED Signature on file DATE 01-12-07	SIGNED Signature on file

PATIENT AND INSURED INFORMATION

FORM 13

APPROVED OMB-0938-0008

PLEASE
DO NOT
STAPLE
IN THIS
AREA

HEALTH INSURANCE CLAIM FORM

PICA [ ][ ]

PICA [ ][ ]

1. MEDICARE · MEDICAID CHAMPUS CHAMPVA GROUP HEALTH PLAN FECA BLK LUNG OTHER	1a. INSURED'S I.D. NUMBER (FOR PROGRAM IN ITEM 1)
[ ] (Medicare #) [ ] (Medicaid #) [ ] (Sponsor's SSN) [ ] (VA File #) [ ] (SSN or ID) [ ] (SSN) [ ] (ID)	

2. PATIENT'S NAME (Last Name, First Name, Middle Initial)

3. PATIENT'S BIRTH DATE MM DD YY   SEX   M [ ] F [ ]

4. INSURED'S NAME (Last Name, First Name, Middle Initial)

5. PATIENT'S ADDRESS (No. Street)

6. PATIENT RELATIONSHIP TO INSURED
Self [ ] Spouse [ ] Child [ ] Other [ ]

7. INSURED'S ADDRESS (No. Street)

CITY   STATE

8. PATIENT STATUS
Single [ ] Married [ ] Other [ ]
Employed [ ] Full-Time Student [ ] Part-Time Student [ ]

CITY   STATE

ZIP CODE   TELEPHONE (Include Area Code)
( )

ZIP CODE   TELEPHONE (INCLUDE AREA CODE)
( )

9. OTHER INSURED'S NAME (Last Name, First Name, Middle Initial)

10. IS PATIENT'S CONDITION RELATED TO:

11. INSURED'S POLICY GROUP OR FECA NUMBER

a. OTHER INSURED'S POLICY OR GROUP NUMBER

a. EMPLOYMENT? (CURRENT OR PREVIOUS)
YES [ ] NO [ ]

a. INSURED'S DATE OF BIRTH MM DD YY   SEX M [ ] F [ ]

b. OTHER INSURED'S DATE OF BIRTH MM DD YY   SEX M [ ] F [ ]

b. AUTO ACCIDENT?   PLACE (State)
YES [ ] NO [ ]

b. EMPLOYER'S NAME OR SCHOOL NAME

c. EMPLOYER'S NAME OR SCHOOL NAME

c. OTHER ACCIDENT?
YES [ ] NO [ ]

c. INSURANCE PLAN NAME OR PROGRAM NAME

d. INSURANCE PLAN NAME OR PROGRAM NAME

10d. RESERVED FOR LOCAL USE

d. IS THERE ANOTHER HEALTH BENEFIT PLAN?
YES [ ] NO [ ] If yes, return to and complete item 9 a – d.

READ BACK OF FORM BEFORE COMPLETING & SIGNING THIS FORM.
12. PATIENT'S OR AUTHORIZED PERSON'S SIGNATURE I authorize the release of any medical or other information necessary to process this claim. I also request payment of government benefits either to myself or to the party who accepts assignment below.

SIGNED _____   DATE _____

13. INSURED'S OR AUTHORIZED PERSON'S SIGNATURE I authorize payment of medical benefits to the undersigned physician or supplier for services described below.

SIGNED _____

14. DATE OF CURRENT: MM DD YY ◄ ILLNESS (First symptom) OR INJURY (Accident) OR PREGNANCY (LMP)

15. IF PATIENT HAS HAD SAME OR SIMILAR ILLNESS, GIVE FIRST DATE MM DD YY

16. DATES PATIENT UNABLE TO WORK IN CURRENT OCCUPATION MM DD YY MM DD YY
FROM   TO

17. NAME OF REFERRING PHYSICIAN OR OTHER SOURCE

17a. I.D. NUMBER OF REFERRING PHYSICIAN

18. HOSPITALIZATION DATES RELATED TO CURRENT SERVICES MM DD YY MM DD YY
FROM   TO

19. RESERVED FOR LOCAL USE

20. OUTSIDE LAB? $ CHARGES
YES [ ] NO [ ]

21. DIAGNOSIS OR NATURE OF ILLNESS OR INJURY. (RELATE ITEMS 1, 2, 3, OR 4 TO ITEM 24E BY LINE)
1. |__.__| 3. |__.__|
2. |__.__| 4. |__.__|

22. MEDICAID RESUBMISSION CODE   ORIGINAL REF. NO.

23. PRIOR AUTHORIZATION NUMBER

24. A DATE(S) OF SERVICE		B Place of Service	C Type of Service	D PROCEDURES, SERVICES, OR SUPPLIES (Explain Unusual Circumstances) CPT/HCPCS MODIFIER	E DIAGNOSIS CODE	F $ CHARGES	G DAYS OR UNITS	H EPSDT Family Plan	I EMG	J COB	K RESERVED FOR LOCAL USE
From MM DD YY	To MM DD YY										
1											
2											
3											
4											
5											
6											

25. FEDERAL TAX I.D. NUMBER   SSN [ ] EIN [ ]

26. PATIENT'S ACCOUNT NO.

27. ACCEPT ASSIGNMENT? (For govt. claims, see back) YES [ ] NO [ ]

28. TOTAL CHARGE $

29. AMOUNT PAID $

30. BALANCE DUE $

31. SIGNATURE OF PHYSICIAN OR SUPPLIER INCLUDING DEGREES OR CREDENTIALS (I certify that the statements on the reverse apply to this bill and are made a part thereof.)

SIGNED _____   DATE _____

32. NAME AND ADDRESS OF FACILITY WHERE SERVICES WERE RENDERED (if other than home or office)

33. PHYSICIAN'S SUPPLIER'S BILLING NAME, ADDRESS, ZIP CODE & PHONE #

PIN#   GRP#

(APPROVED BY AMA COUNCIL ON MEDICAL SERVICE 8/88)

PLEASE PRINT OR TYPE

FORM HCFA-1500 (12-90)
FORM OWCP-1500   FORM RRB-1500
FORM AMA OP050192

FORM 14

Part Five Numbered Forms and Worksheets

EXPLANATION OF BENEFITS
EOB

Hooks Drug Company
845 W. 38th St.
Indianapolis, IN 46222
Group#:   Hook 241

Subscriber: Mr. Kareem Mobutuu
                         315 W. 91st St.
                         Indianapolis, IN 46240

Patient: Miss Aleeshaa Mobutuu

ID#:   61438QR9

Provider: Dr. Harold Beckerman
                         Medical and Dental Associates, P.C.
                         3733 Professional Drive #300
                         Indianapolis, IN 46260

EIN#:   99-9999999

Service:	99213	Plan pays:	$50.00
	71015		
Fee:	$85.00	Co-Insurance:	$35.00
Date:	7/8/--	Total Benefit:	$50.00
Claim No:	3711468	Check No:	C433218

FORM 15

APPROVED OMB-0938-0008

CARRIER

HEALTH INSURANCE CLAIM FORM

PICA □□□

□□ PICA

1. MEDICARE	MEDICAID	CHAMPUS	CHAMPVA	GROUP HEALTH PLAN	FECA BLK LUNG	OTHER	1a. INSURED'S I.D. NUMBER (FOR PROGRAM IN ITEM 1)
□ (Medicare #)	□ (Medicaid #)	□ (Sponsor's SSN)	□ (VA File #)	□ (SSN or ID)	□ (SSN)	□ (ID)	

2. PATIENT'S NAME (Last Name, First Name, Middle Initial)

3. PATIENT'S BIRTH DATE
MM | DD | YY   SEX   M □ F □

4. INSURED'S NAME (Last Name, First Name, Middle Initial)

5. PATIENT'S ADDRESS (No. Street)

6. PATIENT RELATIONSHIP TO INSURED
Self □   Spouse □   Child □   Other □

7. INSURED'S ADDRESS (No. Street)

CITY   STATE

8. PATIENT STATUS
Single □   Married □   Other □
Employed □   Full-Time Student □   Part-Time Student □

CITY   STATE

ZIP CODE   TELEPHONE (Include Area Code)
(   )

ZIP CODE   TELEPHONE (INCLUDE AREA CODE)
(   )

9. OTHER INSURED'S NAME (Last Name, First Name, Middle Initial)

10. IS PATIENT'S CONDITION RELATED TO:

11. INSURED'S POLICY GROUP OR FECA NUMBER

a. OTHER INSURED'S POLICY OR GROUP NUMBER

a. EMPLOYMENT? (CURRENT OR PREVIOUS)
□ YES   □ NO

a. INSURED'S DATE OF BIRTH
MM | DD | YY   SEX   M □ F □

b. OTHER INSURED'S DATE OF BIRTH
MM | DD | YY   SEX   M □ F □

b. AUTO ACCIDENT?   PLACE (State)
□ YES   □ NO

b. EMPLOYER'S NAME OR SCHOOL NAME

c. EMPLOYER'S NAME OR SCHOOL NAME

c. OTHER ACCIDENT?
□ YES   □ NO

c. INSURANCE PLAN NAME OR PROGRAM NAME

d. INSURANCE PLAN NAME OR PROGRAM NAME

10d. RESERVED FOR LOCAL USE

d. IS THERE ANOTHER HEALTH BENEFIT PLAN?
□ YES   □ NO   If yes, return to and complete item 9 a – d.

READ BACK OF FORM BEFORE COMPLETING & SIGNING THIS FORM.
12. PATIENT'S OR AUTHORIZED PERSON'S SIGNATURE I authorize the release of any medical or other information necessary to process this claim. I also request payment of government benefits either to myself or to the party who accepts assignment below.

SIGNED _____   DATE _____

13. INSURED'S OR AUTHORIZED PERSON'S SIGNATURE I authorize payment of medical benefits to the undersigned physician or supplier for services described below.

SIGNED _____

PATIENT AND INSURED INFORMATION

14. DATE OF CURRENT: ILLNESS (First symptom) OR
MM | DD | YY   INJURY (Accident) OR
PREGNANCY (LMP)

15. IF PATIENT HAS HAD SAME OR SIMILAR ILLNESS,
GIVE FIRST DATE   MM | DD | YY

16. DATES PATIENT UNABLE TO WORK IN CURRENT OCCUPATION
MM | DD | YY   MM | DD | YY
FROM   TO

17. NAME OF REFERRING PHYSICIAN OR OTHER SOURCE

17a. I.D. NUMBER OF REFERRING PHYSICIAN

18. HOSPITALIZATION DATES RELATED TO CURRENT SERVICES
MM | DD | YY   MM | DD | YY
FROM   TO

19. RESERVED FOR LOCAL USE

20. OUTSIDE LAB? $ CHARGES
□ YES   □ NO

21. DIAGNOSIS OR NATURE OF ILLNESS OR INJURY. (RELATE ITEMS 1, 2, 3, OR 4 TO ITEM 24E BY LINE)

1. |___|.|__| 3. |___|.|__|

2. |___|.|__| 4. |___|.|__|

22. MEDICAID RESUBMISSION
CODE   ORIGINAL REF. NO.

23. PRIOR AUTHORIZATION NUMBER

24. A DATE(S) OF SERVICE						B Place of Service	C Type of Service	D PROCEDURES, SERVICES, OR SUPPLIES (Explain Unusual Circumstances) CPT/HCPCS MODIFIER	E DIAGNOSIS CODE	F $ CHARGES	G DAYS OR UNITS	H EPSDT Family Plan	I EMG	J COB	K RESERVED FOR LOCAL USE
From MM	DD	YY	To MM	DD	YY										
1															
2															
3															
4															
5															
6															

25. FEDERAL TAX I.D. NUMBER   SSN □ EIN □

26. PATIENT'S ACCOUNT NO.

27. ACCEPT ASSIGNMENT?
(For govt. claims, see back)
□ YES   □ NO

28. TOTAL CHARGE
$

29. AMOUNT PAID
$

30. BALANCE DUE
$

31. SIGNATURE OF PHYSICIAN OR SUPPLIER INCLUDING DEGREES OR CREDENTIALS
(I certify that the statements on the reverse apply to this bill and are made a part thereof.)

SIGNED _____   DATE _____

32. NAME AND ADDRESS OF FACILITY WHERE SERVICES WERE RENDERED (If other than home or office)

33. PHYSICIAN'S SUPPLIER'S BILLING NAME, ADDRESS, ZIP CODE & PHONE #

PIN#   GRP#

PHYSICIAN OR SUPPLIER INFORMATION

(APPROVED BY AMA COUNCIL ON MEDICAL SERVICE 8/88)

PLEASE PRINT OR TYPE

FORM HCFA-1500 (12-90)
FORM OWCP-1500   FORM RRB-1500
FORM AMA OP050192

FORM 16

Part Five Numbered Forms and Worksheets

APPROVED OMB-0938-0008

CARRIER

| | PICA | **HEALTH INSURANCE CLAIM FORM** | PICA | |

| 1. MEDICARE | MEDICAID | CHAMPUS | CHAMPVA | GROUP HEALTH PLAN | FECA BLK LUNG | OTHER | 1a. INSURED'S I.D. NUMBER | (FOR PROGRAM IN ITEM 1) |
| (Medicare #) | (Medicaid #) | (Sponsor's SSN) | (VA File #) | (SSN or ID) | (SSN) | (ID) | | |

2. PATIENT'S NAME (Last Name, First Name, Middle Initial)

3. PATIENT'S BIRTH DATE
MM | DD | YY   SEX   M ☐ F ☐

4. INSURED'S NAME (Last Name, First Name, Middle Initial)

5. PATIENT'S ADDRESS (No. Street)

6. PATIENT RELATIONSHIP TO INSURED
Self ☐ Spouse ☐ Child ☐ Other ☐

7. INSURED'S ADDRESS (No. Street)

CITY   STATE

8. PATIENT STATUS
Single ☐   Married ☐   Other ☐

CITY   STATE

ZIP CODE   TELEPHONE (Include Area Code)
(   )

Employed ☐ Full-Time Student ☐ Part-Time Student ☐

ZIP CODE   TELEPHONE (INCLUDE AREA CODE)
(   )

9. OTHER INSURED'S NAME (Last Name, First Name, Middle Initial)

10. IS PATIENT'S CONDITION RELATED TO:

11. INSURED'S POLICY GROUP OR FECA NUMBER

a. OTHER INSURED'S POLICY OR GROUP NUMBER

a. EMPLOYMENT? (CURRENT OR PREVIOUS)
☐ YES ☐ NO

a. INSURED'S DATE OF BIRTH
MM | DD | YY   SEX   M ☐ F ☐

b. OTHER INSURED'S DATE OF BIRTH
MM | DD | YY   SEX M ☐ F ☐

b. AUTO ACCIDENT?   PLACE (State)
☐ YES ☐ NO

b. EMPLOYER'S NAME OR SCHOOL NAME

c. EMPLOYER'S NAME OR SCHOOL NAME

c. OTHER ACCIDENT?
☐ YES ☐ NO

c. INSURANCE PLAN NAME OR PROGRAM NAME

d. INSURANCE PLAN NAME OR PROGRAM NAME

10d. RESERVED FOR LOCAL USE

d. IS THERE ANOTHER HEALTH BENEFIT PLAN?
☐ YES ☐ NO   If yes, return to and complete item 9 a – d.

READ BACK OF FORM BEFORE COMPLETING & SIGNING THIS FORM.

12. PATIENT'S OR AUTHORIZED PERSON'S SIGNATURE I authorize the release of any medical or other information necessary to process this claim. I also request payment of government benefits either to myself or to the party who accepts assignment below.

SIGNED _____ DATE _____

13. INSURED'S OR AUTHORIZED PERSON'S SIGNATURE I authorize payment of medical benefits to the undersigned physician or supplier for services described below.

SIGNED _____

PATIENT AND INSURED INFORMATION

14. DATE OF CURRENT: ILLNESS (First symptom) OR INJURY (Accident) OR PREGNANCY (LMP)
MM | DD | YY

15. IF PATIENT HAS HAD SAME OR SIMILAR ILLNESS, GIVE FIRST DATE MM | DD | YY

16. DATES PATIENT UNABLE TO WORK IN CURRENT OCCUPATION
FROM MM | DD | YY   TO MM | DD | YY

17. NAME OF REFERRING PHYSICIAN OR OTHER SOURCE

17a. I.D. NUMBER OF REFERRING PHYSICIAN

18. HOSPITALIZATION DATES RELATED TO CURRENT SERVICES
FROM MM | DD | YY   TO MM | DD | YY

19. RESERVED FOR LOCAL USE

20. OUTSIDE LAB? $ CHARGES
☐ YES ☐ NO

21. DIAGNOSIS OR NATURE OF ILLNESS OR INJURY. (RELATE ITEMS 1, 2, 3, OR 4 TO ITEM 24E BY LINE)

1. |___.___| 3. |___.___|

2. |___.___| 4. |___.___|

22. MEDICAID RESUBMISSION CODE   ORIGINAL REF. NO.

23. PRIOR AUTHORIZATION NUMBER

24. A DATE(S) OF SERVICE			B Place of Service	C Type of Service	D PROCEDURES, SERVICES, OR SUPPLIES (Explain Unusual Circumstances)		E DIAGNOSIS CODE	F $ CHARGES	G DAYS OR UNITS	H EPSDT Family Plan	I EMG	J COB	K RESERVED FOR LOCAL USE
From MM DD YY	To MM DD YY				CPT/HCPCS	MODIFIER							
1													
2													
3													
4													
5													
6													

25. FEDERAL TAX I.D. NUMBER   SSN ☐ EIN ☐

26. PATIENT'S ACCOUNT NO.

27. ACCEPT ASSIGNMENT? (For govt. claims, see back)
☐ YES ☐ NO

28. TOTAL CHARGE $

29. AMOUNT PAID $

30. BALANCE DUE $

31. SIGNATURE OF PHYSICIAN OR SUPPLIER INCLUDING DEGREES OR CREDENTIALS
(I certify that the statements on the reverse apply to this bill and are made a part thereof.)

SIGNED _____ DATE _____

32. NAME AND ADDRESS OF FACILITY WHERE SERVICES WERE RENDERED (If other than home or office)

33. PHYSICIAN'S SUPPLIER'S BILLING NAME, ADDRESS, ZIP CODE & PHONE #

PIN#   GRP#

PHYSICIAN OR SUPPLIER INFORMATION

(APPROVED BY AMA COUNCIL ON MEDICAL SERVICE 8/88)

PLEASE PRINT OR TYPE

FORM HCFA-1500 (12-90)
FORM OWCP-1500   FORM RRB-1500
FORM AMA OP050192

FORM 17

HEALTHMEN'S INSURANCE COMPANY
5800 SOUTH GREEN STREET
HAROLD, OHIO 34668

Patient: Timothy Small

Subscriber: Thomas Small

ID#:   425-21-8778

Amount Submitted:	$60.00
Amount Approved:	50.00
Amount Paid:	$25.00

Check No. 696621

(NOT NEGOTIABLE)

Pay to the Order of: MEDICAL & DENTAL ASSOCIATES, P.C. $25.00
_____

TWENTY-FIVE DOLLARS NO/100
_____

(COPY)   _____

FORM 18

APPROVED OMB-0938-0008

CARRIER

☐☐ PICA

HEALTH INSURANCE CLAIM FORM

PICA ☐☐

1. MEDICARE MEDICAID CHAMPUS CHAMPVA GROUP HEALTH PLAN FECA BLK LUNG OTHER	1a. INSURED'S I.D. NUMBER (FOR PROGRAM IN ITEM 1)

☐ (Medicare #) ☐ (Medicaid #) ☐ (Sponsor's SSN) ☐ (VA File #) ☐ (SSN or ID) ☐ (SSN) ☐ (ID)

2. PATIENT'S NAME (Last Name, First Name, Middle Initial)

3. PATIENT'S BIRTH DATE   MM | DD | YY   SEX   M ☐ F ☐

4. INSURED'S NAME (Last Name, First Name, Middle Initial)

5. PATIENT'S ADDRESS (No. Street)

6. PATIENT RELATIONSHIP TO INSURED
Self ☐   Spouse ☐   Child ☐   Other ☐

7. INSURED'S ADDRESS (No. Street)

CITY   STATE

8. PATIENT STATUS
Single ☐   Married ☐   Other ☐
Employed ☐   Full-Time Student ☐   Part-Time Student ☐

CITY   STATE

ZIP CODE   TELEPHONE (Include Area Code) (   )

ZIP CODE   TELEPHONE (INCLUDE AREA CODE) (   )

9. OTHER INSURED'S NAME (Last Name, First Name, Middle Initial)

10. IS PATIENT'S CONDITION RELATED TO:

11. INSURED'S POLICY GROUP OR FECA NUMBER

a. OTHER INSURED'S POLICY OR GROUP NUMBER

a. EMPLOYMENT? (CURRENT OR PREVIOUS)   ☐ YES   ☐ NO

a. INSURED'S DATE OF BIRTH   MM | DD | YY   SEX   M ☐ F ☐

b. OTHER INSURED'S DATE OF BIRTH   MM | DD | YY   SEX   M ☐ F ☐

b. AUTO ACCIDENT?   PLACE (State)   ☐ YES   ☐ NO

b. EMPLOYER'S NAME OR SCHOOL NAME

c. EMPLOYER'S NAME OR SCHOOL NAME

c. OTHER ACCIDENT?   ☐ YES   ☐ NO

c. INSURANCE PLAN NAME OR PROGRAM NAME

d. INSURANCE PLAN NAME OR PROGRAM NAME

10d. RESERVED FOR LOCAL USE

d. IS THERE ANOTHER HEALTH BENEFIT PLAN?
☐ YES   ☐ NO   If yes, return to and complete item 9 a – d.

READ BACK OF FORM BEFORE COMPLETING & SIGNING THIS FORM.

12. PATIENT'S OR AUTHORIZED PERSON'S SIGNATURE I authorize the release of any medical or other information necessary to process this claim. I also request payment of government benefits either to myself or to the party who accepts assignment below.

SIGNED _____   DATE _____

13. INSURED'S OR AUTHORIZED PERSON'S SIGNATURE I authorize payment of medical benefits to the undersigned physician or supplier for services described below.

SIGNED _____

14. DATE OF CURRENT: ILLNESS (First symptom) OR INJURY (Accident) OR PREGNANCY (LMP)   MM | DD | YY

15. IF PATIENT HAS HAD SAME OR SIMILAR ILLNESS, GIVE FIRST DATE   MM | DD | YY

16. DATES PATIENT UNABLE TO WORK IN CURRENT OCCUPATION   FROM MM | DD | YY   TO MM | DD | YY

17. NAME OF REFERRING PHYSICIAN OR OTHER SOURCE

17a. I.D. NUMBER OF REFERRING PHYSICIAN

18. HOSPITALIZATION DATES RELATED TO CURRENT SERVICES   FROM MM | DD | YY   TO MM | DD | YY

19. RESERVED FOR LOCAL USE

20. OUTSIDE LAB?   ☐ YES   ☐ NO $ CHARGES

21. DIAGNOSIS OR NATURE OF ILLNESS OR INJURY. (RELATE ITEMS 1, 2, 3, OR 4 TO ITEM 24E BY LINE)
1. |___.___   3. |___.___
2. |___.___   4. |___.___

22. MEDICAID RESUBMISSION CODE   ORIGINAL REF. NO.

23. PRIOR AUTHORIZATION NUMBER

24. A DATE(S) OF SERVICE						B Place of Service	C Type of Service	D PROCEDURES, SERVICES, OR SUPPLIES (Explain Unusual Circumstances)		E DIAGNOSIS CODE	F $ CHARGES	G DAYS OR UNITS	H EPSDT Family Plan	I EMG	J COB	K RESERVED FOR LOCAL USE
From MM	DD	YY	To MM	DD	YY			CPT/HCPCS	MODIFIER							
1																
2																
3																
4																
5																
6																

25. FEDERAL TAX I.D. NUMBER   SSN ☐ EIN ☐

26. PATIENT'S ACCOUNT NO.

27. ACCEPT ASSIGNMENT? (For govt. claims, see back)   ☐ YES   ☐ NO

28. TOTAL CHARGE $

29. AMOUNT PAID $

30. BALANCE DUE $

31. SIGNATURE OF PHYSICIAN OR SUPPLIER INCLUDING DEGREES OR CREDENTIALS (I certify that the statements on the reverse apply to this bill and are made a part thereof.)

SIGNED _____   DATE _____

32. NAME AND ADDRESS OF FACILITY WHERE SERVICES WERE RENDERED (If other than home or office)

33. PHYSICIAN'S SUPPLIER'S BILLING NAME, ADDRESS, ZIP CODE & PHONE #

PIN# _____   GRP# _____

(APPROVED BY AMA COUNCIL ON MEDICAL SERVICE 8/88)

PLEASE PRINT OR TYPE

FORM HCFA-1500 (12-90)
FORM OWCP-1500   FORM RRB-1500
FORM AMA OP050192

PATIENT AND INSURED INFORMATION

PHYSICIAN OR SUPPLIER INFORMATION

FORM 19

PLEASE
DO NOT
STAPLE
IN THIS
AREA

CARRIER

| | PICA | | | | | **HEALTH INSURANCE CLAIM FORM** | | PICA | | |

1. MEDICARE MEDICAID CHAMPUS CHAMPVA GROUP HEALTH PLAN FECA BLK LUNG OTHER	1a. INSURED'S I.D. NUMBER (FOR PROGRAM IN ITEM 1)
☐ (Medicare #) ☐ (Medicaid #) ☐ (Sponsor's SSN) ☐ (VA File #) ☐ (SSN or ID) ☐ (SSN) ☐ (ID)	

2. PATIENT'S NAME (Last Name, First Name, Middle Initial)	3. PATIENT'S BIRTH DATE MM DD YY SEX M ☐ F ☐	4. INSURED'S NAME (Last Name, First Name, Middle Initial)

5. PATIENT'S ADDRESS (No. Street)	6. PATIENT RELATIONSHIP TO INSURED Self ☐ Spouse ☐ Child ☐ Other ☐	7. INSURED'S ADDRESS (No. Street)

CITY	STATE	8. PATIENT STATUS Single ☐ Married ☐ Other ☐	CITY	STATE

ZIP CODE	TELEPHONE (Include Area Code) ( )	Employed ☐ Full-Time Student ☐ Part-Time Student ☐	ZIP CODE	TELEPHONE (INCLUDE AREA CODE) ( )

9. OTHER INSURED'S NAME (Last Name, First Name, Middle Initial)	10. IS PATIENT'S CONDITION RELATED TO:	11. INSURED'S POLICY GROUP OR FECA NUMBER
a. OTHER INSURED'S POLICY OR GROUP NUMBER	a. EMPLOYMENT? (CURRENT OR PREVIOUS) ☐ YES ☐ NO	a. INSURED'S DATE OF BIRTH MM DD YY SEX M ☐ F ☐
b. OTHER INSURED'S DATE OF BIRTH MM DD YY SEX M ☐ F ☐	b. AUTO ACCIDENT? PLACE (State) ☐ YES ☐ NO	b. EMPLOYER'S NAME OR SCHOOL NAME
c. EMPLOYER'S NAME OR SCHOOL NAME	c. OTHER ACCIDENT? ☐ YES ☐ NO	c. INSURANCE PLAN NAME OR PROGRAM NAME
d. INSURANCE PLAN NAME OR PROGRAM NAME	10d. RESERVED FOR LOCAL USE	d. IS THERE ANOTHER HEALTH BENEFIT PLAN? ☐ YES ☐ NO If yes, return to and complete item 9 a – d.

READ BACK OF FORM BEFORE COMPLETING & SIGNING THIS FORM.

12. PATIENT'S OR AUTHORIZED PERSON'S SIGNATURE I authorize the release of any medical or other information necessary to process this claim. I also request payment of government benefits either to myself or to the party who accepts assignment below.	13. INSURED'S OR AUTHORIZED PERSON'S SIGNATURE I authorize payment of medical benefits to the undersigned physician or supplier for services described below.
SIGNED _____ DATE _____	SIGNED _____

PATIENT AND INSURED INFORMATION

14. DATE OF CURRENT: ILLNESS (First symptom) OR MM DD YY INJURY (Accident) OR PREGNANCY (LMP)	15. IF PATIENT HAS HAD SAME OR SIMILAR ILLNESS, GIVE FIRST DATE MM DD YY	16. DATES PATIENT UNABLE TO WORK IN CURRENT OCCUPATION MM DD YY MM DD YY FROM TO

17. NAME OF REFERRING PHYSICIAN OR OTHER SOURCE	17a. I.D. NUMBER OF REFERRING PHYSICIAN	18. HOSPITALIZATION DATES RELATED TO CURRENT SERVICES MM DD YY MM DD YY FROM TO

19. RESERVED FOR LOCAL USE	20. OUTSIDE LAB? $ CHARGES ☐ YES ☐ NO

21. DIAGNOSIS OR NATURE OF ILLNESS OR INJURY. (RELATE ITEMS 1, 2, 3, OR 4 TO ITEM 24E BY LINE) 1. ___ ___ 3. ___ ___ 2. ___ ___ 4. ___ ___	22. MEDICAID RESUBMISSION CODE ORIGINAL REF. NO.
	23. PRIOR AUTHORIZATION NUMBER

24. A DATE(S) OF SERVICE From To MM DD YY MM DD YY	B Place of Service	C Type of Service	D PROCEDURES, SERVICES, OR SUPPLIES (Explain Unusual Circumstances) CPT/HCPCS MODIFIER	E DIAGNOSIS CODE	F $ CHARGES	G DAYS OR UNITS	H EPSDT Family Plan	I EMG	J COB	K RESERVED FOR LOCAL USE
1										
2										
3										
4										
5										
6										

25. FEDERAL TAX I.D. NUMBER SSN EIN ☐ ☐	26. PATIENT'S ACCOUNT NO.	27. ACCEPT ASSIGNMENT? (For govt. claims, see back) ☐ YES ☐ NO	28. TOTAL CHARGE $	29. AMOUNT PAID $	30. BALANCE DUE $

31. SIGNATURE OF PHYSICIAN OR SUPPLIER INCLUDING DEGREES OR CREDENTIALS (I certify that the statements on the reverse apply to this bill and are made a part thereof.) SIGNED _____ DATE _____	32. NAME AND ADDRESS OF FACILITY WHERE SERVICES WERE RENDERED (If other than home or office)	33. PHYSICIAN'S SUPPLIER'S BILLING NAME, ADDRESS, ZIP CODE & PHONE # PIN# GRP#

PHYSICIAN OR SUPPLIER INFORMATION

(APPROVED BY AMA COUNCIL ON MEDICAL SERVICE 8/88) *PLEASE PRINT OR TYPE*

FORM HCFA-1500 (12-90)
FORM OWCP-1500   FORM RRB-1500
FORM AMA OP050192

FORM 20

Part Five Numbered Forms and Worksheets

APPROVED OMB-0938-0008

| | PICA

HEALTH INSURANCE CLAIM FORM

PICA | |

1. MEDICARE	MEDICAID	CHAMPUS	CHAMPVA	GROUP HEALTH PLAN	FECA BLK LUNG	OTHER	1a. INSURED'S I.D. NUMBER	(FOR PROGRAM IN ITEM 1)
(Medicare #)	(Medicaid #)	(Sponsor's SSN)	(VA File #)	(SSN or ID)	(SSN)	(ID)		

2. PATIENT'S NAME (Last Name, First Name, Middle Initial)

3. PATIENT'S BIRTH DATE   MM DD YY   SEX   M   F

4. INSURED'S NAME (Last Name, First Name, Middle Initial)

5. PATIENT'S ADDRESS (No. Street)

6. PATIENT RELATIONSHIP TO INSURED   Self [ ] Spouse [ ] Child [ ] Other [ ]

7. INSURED'S ADDRESS (No. Street)

CITY   STATE

8. PATIENT STATUS   Single [ ] Married [ ] Other [ ]   Employed [ ] Full-Time Student [ ] Part-Time Student [ ]

CITY   STATE

ZIP CODE   TELEPHONE (Include Area Code) (   )

ZIP CODE   TELEPHONE (INCLUDE AREA CODE) (   )

9. OTHER INSURED'S NAME (Last Name, First Name, Middle Initial)

10. IS PATIENT'S CONDITION RELATED TO:

11. INSURED'S POLICY GROUP OR FECA NUMBER

a. OTHER INSURED'S POLICY OR GROUP NUMBER

a. EMPLOYMENT? (CURRENT OR PREVIOUS)   [ ] YES [ ] NO

a. INSURED'S DATE OF BIRTH   MM DD YY   SEX   M [ ] F [ ]

b. OTHER INSURED'S DATE OF BIRTH   MM DD YY   SEX   M [ ] F [ ]

b. AUTO ACCIDENT?   PLACE (State)   [ ] YES [ ] NO

b. EMPLOYER'S NAME OR SCHOOL NAME

c. EMPLOYER'S NAME OR SCHOOL NAME

c. OTHER ACCIDENT?   [ ] YES [ ] NO

c. INSURANCE PLAN NAME OR PROGRAM NAME

d. INSURANCE PLAN NAME OR PROGRAM NAME

10d. RESERVED FOR LOCAL USE

d. IS THERE ANOTHER HEALTH BENEFIT PLAN?   [ ] YES [ ] NO   If yes, return to and complete item 9 a – d.

READ BACK OF FORM BEFORE COMPLETING & SIGNING THIS FORM.

12. PATIENT'S OR AUTHORIZED PERSON'S SIGNATURE I authorize the release of any medical or other information necessary to process this claim. I also request payment of government benefits either to myself or to the party who accepts assignment below.

SIGNED _____   DATE _____

13. INSURED'S OR AUTHORIZED PERSON'S SIGNATURE I authorize payment of medical benefits to the undersigned physician or supplier for services described below.

SIGNED _____

14. DATE OF CURRENT: ILLNESS (First symptom) OR INJURY (Accident) OR PREGNANCY (LMP) MM DD YY	15. IF PATIENT HAS HAD SAME OR SIMILAR ILLNESS, GIVE FIRST DATE MM DD YY	16. DATES PATIENT UNABLE TO WORK IN CURRENT OCCUPATION FROM MM DD YY TO MM DD YY

17. NAME OF REFERRING PHYSICIAN OR OTHER SOURCE

17a. I.D. NUMBER OF REFERRING PHYSICIAN

18. HOSPITALIZATION DATES RELATED TO CURRENT SERVICES   FROM MM DD YY   TO MM DD YY

19. RESERVED FOR LOCAL USE

20. OUTSIDE LAB?   [ ] YES [ ] NO $ CHARGES

21. DIAGNOSIS OR NATURE OF ILLNESS OR INJURY. (RELATE ITEMS 1, 2, 3, OR 4 TO ITEM 24E BY LINE)

1. |___|___   3. |___|___

2. |___|___   4. |___|___

22. MEDICAID RESUBMISSION CODE   ORIGINAL REF. NO.

23. PRIOR AUTHORIZATION NUMBER

24. A DATE(S) OF SERVICE						B Place of Service	C Type of Service	D PROCEDURES, SERVICES, OR SUPPLIES (Explain Unusual Circumstances) CPT/HCPCS MODIFIER	E DIAGNOSIS CODE	F $ CHARGES	G DAYS OR UNITS	H EPSDT Family Plan	I EMG	J COB	K RESERVED FOR LOCAL USE
From MM DD YY			To MM DD YY												
1															
2															
3															
4															
5															
6															

25. FEDERAL TAX I.D. NUMBER SSN [ ] EIN [ ]	26. PATIENT'S ACCOUNT NO.	27. ACCEPT ASSIGNMENT? (For govt. claims, see back) YES [ ] NO [ ]	28. TOTAL CHARGE $	29. AMOUNT PAID $	30. BALANCE DUE $

31. SIGNATURE OF PHYSICIAN OR SUPPLIER INCLUDING DEGREES OR CREDENTIALS (I certify that the statements on the reverse apply to this bill and are made a part thereof.)

SIGNED _____   DATE _____

32. NAME AND ADDRESS OF FACILITY WHERE SERVICES WERE RENDERED (If other than home or office)

33. PHYSICIAN'S SUPPLIER'S BILLING NAME, ADDRESS, ZIP CODE & PHONE #

PIN#   GRP#

(APPROVED BY AMA COUNCIL ON MEDICAL SERVICE 8/88)

PLEASE PRINT OR TYPE

FORM HCFA-1500 (12-90)
FORM OWCP-1500   FORM RRB-1500
FORM AMA OP050192

CARRIER

PATIENT AND INSURED INFORMATION

PHYSICIAN OR SUPPLIER INFORMATION

FORM 21

APPROVED OMB-0938-0008

CARRIER

HEALTH INSURANCE CLAIM FORM

| | PICA | | | | | | | PICA | | |

1. MEDICARE ☐ (Medicare #) MEDICAID ☐ (Medicaid #) CHAMPUS ☐ (Sponsor's SSN) CHAMPVA ☐ (VA File #) GROUP HEALTH PLAN ☐ (SSN or ID) FECA BLK LUNG ☐ (SSN) OTHER ☐ (ID)

1a. INSURED'S I.D. NUMBER (FOR PROGRAM IN ITEM 1)

2. PATIENT'S NAME (Last Name, First Name, Middle Initial)

3. PATIENT'S BIRTH DATE   MM ┊ DD ┊ YY   SEX   M ☐   F ☐

4. INSURED'S NAME (Last Name, First Name, Middle Initial)

5. PATIENT'S ADDRESS (No. Street)

6. PATIENT RELATIONSHIP TO INSURED   Self ☐   Spouse ☐   Child ☐   Other ☐

7. INSURED'S ADDRESS (No. Street)

CITY   STATE

8. PATIENT STATUS   Single ☐   Married ☐   Other ☐   Employed ☐   Full-Time Student ☐   Part-Time Student ☐

CITY   STATE

ZIP CODE   TELEPHONE (Include Area Code) (   )

ZIP CODE   TELEPHONE (INCLUDE AREA CODE) (   )

9. OTHER INSURED'S NAME (Last Name, First Name, Middle Initial)

10. IS PATIENT'S CONDITION RELATED TO:

11. INSURED'S POLICY GROUP OR FECA NUMBER

a. OTHER INSURED'S POLICY OR GROUP NUMBER

a. EMPLOYMENT? (CURRENT OR PREVIOUS)   YES ☐   NO ☐

a. INSURED'S DATE OF BIRTH   MM ┊ DD ┊ YY   SEX   M ☐   F ☐

b. OTHER INSURED'S DATE OF BIRTH   MM ┊ DD ┊ YY   SEX   M ☐   F ☐

b. AUTO ACCIDENT?   PLACE (State)   YES ☐   NO ☐

b. EMPLOYER'S NAME OR SCHOOL NAME

c. EMPLOYER'S NAME OR SCHOOL NAME

c. OTHER ACCIDENT?   YES ☐   NO ☐

c. INSURANCE PLAN NAME OR PROGRAM NAME

d. INSURANCE PLAN NAME OR PROGRAM NAME

10d. RESERVED FOR LOCAL USE

d. IS THERE ANOTHER HEALTH BENEFIT PLAN?   YES ☐   NO ☐   If yes, return to and complete item 9 a – d.

READ BACK OF FORM BEFORE COMPLETING & SIGNING THIS FORM.
12. PATIENT'S OR AUTHORIZED PERSON'S SIGNATURE I authorize the release of any medical or other information necessary to process this claim. I also request payment of government benefits either to myself or to the party who accepts assignment below.

SIGNED _____   DATE _____

13. INSURED'S OR AUTHORIZED PERSON'S SIGNATURE I authorize payment of medical benefits to the undersigned physician or supplier for services described below.

SIGNED _____

PATIENT AND INSURED INFORMATION

14. DATE OF CURRENT: ILLNESS (First symptom) OR INJURY (Accident) OR PREGNANCY (LMP)   MM ┊ DD ┊ YY

15. IF PATIENT HAS HAD SAME OR SIMILAR ILLNESS, GIVE FIRST DATE   MM ┊ DD ┊ YY

16. DATES PATIENT UNABLE TO WORK IN CURRENT OCCUPATION   FROM MM ┊ DD ┊ YY   TO MM ┊ DD ┊ YY

17. NAME OF REFERRING PHYSICIAN OR OTHER SOURCE

17a. I.D. NUMBER OF REFERRING PHYSICIAN

18. HOSPITALIZATION DATES RELATED TO CURRENT SERVICES   FROM MM ┊ DD ┊ YY   TO MM ┊ DD ┊ YY

19. RESERVED FOR LOCAL USE

20. OUTSIDE LAB?   YES ☐   NO ☐ $ CHARGES

21. DIAGNOSIS OR NATURE OF ILLNESS OR INJURY. (RELATE ITEMS 1, 2, 3, OR 4 TO ITEM 24E BY LINE)
1. ┕___ . ___   3. ┕___ . ___
2. ┕___ . ___   4. ┕___ . ___

22. MEDICAID RESUBMISSION CODE   ORIGINAL REF. NO.

23. PRIOR AUTHORIZATION NUMBER

24. A DATE(S) OF SERVICE						B Place of Service	C Type of Service	D PROCEDURES, SERVICES, OR SUPPLIES (Explain Unusual Circumstances)		E DIAGNOSIS CODE	F $ CHARGES	G DAYS OR UNITS	H EPSDT Family Plan	I EMG	J COB	K RESERVED FOR LOCAL USE
From MM	DD	YY	To MM	DD	YY			CPT/HCPCS	MODIFIER							
1																
2																
3																
4																
5																
6																

25. FEDERAL TAX I.D. NUMBER   SSN ☐   EIN ☐

26. PATIENT'S ACCOUNT NO.

27. ACCEPT ASSIGNMENT? (For govt. claims, see back)   YES ☐   NO ☐

28. TOTAL CHARGE $

29. AMOUNT PAID $

30. BALANCE DUE $

31. SIGNATURE OF PHYSICIAN OR SUPPLIER INCLUDING DEGREES OR CREDENTIALS (I certify that the statements on the reverse apply to this bill and are made a part thereof.)

SIGNED _____   DATE _____

32. NAME AND ADDRESS OF FACILITY WHERE SERVICES WERE RENDERED (If other than home or office)

33. PHYSICIAN'S SUPPLIER'S BILLING NAME, ADDRESS, ZIP CODE & PHONE #

PIN# _____   GRP# _____

PHYSICIAN OR SUPPLIER INFORMATION

(APPROVED BY AMA COUNCIL ON MEDICAL SERVICE 8/88)

PLEASE PRINT OR TYPE

FORM HCFA-1500 (12-90)
FORM OWCP-1500   FORM RRB-1500
FORM AMA OP050192

FORM 22

MEDICAID COVERAGE

medicare
c/o Blue cross/blue shield
1500 E 10th
Indpls. 46215

HEALTH INSURANCE CLAIM FORM

| | | PICA | | | | | | | | | PICA | | |

1. MEDICARE ☒ (Medicare #) MEDICAID ☐ (Medicaid #) CHAMPUS ☐ (Sponsor's SSN) CHAMPVA ☐ (VA File #) GROUP HEALTH PLAN ☐ (SSN or ID) FECA BLK LUNG ☐ (SSN) OTHER ☐ (ID)

1a. INSURED'S I.D. NUMBER (FOR PROGRAM IN ITEM 1)
482-40-1640 AB

2. PATIENT'S NAME (Last Name, First Name, Middle Initial)
OLEARY BARBARA M

3. PATIENT'S BIRTH DATE MM 6 DD 23 YY SEX M ☐ F ☐

4. INSURED'S NAME (Last Name, First Name, Middle Initial)
SAME

5. PATIENT'S ADDRESS (No. Street)
59986 10 St
CITY Indpls STATE IN
ZIP CODE 46294 TELEPHONE (Include Area Code) ( )

6. PATIENT RELATIONSHIP TO INSURED
Self ☒ Spouse ☐ Child ☐ Other ☐

8. PATIENT STATUS
Single ☐ Married ☒ Other ☐
Employed ☐ Full-Time Student ☐ Part-Time Student ☐

7. INSURED'S ADDRESS (No. Street)
SAME
CITY STATE
ZIP CODE TELEPHONE (INCLUDE AREA CODE) ( )

9. OTHER INSURED'S NAME (Last Name, First Name, Middle Initial)
none

10. IS PATIENT'S CONDITION RELATED TO:

11. INSURED'S POLICY GROUP OR FECA NUMBER

a. OTHER INSURED'S POLICY OR GROUP NUMBER

a. EMPLOYMENT? (CURRENT OR PREVIOUS) ☐ YES ☒ NO

a. INSURED'S DATE OF BIRTH MM DD YY SEX M ☐ F ☐

b. OTHER INSURED'S DATE OF BIRTH MM DD YY SEX M ☐ F ☐

b. AUTO ACCIDENT? ☐ YES ☒ NO PLACE (State)

b. EMPLOYER'S NAME OR SCHOOL NAME

c. EMPLOYER'S NAME OR SCHOOL NAME

c. OTHER ACCIDENT? ☐ YES ☒ NO

c. INSURANCE PLAN NAME OR PROGRAM NAME

d. INSURANCE PLAN NAME OR PROGRAM NAME

10d. RESERVED FOR LOCAL USE

d. IS THERE ANOTHER HEALTH BENEFIT PLAN? ☐ YES ☒ NO If yes, return to and complete item 9 a - d.

READ BACK OF FORM BEFORE COMPLETING & SIGNING THIS FORM.
12. PATIENT'S OR AUTHORIZED PERSON'S SIGNATURE I authorize the release of any medical or other information necessary to process this claim. I also request payment of government benefits either to myself or to the party who accepts assignment below.
SIGNED Signature on file DATE Today

13. INSURED'S OR AUTHORIZED PERSON'S SIGNATURE I authorize payment of medical benefits to the undersigned physician or supplier for services described below.
SIGNED Signature on file

14. DATE OF CURRENT: ILLNESS (First symptom) OR INJURY (Accident) OR PREGNANCY (LMP) MM 12 DD 01 YY OR

15. IF PATIENT HAS HAD SAME OR SIMILAR ILLNESS, GIVE FIRST DATE MM DD YY

16. DATES PATIENT UNABLE TO WORK IN CURRENT OCCUPATION FROM MM DD YY TO MM DD YY

17. NAME OF REFERRING PHYSICIAN OR OTHER SOURCE
DR. Geovry

17a. I.D. NUMBER OF REFERRING PHYSICIAN
99-9999999

18. HOSPITALIZATION DATES RELATED TO CURRENT SERVICES FROM MM DD YY TO MM DD YY

19. RESERVED FOR LOCAL USE

20. OUTSIDE LAB? ☒ YES ☐ NO $ CHARGES

21. DIAGNOSIS OR NATURE OF ILLNESS OR INJURY. (RELATE ITEMS 1, 2, 3, OR 4 TO ITEM 24E BY LINE)
1. 99214
2. 90704
3. V80.2
4.

22. MEDICAID RESUBMISSION CODE ORIGINAL REF. NO.

23. PRIOR AUTHORIZATION NUMBER

24.

A DATE(S) OF SERVICE						B Place of Service	C Type of Service	D PROCEDURES, SERVICES, OR SUPPLIES (Explain Unusual Circumstances) CPT/HCPCS MODIFIER	E DIAGNOSIS CODE	F $ CHARGES	G DAYS OR UNITS	H EPSDT Family Plan	I EMG	J COB	K RESERVED FOR LOCAL USE
From MM 01	DD 12	YY	To MM	DD	YY	11		99214	V20.2	20 00					
								90704							

25. FEDERAL TAX I.D. NUMBER 99-9999999 SSN ☐ EIN ☐

26. PATIENT'S ACCOUNT NO.

27. ACCEPT ASSIGNMENT? (For govt. claims, see back) YES ☐ NO ☐

28. TOTAL CHARGE $ 20.00

29. AMOUNT PAID $

30. BALANCE DUE $

31. SIGNATURE OF PHYSICIAN OR SUPPLIER INCLUDING DEGREES OR CREDENTIALS (I certify that the statements on the reverse apply to this bill and are made a part thereof.)
SIGNED Dr. George DATE 12/1

32. NAME AND ADDRESS OF FACILITY WHERE SERVICES WERE RENDERED (If other than home or office)
3733 Professional Dr #300
Indpls IN, 46260

33. PHYSICIAN'S SUPPLIER'S BILLING NAME, ADDRESS, ZIP CODE & PHONE #
Linda Georgi N.D
3733 Professional Dr #300
Indpls. IN 46260 medicare
CDIN # 1336900
PIN# GRP# 314677823

FORM 23

272

APPROVED OMB-0938-0008

CARRIER

HEALTH INSURANCE CLAIM FORM

| | PICA | | | PICA | | |

| 1. MEDICARE | MEDICAID | CHAMPUS | CHAMPVA | GROUP HEALTH PLAN (SSN or ID) | FECA BLK LUNG (SSN) | OTHER (ID) | 1a. INSURED'S I.D. NUMBER (FOR PROGRAM IN ITEM 1) |

(Medicare #) (Medicaid #) (Sponsor's SSN) (VA File #)

| 2. PATIENT'S NAME (Last Name, First Name, Middle Initial) | 3. PATIENT'S BIRTH DATE MM | DD | YY   SEX M F | 4. INSURED'S NAME (Last Name, First Name, Middle Initial) |

| 5. PATIENT'S ADDRESS (No. Street) | 6. PATIENT RELATIONSHIP TO INSURED Self Spouse Child Other | 7. INSURED'S ADDRESS (No. Street) |

| CITY | STATE | 8. PATIENT STATUS Single Married Other | CITY | STATE |

| ZIP CODE | TELEPHONE (Include Area Code) ( ) | Employed Full-Time Student Part-Time Student | ZIP CODE | TELEPHONE (INCLUDE AREA CODE) ( ) |

| 9. OTHER INSURED'S NAME (Last Name, First Name, Middle Initial) | 10. IS PATIENT'S CONDITION RELATED TO: | 11. INSURED'S POLICY GROUP OR FECA NUMBER |

| a. OTHER INSURED'S POLICY OR GROUP NUMBER | a. EMPLOYMENT? (CURRENT OR PREVIOUS) YES NO | a. INSURED'S DATE OF BIRTH MM | DD | YY   SEX M F |

| b. OTHER INSURED'S DATE OF BIRTH MM | DD | YY   SEX M F | b. AUTO ACCIDENT?   PLACE (State) YES NO | b. EMPLOYER'S NAME OR SCHOOL NAME |

| c. EMPLOYER'S NAME OR SCHOOL NAME | c. OTHER ACCIDENT? YES NO | c. INSURANCE PLAN NAME OR PROGRAM NAME |

| d. INSURANCE PLAN NAME OR PROGRAM NAME | 10d. RESERVED FOR LOCAL USE | d. IS THERE ANOTHER HEALTH BENEFIT PLAN? YES NO   If yes, return to and complete Item 9 a – d. |

READ BACK OF FORM BEFORE COMPLETING & SIGNING THIS FORM.
12. PATIENT'S OR AUTHORIZED PERSON'S SIGNATURE I authorize the release of any medical or other information necessary to process this claim. I also request payment of government benefits either to myself or to the party who accepts assignment below.

SIGNED _____   DATE _____

13. INSURED'S OR AUTHORIZED PERSON'S SIGNATURE I authorize payment of medical benefits to the undersigned physician or supplier for services described below.

SIGNED _____

PATIENT AND INSURED INFORMATION

| 14. DATE OF CURRENT: MM | DD | YY   ILLNESS (First symptom) OR INJURY (Accident) OR PREGNANCY (LMP) | 15. IF PATIENT HAS HAD SAME OR SIMILAR ILLNESS, GIVE FIRST DATE MM | DD | YY | 16. DATES PATIENT UNABLE TO WORK IN CURRENT OCCUPATION MM | DD | YY   MM | DD | YY FROM   TO |

| 17. NAME OF REFERRING PHYSICIAN OR OTHER SOURCE | 17a. I.D. NUMBER OF REFERRING PHYSICIAN | 18. HOSPITALIZATION DATES RELATED TO CURRENT SERVICES MM | DD | YY   MM | DD | YY FROM   TO |

| 19. RESERVED FOR LOCAL USE | 20. OUTSIDE LAB? YES NO $ CHARGES |

21. DIAGNOSIS OR NATURE OF ILLNESS OR INJURY. (RELATE ITEMS 1, 2, 3, OR 4 TO ITEM 24E BY LINE)

1. |___.___| 3. |___.___|

2. |___.___| 4. |___.___|

| 22. MEDICAID RESUBMISSION CODE   ORIGINAL REF. NO. |

| 23. PRIOR AUTHORIZATION NUMBER |

24. A DATE(S) OF SERVICE						B Place of Service	C Type of Service	D PROCEDURES, SERVICES, OR SUPPLIES (Explain Unusual Circumstances) CPT/HCPCS	MODIFIER	E DIAGNOSIS CODE	F $ CHARGES	G DAYS OR UNITS	H EPSDT Family Plan	I EMG	J COB	K RESERVED FOR LOCAL USE
From MM	DD	YY	To MM	DD	YY											
1																
2																
3																
4																
5																
6																

| 25. FEDERAL TAX I.D. NUMBER   SSN EIN | 26. PATIENT'S ACCOUNT NO. | 27. ACCEPT ASSIGNMENT? (For govt. claims, see back) YES NO | 28. TOTAL CHARGE $ | 29. AMOUNT PAID $ | 30. BALANCE DUE $ |

| 31. SIGNATURE OF PHYSICIAN OR SUPPLIER INCLUDING DEGREES OR CREDENTIALS (I certify that the statements on the reverse apply to this bill and are made a part thereof.)

SIGNED _____ DATE _____ | 32. NAME AND ADDRESS OF FACILITY WHERE SERVICES WERE RENDERED (If other than home or office) | 33. PHYSICIAN'S SUPPLIER'S BILLING NAME, ADDRESS, ZIP CODE & PHONE #

PIN#   GRP# |

PHYSICIAN OR SUPPLIER INFORMATION

(APPROVED BY AMA COUNCIL ON MEDICAL SERVICE 8/88)

PLEASE PRINT OR TYPE

FORM HCFA-1500 (12-90)
FORM OWCP-1500   FORM RRB-1500
FORM AMA OP050192

FORM 24

APPROVED OMB-0938-0008

CARRIER

| | PICA | | **HEALTH INSURANCE CLAIM FORM** | PICA | |

| 1. MEDICARE | MEDICAID | CHAMPUS | CHAMPVA | GROUP HEALTH PLAN | FECA BLK LUNG | OTHER | 1a. INSURED'S I.D. NUMBER | (FOR PROGRAM IN ITEM 1) |
| [ ] (Medicare #) | [ ] (Medicaid #) | [ ] (Sponsor's SSN) | [ ] (VA File #) | [ ] (SSN or ID) | [ ] (SSN) | [ ] (ID) | | |

2. PATIENT'S NAME (Last Name, First Name, Middle Initial)

3. PATIENT'S BIRTH DATE   MM DD YY   SEX   M [ ] F [ ]

4. INSURED'S NAME (Last Name, First Name, Middle Initial)

5. PATIENT'S ADDRESS (No. Street)

6. PATIENT RELATIONSHIP TO INSURED   Self [ ] Spouse [ ] Child [ ] Other [ ]

7. INSURED'S ADDRESS (No. Street)

CITY   STATE

8. PATIENT STATUS   Single [ ] Married [ ] Other [ ]
Employed [ ] Full-Time Student [ ] Part-Time Student [ ]

CITY   STATE

ZIP CODE   TELEPHONE (Include Area Code) (   )

ZIP CODE   TELEPHONE (INCLUDE AREA CODE) (   )

9. OTHER INSURED'S NAME (Last Name, First Name, Middle Initial)

10. IS PATIENT'S CONDITION RELATED TO:

11. INSURED'S POLICY GROUP OR FECA NUMBER

a. OTHER INSURED'S POLICY OR GROUP NUMBER

a. EMPLOYMENT? (CURRENT OR PREVIOUS)   YES [ ] NO [ ]

a. INSURED'S DATE OF BIRTH   MM DD YY   SEX   M [ ] F [ ]

b. OTHER INSURED'S DATE OF BIRTH   MM DD YY   SEX   M [ ] F [ ]

b. AUTO ACCIDENT?   PLACE (State)   YES [ ] NO [ ]

b. EMPLOYER'S NAME OR SCHOOL NAME

c. EMPLOYER'S NAME OR SCHOOL NAME

c. OTHER ACCIDENT?   YES [ ] NO [ ]

c. INSURANCE PLAN NAME OR PROGRAM NAME

d. INSURANCE PLAN NAME OR PROGRAM NAME

10d. RESERVED FOR LOCAL USE

d. IS THERE ANOTHER HEALTH BENEFIT PLAN?   YES [ ] NO [ ] If yes, return to and complete item 9 a – d.

READ BACK OF FORM BEFORE COMPLETING & SIGNING THIS FORM.
12. PATIENT'S OR AUTHORIZED PERSON'S SIGNATURE I authorize the release of any medical or other information necessary to process this claim. I also request payment of government benefits either to myself or to the party who accepts assignment below.

SIGNED _____   DATE _____

13. INSURED'S OR AUTHORIZED PERSON'S SIGNATURE I authorize payment of medical benefits to the undersigned physician or supplier for services described below.

SIGNED _____

PATIENT AND INSURED INFORMATION

14. DATE OF CURRENT: MM DD YY   ILLNESS (First symptom) OR INJURY (Accident) OR PREGNANCY (LMP)

15. IF PATIENT HAS HAD SAME OR SIMILAR ILLNESS, GIVE FIRST DATE   MM DD YY

16. DATES PATIENT UNABLE TO WORK IN CURRENT OCCUPATION   MM DD YY   FROM   TO   MM DD YY

17. NAME OF REFERRING PHYSICIAN OR OTHER SOURCE

17a. I.D. NUMBER OF REFERRING PHYSICIAN

18. HOSPITALIZATION DATES RELATED TO CURRENT SERVICES   MM DD YY   FROM   TO   MM DD YY

19. RESERVED FOR LOCAL USE

20. OUTSIDE LAB? $ CHARGES   YES [ ] NO [ ]

21. DIAGNOSIS OR NATURE OF ILLNESS OR INJURY. (RELATE ITEMS 1, 2, 3, OR 4 TO ITEM 24E BY LINE)
1. |___.___   3. |___.___
2. |___.___   4. |___.___

22. MEDICAID RESUBMISSION CODE   ORIGINAL REF. NO.

23. PRIOR AUTHORIZATION NUMBER

24. A						B	C	D		E	F	G	H	I	J	K
DATE(S) OF SERVICE						Place of Service	Type of Service	PROCEDURES, SERVICES, OR SUPPLIES (Explain Unusual Circumstances)		DIAGNOSIS CODE	$ CHARGES	DAYS OR UNITS	EPSDT Family Plan	EMG	COB	RESERVED FOR LOCAL USE
From			To					CPT/HCPCS	MODIFIER							
MM	DD	YY	MM	DD	YY											
1																
2																
3																
4																
5																
6																

25. FEDERAL TAX I.D. NUMBER   SSN [ ] EIN [ ]

26. PATIENT'S ACCOUNT NO.

27. ACCEPT ASSIGNMENT? (For govt. claims, see back)   YES [ ] NO [ ]

28. TOTAL CHARGE $

29. AMOUNT PAID $

30. BALANCE DUE $

31. SIGNATURE OF PHYSICIAN OR SUPPLIER INCLUDING DEGREES OR CREDENTIALS (I certify that the statements on the reverse apply to this bill and are made a part thereof.)

SIGNED _____   DATE _____

32. NAME AND ADDRESS OF FACILITY WHERE SERVICES WERE RENDERED (If other than home or office)

33. PHYSICIAN'S SUPPLIER'S BILLING NAME, ADDRESS, ZIP CODE & PHONE #

PIN#   GRP#

PHYSICIAN OR SUPPLIER INFORMATION

(APPROVED BY AMA COUNCIL ON MEDICAL SERVICE 8/88)   *PLEASE PRINT OR TYPE*

FORM HCFA-1500 (12-90)
FORM OWCP-1500   FORM RRB-1500
FORM AMA OP050192

FORM 25

PLEASE
DO NOT
STAPLE
IN THIS
AREA

CARRIER

| | PICA

HEALTH INSURANCE CLAIM FORM

PICA | |

| 1. MEDICARE MEDICAID CHAMPUS CHAMPVA GROUP FECA OTHER | 1a. INSURED'S I.D. NUMBER (FOR PROGRAM IN ITEM 1) |
| | |

☐ (Medicare #) ☐ (Medicaid #) ☐ (Sponsor's SSN) ☐ (VA File #) HEALTH PLAN ☐ BLK LUNG ☐ (ID)
(SSN or ID) (SSN)

2. PATIENT'S NAME (Last Name, First Name, Middle Initial)

3. PATIENT'S BIRTH DATE SEX
MM DD YY M ☐ F ☐

4. INSURED'S NAME (Last Name, First Name, Middle Initial)

5. PATIENT'S ADDRESS (No. Street)

6. PATIENT RELATIONSHIP TO INSURED
Self ☐ Spouse ☐ Child ☐ Other ☐

7. INSURED'S ADDRESS (No. Street)

CITY   STATE

8. PATIENT STATUS
Single ☐ Married ☐ Other ☐

Employed ☐ Full-Time Student ☐ Part-Time Student ☐

CITY   STATE

ZIP CODE   TELEPHONE (Include Area Code)
( )

ZIP CODE   TELEPHONE (INCLUDE AREA CODE)
( )

9. OTHER INSURED'S NAME (Last Name, First Name, Middle Initial)

10. IS PATIENT'S CONDITION RELATED TO:

11. INSURED'S POLICY GROUP OR FECA NUMBER

a. OTHER INSURED'S POLICY OR GROUP NUMBER

a. EMPLOYMENT? (CURRENT OR PREVIOUS)
☐ YES ☐ NO

a. INSURED'S DATE OF BIRTH SEX
MM DD YY M ☐ F ☐

b. OTHER INSURED'S DATE OF BIRTH SEX
MM DD YY M ☐ F ☐

b. AUTO ACCIDENT? PLACE (State)
☐ YES ☐ NO

b. EMPLOYER'S NAME OR SCHOOL NAME

c. EMPLOYER'S NAME OR SCHOOL NAME

c. OTHER ACCIDENT?
☐ YES ☐ NO

c. INSURANCE PLAN NAME OR PROGRAM NAME

d. INSURANCE PLAN NAME OR PROGRAM NAME

10d. RESERVED FOR LOCAL USE

d. IS THERE ANOTHER HEALTH BENEFIT PLAN?
☐ YES ☐ NO If yes, return to and complete item 9 a – d.

READ BACK OF FORM BEFORE COMPLETING & SIGNING THIS FORM.
12. PATIENT'S OR AUTHORIZED PERSON'S SIGNATURE I authorize the release of any medical or other information necessary to process this claim. I also request payment of government benefits either to myself or to the party who accepts assignment below.

SIGNED _____ DATE _____

13. INSURED'S OR AUTHORIZED PERSON'S SIGNATURE I authorize payment of medical benefits to the undersigned physician or supplier for services described below.

SIGNED _____

PATIENT AND INSURED INFORMATION

14. DATE OF CURRENT: ILLNESS (First symptom) OR
MM DD YY INJURY (Accident) OR
PREGNANCY (LMP)

15. IF PATIENT HAS HAD SAME OR SIMILAR ILLNESS, GIVE FIRST DATE MM DD YY

16. DATES PATIENT UNABLE TO WORK IN CURRENT OCCUPATION
MM DD YY MM DD YY
FROM TO

17. NAME OF REFERRING PHYSICIAN OR OTHER SOURCE

17a. I.D. NUMBER OF REFERRING PHYSICIAN

18. HOSPITALIZATION DATES RELATED TO CURRENT SERVICES
MM DD YY MM DD YY
FROM TO

19. RESERVED FOR LOCAL USE

20. OUTSIDE LAB? $ CHARGES
☐ YES ☐ NO

21. DIAGNOSIS OR NATURE OF ILLNESS OR INJURY. (RELATE ITEMS 1, 2, 3, OR 4 TO ITEM 24E BY LINE)

1. |___.___   3. |___.___

2. |___.___   4. |___.___

22. MEDICAID RESUBMISSION
CODE   ORIGINAL REF. NO.

23. PRIOR AUTHORIZATION NUMBER

24. A DATE(S) OF SERVICE			B Place of Service	C Type of Service	D PROCEDURES, SERVICES, OR SUPPLIES (Explain Unusual Circumstances) CPT/HCPCS MODIFIER	E DIAGNOSIS CODE	F $ CHARGES	G DAYS OR UNITS	H EPSDT Family Plan	I EMG	J COB	K RESERVED FOR LOCAL USE
From MM DD YY	To MM DD YY											
1												
2												
3												
4												
5												
6												

25. FEDERAL TAX I.D. NUMBER SSN EIN
☐ ☐

26. PATIENT'S ACCOUNT NO.

27. ACCEPT ASSIGNMENT?
(For govt. claims, see back)
☐ YES ☐ NO

28. TOTAL CHARGE
$

29. AMOUNT PAID
$

30. BALANCE DUE
$

31. SIGNATURE OF PHYSICIAN OR SUPPLIER INCLUDING DEGREES OR CREDENTIALS
(I certify that the statements on the reverse apply to this bill and are made a part thereof.)

SIGNED _____ DATE _____

32. NAME AND ADDRESS OF FACILITY WHERE SERVICES WERE RENDERED (If other than home or office)

33. PHYSICIAN'S SUPPLIER'S BILLING NAME, ADDRESS, ZIP CODE & PHONE #

PIN#   GRP#

PHYSICIAN OR SUPPLIER INFORMATION

(APPROVED BY AMA COUNCIL ON MEDICAL SERVICE 8/88)

PLEASE PRINT OR TYPE

FORM HCFA-1500 (12-90)
FORM OWCP-1500 FORM RRB-1500
FORM AMA OP050192

FORM 26

Medicare- Medigap Claim Form

PLEASE
DO NOT
STAPLE
IN THIS
AREA

metro medigap
10 market st
city, 46201

CARRIER

| | PICA

HEALTH INSURANCE CLAIM FORM

PICA | |

1.	MEDICARE	MEDICAID	CHAMPUS	CHAMPVA	GROUP HEALTH PLAN (SSN or ID)	FECA BLK LUNG (SSN)	OTHER (ID)	1a. INSURED'S I.D. NUMBER (FOR PROGRAM IN ITEM 1)
	☒ (Medicare #)	☐ (Medicaid #)	☐ (Sponsor's SSN)	☐ (VA File #)	☐	☐	☐	211-88-5244 (B3)

2. PATIENT'S NAME (Last Name, First Name, Middle Initial)
Steinbert Gerald

3. PATIENT'S BIRTH DATE MM DD YY 2 2   SEX M ☒ F ☐

4. INSURED'S NAME (Last Name, First Name, Middle Initial)
Steinbert, Gerald

5. PATIENT'S ADDRESS (No. Street)
110 S. State St

6. PATIENT RELATIONSHIP TO INSURED
Self ☒ Spouse ☐ Child ☐ Other ☐

7. INSURED'S ADDRESS (No. Street)

CITY City Indpls.   STATE IN

8. PATIENT STATUS
Single ☒ Married ☐ Other ☒
Employed ☐ Full-Time Student ☐ Part-Time Student ☐

CITY   STATE

ZIP CODE 46203

TELEPHONE (Include Area Code) ( )

ZIP CODE

TELEPHONE (INCLUDE AREA CODE) ( )

9. OTHER INSURED'S NAME (Last Name, First Name, Middle Initial)
Same

a. OTHER INSURED'S POLICY OR GROUP NUMBER
#7707 medigap 5244AB

b. OTHER INSURED'S DATE OF BIRTH MM DD YY 82 021 SEX M ☒ F ☐

c. EMPLOYER'S NAME OR SCHOOL NAME
10 market St. IN 46201

d. INSURANCE PLAN NAME OR PROGRAM NAME
metro medigap

10. IS PATIENT'S CONDITION RELATED TO:

a. EMPLOYMENT? (CURRENT OR PREVIOUS) YES ☐ NO ☒

b. AUTO ACCIDENT? YES ☐ NO ☒   PLACE (State)

c. OTHER ACCIDENT? YES ☐ NO ☒

10d. RESERVED FOR LOCAL USE
211-88-5244 BC

11. INSURED'S POLICY GROUP OR FECA NUMBER

a. INSURED'S DATE OF BIRTH MM DD YY SEX M ☐ F ☐

b. EMPLOYER'S NAME OR SCHOOL NAME

c. INSURANCE PLAN NAME OR PROGRAM NAME

d. IS THERE ANOTHER HEALTH BENEFIT PLAN?
YES ☒ NO ☐   If yes, return to and complete item 9 a - d.

12. PATIENT'S OR AUTHORIZED PERSON'S SIGNATURE I authorize the release of any medical or other information necessary to process this claim. I also request payment of government benefits either to myself or to the party who accepts assignment below.
SIGNED Signature on file   DATE Today

13. INSURED'S OR AUTHORIZED PERSON'S SIGNATURE I authorize payment of medical benefits to the undersigned physician or supplier for services described below.
SIGNED Signature on file

14. DATE OF CURRENT: ILLNESS (First symptom) OR INJURY (Accident) OR PREGNANCY (LMP) MM DD YY

15. IF PATIENT HAS HAD SAME OR SIMILAR ILLNESS, GIVE FIRST DATE MM DD YY

16. DATES PATIENT UNABLE TO WORK IN CURRENT OCCUPATION MM DD YY FROM TO MM DD YY

17. NAME OF REFERRING PHYSICIAN OR OTHER SOURCE

17a. I.D. NUMBER OF REFERRING PHYSICIAN
99-9999999

18. HOSPITALIZATION DATES RELATED TO CURRENT SERVICES MM DD YY FROM TO MM DD YY

19. RESERVED FOR LOCAL USE

20. OUTSIDE LAB? YES ☐ NO ☐ $ CHARGES

21. DIAGNOSIS OR NATURE OF ILLNESS OR INJURY. (RELATE ITEMS 1, 2, 3, OR 4 TO ITEM 24E BY LINE)
1. 786.50
2. 600.00
3. ____
4. ____

22. MEDICAID RESUBMISSION CODE   ORIGINAL REF. NO.

23. PRIOR AUTHORIZATION NUMBER

24. A	DATE(S) OF SERVICE					B Place of Service	C Type of Service	D PROCEDURES, SERVICES, OR SUPPLIES (Explain Unusual Circumstances) CPT/HCPCS MODIFIER	E DIAGNOSIS CODE	F $ CHARGES	G DAYS OR UNITS	H EPSDT Family Plan	I EMG	J COB	K RESERVED FOR LOCAL USE
	From MM	DD	YY	To MM	DD	YY										
1	9	4					11	2	99214		48 00	1				
2	9	4					11	1	7015		45 00	1				
3																
4																
5																
6																

25. FEDERAL TAX I.D. NUMBER 99-9999999 SSN ☐ EIN ☒

26. PATIENT'S ACCOUNT NO.

27. ACCEPT ASSIGNMENT? (For govt. claims, see back) YES ☒ NO ☐

28. TOTAL CHARGE $ 93 00

29. AMOUNT PAID $ ___

30. BALANCE DUE $93.00

31. SIGNATURE OF PHYSICIAN OR SUPPLIER INCLUDING DEGREES OR CREDENTIALS (I certify that the statements on the reverse apply to this bill and are made a part thereof.)
SIGNED ___ DATE 7/?

32. NAME AND ADDRESS OF FACILITY WHERE SERVICES WERE RENDERED (If other than home or office)

33. PHYSICIAN'S SUPPLIER'S BILLING NAME, ADDRESS, ZIP CODE & PHONE #
Linda R. Gregory, MD 300
3733 Professional Dr # 300
Indpls, IN 46260
PIN# 6593060   GRP# MDA 80800

(APPROVED BY AMA COUNCIL ON MEDICAL SERVICE 8/88)

PLEASE PRINT OR TYPE

FORM HCFA-1500 (12-90)
FORM OWCP-1500 FORM RRB-1500
FORM AMA OP050192

PATIENT AND INSURED INFORMATION

PHYSICIAN OR SUPPLIER INFORMATION

FORM 27

PLEASE
DO NOT
STAPLE
IN THIS
AREA

CARRIER

□□ PICA

HEALTH INSURANCE CLAIM FORM

PICA □□

1. MEDICARE	MEDICAID	CHAMPUS	CHAMPVA	GROUP HEALTH PLAN	FECA BLK LUNG	OTHER	1a. INSURED'S I.D. NUMBER (FOR PROGRAM IN ITEM 1)
□ (Medicare #)	□ (Medicaid #)	□ (Sponsor's SSN)	□ (VA File #)	□ (SSN or ID)	□ (SSN)	□ (ID)	

2. PATIENT'S NAME (Last Name, First Name, Middle Initial)

3. PATIENT'S BIRTH DATE MM | DD | YY   SEX   M □   F □

4. INSURED'S NAME (Last Name, First Name, Middle Initial)

5. PATIENT'S ADDRESS (No. Street)

6. PATIENT RELATIONSHIP TO INSURED   Self □   Spouse □   Child □   Other □

7. INSURED'S ADDRESS (No. Street)

CITY   STATE

8. PATIENT STATUS   Single □   Married □   Other □

CITY   STATE

ZIP CODE   TELEPHONE (Include Area Code) (   )

Employed □   Full-Time Student □   Part-Time Student □

ZIP CODE   TELEPHONE (INCLUDE AREA CODE) (   )

9. OTHER INSURED'S NAME (Last Name, First Name, Middle Initial)

10. IS PATIENT'S CONDITION RELATED TO:

11. INSURED'S POLICY GROUP OR FECA NUMBER

a. OTHER INSURED'S POLICY OR GROUP NUMBER

a. EMPLOYMENT? (CURRENT OR PREVIOUS)   □ YES   □ NO

a. INSURED'S DATE OF BIRTH MM | DD | YY   SEX   M □   F □

b. OTHER INSURED'S DATE OF BIRTH MM | DD | YY   SEX   M □   F □

b. AUTO ACCIDENT?   PLACE (State)   □ YES   □ NO

b. EMPLOYER'S NAME OR SCHOOL NAME

c. EMPLOYER'S NAME OR SCHOOL NAME

c. OTHER ACCIDENT?   □ YES   □ NO

c. INSURANCE PLAN NAME OR PROGRAM NAME

d. INSURANCE PLAN NAME OR PROGRAM NAME

10d. RESERVED FOR LOCAL USE

d. IS THERE ANOTHER HEALTH BENEFIT PLAN?   □ YES   □ NO   If yes, return to and complete item 9 a – d.

READ BACK OF FORM BEFORE COMPLETING & SIGNING THIS FORM.
12. PATIENT'S OR AUTHORIZED PERSON'S SIGNATURE I authorize the release of any medical or other information necessary to process this claim. I also request payment of government benefits either to myself or to the party who accepts assignment below.

SIGNED _____   DATE _____

13. INSURED'S OR AUTHORIZED PERSON'S SIGNATURE I authorize payment of medical benefits to the undersigned physician or supplier for services described below.

SIGNED _____

PATIENT AND INSURED INFORMATION

14. DATE OF CURRENT: MM | DD | YY   ◄ ILLNESS (First symptom) OR INJURY (Accident) OR PREGNANCY (LMP)

15. IF PATIENT HAS HAD SAME OR SIMILAR ILLNESS, GIVE FIRST DATE MM | DD | YY

16. DATES PATIENT UNABLE TO WORK IN CURRENT OCCUPATION MM | DD | YY   FROM   TO   MM | DD | YY

17. NAME OF REFERRING PHYSICIAN OR OTHER SOURCE

17a. I.D. NUMBER OF REFERRING PHYSICIAN

18. HOSPITALIZATION DATES RELATED TO CURRENT SERVICES MM | DD | YY   FROM   TO   MM | DD | YY

19. RESERVED FOR LOCAL USE

20. OUTSIDE LAB?   □ YES   □ NO $ CHARGES

21. DIAGNOSIS OR NATURE OF ILLNESS OR INJURY. (RELATE ITEMS 1, 2, 3, OR 4 TO ITEM 24E BY LINE)
1. └──.──
2. └──.──
3. └──.──
4. └──.──

22. MEDICAID RESUBMISSION CODE   ORIGINAL REF. NO.

23. PRIOR AUTHORIZATION NUMBER

24. A DATE(S) OF SERVICE						B Place of Service	C Type of Service	D PROCEDURES, SERVICES, OR SUPPLIES (Explain Unusual Circumstances) CPT/HCPCS	MODIFIER	E DIAGNOSIS CODE	F $ CHARGES	G DAYS OR UNITS	H EPSDT Family Plan	I EMG	J COB	K RESERVED FOR LOCAL USE
From MM	DD	YY	To MM	DD	YY											
1																
2																
3																
4																
5																
6																

25. FEDERAL TAX I.D. NUMBER   SSN □ EIN □

26. PATIENT'S ACCOUNT NO.

27. ACCEPT ASSIGNMENT? (For govt. claims, see back)   □ YES   □ NO

28. TOTAL CHARGE $

29. AMOUNT PAID $

30. BALANCE DUE $

31. SIGNATURE OF PHYSICIAN OR SUPPLIER INCLUDING DEGREES OR CREDENTIALS (I certify that the statements on the reverse apply to this bill and are made a part thereof.)

SIGNED _____   DATE _____

32. NAME AND ADDRESS OF FACILITY WHERE SERVICES WERE RENDERED (If other than home or office)

33. PHYSICIAN'S SUPPLIER'S BILLING NAME, ADDRESS, ZIP CODE & PHONE #

PIN#   GRP#

PHYSICIAN OR SUPPLIER INFORMATION

(APPROVED BY AMA COUNCIL ON MEDICAL SERVICE 8/88)

PLEASE PRINT OR TYPE

FORM HCFA-1500 (12-90)
FORM OWCP-1500   FORM RRB-1500
FORM AMA OP050192

FORM 28

Medicaid

Medicaid
P.O. Box 68A888
Indpls. IN
46288

HEALTH INSURANCE CLAIM FORM

PLEASE DO NOT STAPLE IN THIS AREA

☐☐☐ PICA

PICA ☐☐☐

| 1. MEDICARE ☐ (Medicare #) | MEDICAID ☒ (Medicaid #) | CHAMPUS ☐ (Sponsor's SSN) | CHAMPVA ☐ (VA File #) | GROUP HEALTH PLAN ☐ (SSN or ID) | FECA BLK LUNG ☐ (SSN) | OTHER ☐ (ID) | 1a. INSURED'S I.D. NUMBER (FOR PROGRAM IN ITEM 1) 42-394166571-5 |

| 2. PATIENT'S NAME (Last Name, First Name, Middle Initial) Hieson Diana | 3. PATIENT'S BIRTH DATE MM 09 DD 15 YY SEX M ☐ F ☒ | 4. INSURED'S NAME (Last Name, First Name, Middle Initial) |

| 5. PATIENT'S ADDRESS (No. Street) 31 Glenna Lane | 6. PATIENT RELATIONSHIP TO INSURED Self ☐ Spouse ☐ Child ☐ Other ☐ | 7. INSURED'S ADDRESS (No. Street) |

| CITY Indpls | STATE IN | 8. PATIENT STATUS Single ☐ Married ☐ Other ☐ | CITY | STATE |

| ZIP CODE 46239 | TELEPHONE (Include Area Code) ( ) | Employed ☐ Full-Time Student ☐ Part-Time Student ☐ | ZIP CODE | TELEPHONE (INCLUDE AREA CODE) ( ) |

| 9. OTHER INSURED'S NAME (Last Name, First Name, Middle Initial) | 10. IS PATIENT'S CONDITION RELATED TO: | 11. INSURED'S POLICY GROUP OR FECA NUMBER |

| a. OTHER INSURED'S POLICY OR GROUP NUMBER | a. EMPLOYMENT? (CURRENT OR PREVIOUS) YES ☐ NO ☒ | a. INSURED'S DATE OF BIRTH MM DD YY SEX M ☐ F ☐ |

| b. OTHER INSURED'S DATE OF BIRTH MM DD YY SEX M ☐ F ☐ | b. AUTO ACCIDENT? PLACE (State) YES ☐ NO ☒ | b. EMPLOYER'S NAME OR SCHOOL NAME |

| c. EMPLOYER'S NAME OR SCHOOL NAME | c. OTHER ACCIDENT? YES ☐ NO ☒ | c. INSURANCE PLAN NAME OR PROGRAM NAME |

| d. INSURANCE PLAN NAME OR PROGRAM NAME | 10d. RESERVED FOR LOCAL USE | d. IS THERE ANOTHER HEALTH BENEFIT PLAN? YES ☐ NO ☒ If yes, return to and complete item 9 a – d. |

READ BACK OF FORM BEFORE COMPLETING & SIGNING THIS FORM.
12. PATIENT'S OR AUTHORIZED PERSON'S SIGNATURE I authorize the release of any medical or other information necessary to process this claim. I also request payment of government benefits either to myself or to the party who accepts assignment below.

SIGNED _____ DATE Today

13. INSURED'S OR AUTHORIZED PERSON'S SIGNATURE I authorize payment of medical benefits to the undersigned physician or supplier for services described below.

SIGNED _____

| 14. DATE OF CURRENT: MM DD YY ◄ ILLNESS (First symptom) OR INJURY (Accident) OR PREGNANCY (LMP) | 15. IF PATIENT HAS HAD SAME OR SIMILAR ILLNESS, GIVE FIRST DATE MM DD YY | 16. DATES PATIENT UNABLE TO WORK IN CURRENT OCCUPATION FROM MM DD YY TO MM DD YY |

| 17. NAME OF REFERRING PHYSICIAN OR OTHER SOURCE | 17a. I.D. NUMBER OF REFERRING PHYSICIAN 99-9999999 | 18. HOSPITALIZATION DATES RELATED TO CURRENT SERVICES FROM MM DD YY TO MM DD YY |

| 19. RESERVED FOR LOCAL USE | | 20. OUTSIDE LAB? YES ☐ NO ☒ $ CHARGES |

21. DIAGNOSIS OR NATURE OF ILLNESS OR INJURY. (RELATE ITEMS 1, 2, 3, OR 4 TO ITEM 24E BY LINE)
1. B71 50
3.
2.
4.

22. MEDICAID RESUBMISSION CODE ORIGINAL REF. NO.

23. PRIOR AUTHORIZATION NUMBER

24. A. DATE(S) OF SERVICE From MM DD YY	To MM DD YY	B. Place of Service	C. Type of Service	D. PROCEDURES, SERVICES, OR SUPPLIES (Explain Unusual Circumstances) CPT/HCPCS MODIFIER	E. DIAGNOSIS CODE	F. $ CHARGES	G. DAYS OR UNITS	H. EPSDT Family Plan	I. EMG	J. COB	K. RESERVED FOR LOCAL USE
2 10		11		99203	1	60 00	1				219990218

| 25. FEDERAL TAX I.D. NUMBER SSN ☐ EIN ☐ | 26. PATIENT'S ACCOUNT NO. | 27. ACCEPT ASSIGNMENT? (For govt. claims, see back) YES ☐ NO ☐ | 28. TOTAL CHARGE $ 60 00 | 29. AMOUNT PAID $ | 30. BALANCE DUE $ |

31. SIGNATURE OF PHYSICIAN OR SUPPLIER INCLUDING DEGREES OR CREDENTIALS (I certify that the statements on the reverse apply to this bill and are made a part thereof.)

SIGNED _____ DATE _____

32. NAME AND ADDRESS OF FACILITY WHERE SERVICES WERE RENDERED (If other than home or office)

33. PHYSICIAN'S SUPPLIER'S BILLING NAME, ADDRESS, ZIP CODE & PHONE #
James P Cartman MD
3733 Professional Dr #300
Indpls IN 46260
PIN# 219990218   GRP# 21886

(APPROVED BY AMA COUNCIL ON MEDICAL SERVICE 8/88)

PLEASE PRINT OR TYPE

FORM HCFA-1500 (12-90)
FORM OWCP-1500   FORM RRB-1500
FORM AMA OP050192

FORM 29

APPROVED OMB-0938-0008

CARRIER

| | PICA | | **HEALTH INSURANCE CLAIM FORM** | PICA | | |

| 1. MEDICARE   MEDICAID   CHAMPUS   CHAMPVA   GROUP HEALTH PLAN   FECA BLK LUNG   OTHER | 1a. INSURED'S I.D. NUMBER   (FOR PROGRAM IN ITEM 1) |

(Medicare #) (Medicaid #) (Sponsor's SSN) (VA File #) (SSN or ID) (SSN) (ID)

| 2. PATIENT'S NAME (Last Name, First Name, Middle Initial) | 3. PATIENT'S BIRTH DATE MM | DD | YY   SEX M   F | 4. INSURED'S NAME (Last Name, First Name, Middle Initial) |

| 5. PATIENT'S ADDRESS (No. Street) | 6. PATIENT RELATIONSHIP TO INSURED Self   Spouse   Child   Other | 7. INSURED'S ADDRESS (No. Street) |

| CITY | STATE | 8. PATIENT STATUS   Single   Married   Other | CITY | STATE |

| ZIP CODE   TELEPHONE (Include Area Code) ( ) | Employed   Full-Time Student   Part-Time Student | ZIP CODE   TELEPHONE (INCLUDE AREA CODE) ( ) |

| 9. OTHER INSURED'S NAME (Last Name, First Name, Middle Initial) | 10. IS PATIENT'S CONDITION RELATED TO: | 11. INSURED'S POLICY GROUP OR FECA NUMBER |

| a. OTHER INSURED'S POLICY OR GROUP NUMBER | a. EMPLOYMENT? (CURRENT OR PREVIOUS)   YES   NO | a. INSURED'S DATE OF BIRTH MM | DD | YY   SEX M   F |

| b. OTHER INSURED'S DATE OF BIRTH MM | DD | YY   SEX M   F | b. AUTO ACCIDENT?   PLACE (State)   YES   NO | b. EMPLOYER'S NAME OR SCHOOL NAME |

| c. EMPLOYER'S NAME OR SCHOOL NAME | c. OTHER ACCIDENT?   YES   NO | c. INSURANCE PLAN NAME OR PROGRAM NAME |

| d. INSURANCE PLAN NAME OR PROGRAM NAME | 10d. RESERVED FOR LOCAL USE | d. IS THERE ANOTHER HEALTH BENEFIT PLAN?   YES   NO   If yes, return to and complete item 9 a – d. |

READ BACK OF FORM BEFORE COMPLETING & SIGNING THIS FORM.
12. PATIENT'S OR AUTHORIZED PERSON'S SIGNATURE I authorize the release of any medical or other information necessary to process this claim. I also request payment of government benefits either to myself or to the party who accepts assignment below.

SIGNED _____ DATE _____

13. INSURED'S OR AUTHORIZED PERSON'S SIGNATURE I authorize payment of medical benefits to the undersigned physician or supplier for services described below.

SIGNED _____

PATIENT AND INSURED INFORMATION

| 14. DATE OF CURRENT: ILLNESS (First symptom) OR INJURY (Accident) OR PREGNANCY (LMP) MM | DD | YY | 15. IF PATIENT HAS HAD SAME OR SIMILAR ILLNESS, GIVE FIRST DATE MM | DD | YY | 16. DATES PATIENT UNABLE TO WORK IN CURRENT OCCUPATION MM | DD | YY   MM | DD | YY FROM   TO |

| 17. NAME OF REFERRING PHYSICIAN OR OTHER SOURCE | 17a. I.D. NUMBER OF REFERRING PHYSICIAN | 18. HOSPITALIZATION DATES RELATED TO CURRENT SERVICES MM | DD | YY   MM | DD | YY FROM   TO |

| 19. RESERVED FOR LOCAL USE | 20. OUTSIDE LAB? $ CHARGES   YES   NO |

| 21. DIAGNOSIS OR NATURE OF ILLNESS OR INJURY. (RELATE ITEMS 1, 2, 3, OR 4 TO ITEM 24E BY LINE)
1. |___.___   3. |___.___
2. |___.___   4. |___.___ | 22. MEDICAID RESUBMISSION CODE   ORIGINAL REF. NO. |
| | 23. PRIOR AUTHORIZATION NUMBER |

24. A. DATE(S) OF SERVICE From MM DD YY To MM DD YY	B. Place of Service	C. Type of Service	D. PROCEDURES, SERVICES, OR SUPPLIES (Explain Unusual Circumstances) CPT/HCPCS	MODIFIER	E. DIAGNOSIS CODE	F. $ CHARGES	G. DAYS OR UNITS	H. EPSDT Family Plan	I. EMG	J. COB	K. RESERVED FOR LOCAL USE
1											
2											
3											
4											
5											
6											

| 25. FEDERAL TAX I.D. NUMBER   SSN   EIN | 26. PATIENT'S ACCOUNT NO. | 27. ACCEPT ASSIGNMENT? (For govt. claims, see back)   YES   NO | 28. TOTAL CHARGE $ | 29. AMOUNT PAID $ | 30. BALANCE DUE $ |

| 31. SIGNATURE OF PHYSICIAN OR SUPPLIER INCLUDING DEGREES OR CREDENTIALS (I certify that the statements on the reverse apply to this bill and are made a part thereof.)

SIGNED _____ DATE _____ | 32. NAME AND ADDRESS OF FACILITY WHERE SERVICES WERE RENDERED (If other than home or office) | 33. PHYSICIAN'S SUPPLIER'S BILLING NAME, ADDRESS, ZIP CODE & PHONE #

PIN#   GRP# |

PHYSICIAN OR SUPPLIER INFORMATION

(APPROVED BY AMA COUNCIL ON MEDICAL SERVICE 8/88)   *PLEASE PRINT OR TYPE*   FORM HCFA-1500 (12-90)
FORM OWCP-1500   FORM RRB-1500
FORM AMA OP050192

FORM 30

APPROVED OMB-0938-0008

☐☐ PICA

HEALTH INSURANCE CLAIM FORM

PICA ☐☐

| 1. MEDICARE MEDICAID CHAMPUS CHAMPVA GROUP HEALTH PLAN FECA BLK LUNG OTHER | 1a. INSURED'S I.D. NUMBER (FOR PROGRAM IN ITEM 1) |

☐ (Medicare #) ☐ (Medicaid #) ☐ (Sponsor's SSN) ☐ (VA File #) ☐ (SSN or ID) ☐ (SSN) ☐ (ID)

2. PATIENT'S NAME (Last Name, First Name, Middle Initial)

3. PATIENT'S BIRTH DATE MM DD YY SEX M ☐ F ☐

4. INSURED'S NAME (Last Name, First Name, Middle Initial)

5. PATIENT'S ADDRESS (No. Street)

6. PATIENT RELATIONSHIP TO INSURED Self ☐ Spouse ☐ Child ☐ Other ☐

7. INSURED'S ADDRESS (No. Street)

CITY   STATE

8. PATIENT STATUS Single ☐ Married ☐ Other ☐

CITY   STATE

ZIP CODE   TELEPHONE (Include Area Code) (   )

Employed ☐ Full-Time Student ☐ Part-Time Student ☐

ZIP CODE   TELEPHONE (INCLUDE AREA CODE) (   )

9. OTHER INSURED'S NAME (Last Name, First Name, Middle Initial)

10. IS PATIENT'S CONDITION RELATED TO:

11. INSURED'S POLICY GROUP OR FECA NUMBER

a. OTHER INSURED'S POLICY OR GROUP NUMBER

a. EMPLOYMENT? (CURRENT OR PREVIOUS) ☐ YES ☐ NO

a. INSURED'S DATE OF BIRTH MM DD YY SEX M ☐ F ☐

b. OTHER INSURED'S DATE OF BIRTH MM DD YY SEX M ☐ F ☐

b. AUTO ACCIDENT? PLACE (State) ☐ YES ☐ NO

b. EMPLOYER'S NAME OR SCHOOL NAME

c. EMPLOYER'S NAME OR SCHOOL NAME

c. OTHER ACCIDENT? ☐ YES ☐ NO

c. INSURANCE PLAN NAME OR PROGRAM NAME

d. INSURANCE PLAN NAME OR PROGRAM NAME

10d. RESERVED FOR LOCAL USE

d. IS THERE ANOTHER HEALTH BENEFIT PLAN? ☐ YES ☐ NO If yes, return to and complete item 9 a – d.

READ BACK OF FORM BEFORE COMPLETING & SIGNING THIS FORM.
12. PATIENT'S OR AUTHORIZED PERSON'S SIGNATURE I authorize the release of any medical or other information necessary to process this claim. I also request payment of government benefits either to myself or to the party who accepts assignment below.

SIGNED _____   DATE _____

13. INSURED'S OR AUTHORIZED PERSON'S SIGNATURE I authorize payment of medical benefits to the undersigned physician or supplier for services described below.

SIGNED _____

14. DATE OF CURRENT: MM DD YY ILLNESS (First symptom) OR INJURY (Accident) OR PREGNANCY (LMP)

15. IF PATIENT HAS HAD SAME OR SIMILAR ILLNESS, GIVE FIRST DATE MM DD YY

16. DATES PATIENT UNABLE TO WORK IN CURRENT OCCUPATION MM DD YY MM DD YY FROM TO

17. NAME OF REFERRING PHYSICIAN OR OTHER SOURCE

17a. I.D. NUMBER OF REFERRING PHYSICIAN

18. HOSPITALIZATION DATES RELATED TO CURRENT SERVICES MM DD YY MM DD YY FROM TO

19. RESERVED FOR LOCAL USE

20. OUTSIDE LAB? ☐ YES ☐ NO $ CHARGES

21. DIAGNOSIS OR NATURE OF ILLNESS OR INJURY. (RELATE ITEMS 1, 2, 3, OR 4 TO ITEM 24E BY LINE)

1. |___.___| 3. |___.___|

2. |___.___| 4. |___.___|

22. MEDICAID RESUBMISSION CODE   ORIGINAL REF. NO.

23. PRIOR AUTHORIZATION NUMBER

24. A DATE(S) OF SERVICE		B Place of Service	C Type of Service	D PROCEDURES, SERVICES, OR SUPPLIES (Explain Unusual Circumstances)		E DIAGNOSIS CODE	F $ CHARGES	G DAYS OR UNITS	H EPSDT Family Plan	I EMG	J COB	K RESERVED FOR LOCAL USE
From MM DD YY	To MM DD YY			CPT/HCPCS	MODIFIER							
1												
2												
3												
4												
5												
6												

25. FEDERAL TAX I.D. NUMBER ☐ SSN ☐ EIN

26. PATIENT'S ACCOUNT NO.

27. ACCEPT ASSIGNMENT? (For govt. claims, see back) ☐ YES ☐ NO

28. TOTAL CHARGE $

29. AMOUNT PAID $

30. BALANCE DUE $

31. SIGNATURE OF PHYSICIAN OR SUPPLIER INCLUDING DEGREES OR CREDENTIALS (I certify that the statements on the reverse apply to this bill and are made a part thereof.)

SIGNED _____   DATE _____

32. NAME AND ADDRESS OF FACILITY WHERE SERVICES WERE RENDERED (If other than home or office)

33. PHYSICIAN'S SUPPLIER'S BILLING NAME, ADDRESS, ZIP CODE & PHONE #

PIN#   GRP#

(APPROVED BY AMA COUNCIL ON MEDICAL SERVICE 8/88)

PLEASE PRINT OR TYPE

FORM HCFA-1500 (12-90)
FORM OWCP-1500   FORM RRB-1500
FORM AMA OP050192

CARRIER

PATIENT AND INSURED INFORMATION

PHYSICIAN OR SUPPLIER INFORMATION

FORM 31

Worker's Compensation

CARRIER

Champus
BC / BS of R.I.
P.O. B 33
Providence RF
02901

HEALTH INSURANCE CLAIM FORM

PLEASE
DO NOT
STAPLE
IN THIS
AREA

☐☐ PICA   PICA ☐☐

1. MEDICARE	MEDICAID	CHAMPUS	CHAMPVA	GROUP HEALTH PLAN	FECA BLK LUNG	OTHER	1a. INSURED'S I.D. NUMBER (FOR PROGRAM IN ITEM 1)

1. MEDICARE ☐ (Medicare #) MEDICAID ☐ (Medicaid #) CHAMPUS ☒ (Sponsor's SSN) CHAMPVA ☐ (VA File #) GROUP HEALTH PLAN ☐ (SSN or ID) FECA BLK LUNG ☐ (SSN) OTHER ☐ (ID)

1a. INSURED'S I.D. NUMBER (FOR PROGRAM IN ITEM 1)
132.60 - 800

2. PATIENT'S NAME (Last Name, First Name, Middle Initial)
Ebner Donald

3. PATIENT'S BIRTH DATE MM 12 DD 13 YY   SEX M ☐ F ☐

4. INSURED'S NAME (Last Name, First Name, Middle Initial)
Ebner, Donald

5. PATIENT'S ADDRESS (No. Street)
6018 Orchard Lane

6. PATIENT RELATIONSHIP TO INSURED
Self ☐ Spouse ☐ Child ☐ Other ☐

7. INSURED'S ADDRESS (No. Street)
Same

CITY Bltgn   STATE IN

8. PATIENT STATUS
Single ☐ Married ☐ Other ☐
Employed ☒ Full-Time Student ☐ Part-Time Student ☐

CITY   STATE

ZIP CODE 47437-1237   TELEPHONE (Include Area Code) (   )

ZIP CODE   TELEPHONE (INCLUDE AREA CODE) (   )

9. OTHER INSURED'S NAME (Last Name, First Name, Middle Initial)

10. IS PATIENT'S CONDITION RELATED TO:

11. INSURED'S POLICY GROUP OR FECA NUMBER
USN (GR) RET

a. OTHER INSURED'S POLICY OR GROUP NUMBER

a. EMPLOYMENT? (CURRENT OR PREVIOUS)
☒ YES ☐ NO

a. INSURED'S DATE OF BIRTH MM DD YY   SEX M ☐ F ☐

b. OTHER INSURED'S DATE OF BIRTH MM DD YY   SEX M ☐ F ☐

b. AUTO ACCIDENT?   PLACE (State)
☐ YES ☐ NO

b. EMPLOYER'S NAME OR SCHOOL NAME

c. EMPLOYER'S NAME OR SCHOOL NAME

c. OTHER ACCIDENT?
☐ YES ☐ NO

c. INSURANCE PLAN NAME OR PROGRAM NAME

d. INSURANCE PLAN NAME OR PROGRAM NAME

10d. RESERVED FOR LOCAL USE

d. IS THERE ANOTHER HEALTH BENEFIT PLAN?
☐ YES ☐ NO If yes, return to and complete item 9 a – d.

READ BACK OF FORM BEFORE COMPLETING & SIGNING THIS FORM.
12. PATIENT'S OR AUTHORIZED PERSON'S SIGNATURE I authorize the release of any medical or other information necessary to process this claim. I also request payment of government benefits either to myself or to the party who accepts assignment below.
SIGNED Signature on file   DATE Today

13. INSURED'S OR AUTHORIZED PERSON'S SIGNATURE I authorize payment of medical benefits to the undersigned physician or supplier for services described below.
SIGNED Signature on file

14. DATE OF CURRENT: ILLNESS (First symptom) OR INJURY (Accident) OR PREGNANCY (LMP) MM DD YY

15. IF PATIENT HAS HAD SAME OR SIMILAR ILLNESS, GIVE FIRST DATE MM DD YY

16. DATES PATIENT UNABLE TO WORK IN CURRENT OCCUPATION FROM MM DD YY TO MM DD YY

17. NAME OF REFERRING PHYSICIAN OR OTHER SOURCE

17a. I.D. NUMBER OF REFERRING PHYSICIAN

18. HOSPITALIZATION DATES RELATED TO CURRENT SERVICES FROM MM DD YY TO MM DD YY

19. RESERVED FOR LOCAL USE

20. OUTSIDE LAB? $ CHARGES
☒ YES ☐ NO

21. DIAGNOSIS OR NATURE OF ILLNESS OR INJURY. (RELATE ITEMS 1, 2, 3, OR 4 TO ITEM 24E BY LINE)
1. 600.01 (code)
2. 788.29
3.
4.

22. MEDICAID RESUBMISSION CODE   ORIGINAL REF. NO.

23. PRIOR AUTHORIZATION NUMBER

24. A DATE(S) OF SERVICE		B Place of Service	C Type of Service	D PROCEDURES, SERVICES, OR SUPPLIES (Explain Unusual Circumstances)		E DIAGNOSIS CODE	F $ CHARGES	G DAYS OR UNITS	H EPSDT Family Plan	I EMG	J COB	K RESERVED FOR LOCAL USE
From MM DD YY	To MM DD YY			CPT/HCPCS	MODIFIER							
03 18		11		52000		1, 2	200 00	1				
03 18		22		32601		2	1800 00	1				

25. FEDERAL TAX I.D. NUMBER SSN ☐ EIN ☒
04-9999999

26. PATIENT'S ACCOUNT NO.

27. ACCEPT ASSIGNMENT? (For govt. claims, see back)
YES ☐ NO ☐

28. TOTAL CHARGE $ 2000.00

29. AMOUNT PAID $

30. BALANCE DUE $

31. SIGNATURE OF PHYSICIAN OR SUPPLIER INCLUDING DEGREES OR CREDENTIALS (I certify that the statements on the reverse apply to this bill and are made a part thereof.)
SIGNED Linda Gregory, MD   DATE

32. NAME AND ADDRESS OF FACILITY WHERE SERVICES WERE RENDERED (If other than home or office)
Good Samaritan Hos,
1212 W. 88 St.
Indpls. IN. 46260

33. PHYSICIAN'S SUPPLIER'S BILLING NAME, ADDRESS, ZIP CODE & PHONE #
Linda Gregory m.D
3733 Professional Dr. # 300
Indpls IN 46260
PIN# 7765003   GRP#

(APPROVED BY AMA COUNCIL ON MEDICAL SERVICE 8/88)   PLEASE PRINT OR TYPE

FORM HCFA-1500 (12-90)
FORM OWCP-1500 FORM RRB-1500
FORM AMA OP050192

FORM 32

APPROVED OMB-0938-0008

CARRIER

| | PICA | | | | **HEALTH INSURANCE CLAIM FORM** | | PICA | | |

HEALTH INSURANCE CLAIM FORM

1. MEDICARE	MEDICAID	CHAMPUS	CHAMPVA	GROUP HEALTH PLAN	FECA BLK LUNG	OTHER	1a. INSURED'S I.D. NUMBER	(FOR PROGRAM IN ITEM 1)
☐ (Medicare #)	☐ (Medicaid #)	☐ (Sponsor's SSN)	☐ (VA File #)	☐ (SSN or ID)	☐ (SSN)	☐ (ID)		

2. PATIENT'S NAME (Last Name, First Name, Middle Initial)

3. PATIENT'S BIRTH DATE   MM   DD   YY   SEX   M ☐   F ☐

4. INSURED'S NAME (Last Name, First Name, Middle Initial)

5. PATIENT'S ADDRESS (No. Street)

6. PATIENT RELATIONSHIP TO INSURED   Self ☐   Spouse ☐   Child ☐   Other ☐

7. INSURED'S ADDRESS (No. Street)

CITY   STATE

8. PATIENT STATUS   Single ☐   Married ☐   Other ☐

CITY   STATE

ZIP CODE   TELEPHONE (Include Area Code) ( )

Employed ☐   Full-Time Student ☐   Part-Time Student ☐

ZIP CODE   TELEPHONE (INCLUDE AREA CODE) ( )

9. OTHER INSURED'S NAME (Last Name, First Name, Middle Initial)

10. IS PATIENT'S CONDITION RELATED TO:

11. INSURED'S POLICY GROUP OR FECA NUMBER

a. OTHER INSURED'S POLICY OR GROUP NUMBER

a. EMPLOYMENT? (CURRENT OR PREVIOUS)   ☐ YES   ☐ NO

a. INSURED'S DATE OF BIRTH   MM   DD   YY   SEX   M ☐   F ☐

b. OTHER INSURED'S DATE OF BIRTH   MM   DD   YY   SEX   M ☐   F ☐

b. AUTO ACCIDENT?   PLACE (State)   ☐ YES   ☐ NO

b. EMPLOYER'S NAME OR SCHOOL NAME

c. EMPLOYER'S NAME OR SCHOOL NAME

c. OTHER ACCIDENT?   ☐ YES   ☐ NO

c. INSURANCE PLAN NAME OR PROGRAM NAME

d. INSURANCE PLAN NAME OR PROGRAM NAME

10d. RESERVED FOR LOCAL USE

d. IS THERE ANOTHER HEALTH BENEFIT PLAN?   ☐ YES   ☐ NO   If yes, return to and complete item 9 a – d.

READ BACK OF FORM BEFORE COMPLETING & SIGNING THIS FORM.
12. PATIENT'S OR AUTHORIZED PERSON'S SIGNATURE I authorize the release of any medical or other information necessary to process this claim. I also request payment of government benefits either to myself or to the party who accepts assignment below.

SIGNED _____   DATE _____

13. INSURED'S OR AUTHORIZED PERSON'S SIGNATURE I authorize payment of medical benefits to the undersigned physician or supplier for services described below.

SIGNED _____

PATIENT AND INSURED INFORMATION

14. DATE OF CURRENT: ◄ ILLNESS (First symptom) OR   MM   DD   YY   INJURY (Accident) OR   PREGNANCY (LMP)

15. IF PATIENT HAS HAD SAME OR SIMILAR ILLNESS, GIVE FIRST DATE   MM   DD   YY

16. DATES PATIENT UNABLE TO WORK IN CURRENT OCCUPATION   MM   DD   YY   MM   DD   YY   FROM   TO

17. NAME OF REFERRING PHYSICIAN OR OTHER SOURCE

17a. I.D. NUMBER OF REFERRING PHYSICIAN

18. HOSPITALIZATION DATES RELATED TO CURRENT SERVICES   MM   DD   YY   MM   DD   YY   FROM   TO

19. RESERVED FOR LOCAL USE

20. OUTSIDE LAB?   ☐ YES   ☐ NO $ CHARGES

21. DIAGNOSIS OR NATURE OF ILLNESS OR INJURY. (RELATE ITEMS 1, 2, 3, OR 4 TO ITEM 24E BY LINE)

1. └___ . __   3. └___ . __

2. └___ . __   4. └___ . __

22. MEDICAID RESUBMISSION CODE   ORIGINAL REF. NO.

23. PRIOR AUTHORIZATION NUMBER

24. A DATE(S) OF SERVICE						B Place of Service	C Type of Service	D PROCEDURES, SERVICES, OR SUPPLIES (Explain Unusual Circumstances)		E DIAGNOSIS CODE	F $ CHARGES	G DAYS OR UNITS	H EPSDT Family Plan	I EMG	J COB	K RESERVED FOR LOCAL USE
From MM	DD	YY	To MM	DD	YY			CPT/HCPCS	MODIFIER							
1																
2																
3																
4																
5																
6																

25. FEDERAL TAX I.D. NUMBER   SSN ☐ EIN ☐

26. PATIENT'S ACCOUNT NO.

27. ACCEPT ASSIGNMENT? (For govt. claims, see back)   ☐ YES   ☐ NO

28. TOTAL CHARGE $

29. AMOUNT PAID $

30. BALANCE DUE $

31. SIGNATURE OF PHYSICIAN OR SUPPLIER INCLUDING DEGREES OR CREDENTIALS (I certify that the statements on the reverse apply to this bill and are made a part thereof.)

SIGNED _____   DATE _____

32. NAME AND ADDRESS OF FACILITY WHERE SERVICES WERE RENDERED (If other than home or office)

33. PHYSICIAN'S SUPPLIER'S BILLING NAME, ADDRESS, ZIP CODE & PHONE #

PIN#   GRP#

PHYSICIAN OR SUPPLIER INFORMATION

(APPROVED BY AMA COUNCIL ON MEDICAL SERVICE 8/88)

PLEASE PRINT OR TYPE

FORM HCFA-1500 (12-90)
FORM OWCP-1500   FORM RRB-1500
FORM AMA OP050192

FORM 33

282

PLEASE
DO NOT
STAPLE
IN THIS
AREA

CARRIER

HEALTH INSURANCE CLAIM FORM

| | PICA | | | PICA | | |

1.
| MEDICARE | MEDICAID | CHAMPUS | CHAMPVA | GROUP HEALTH PLAN | FECA BLK LUNG | OTHER | 1a. INSURED'S I.D. NUMBER (FOR PROGRAM IN ITEM 1) |
| (Medicare #) | (Medicaid #) | (Sponsor's SSN) | (VA File #) | (SSN or ID) | (SSN) | (ID) | |

2. PATIENT'S NAME (Last Name, First Name, Middle Initial)

3. PATIENT'S BIRTH DATE
MM DD YY   SEX   M☐   F☐

4. INSURED'S NAME (Last Name, First Name, Middle Initial)

5. PATIENT'S ADDRESS (No. Street)

6. PATIENT RELATIONSHIP TO INSURED
Self ☐   Spouse ☐   Child ☐   Other ☐

7. INSURED'S ADDRESS (No. Street)

CITY   STATE

8. PATIENT STATUS
Single ☐   Married ☐   Other ☐
Employed ☐   Full-Time Student ☐   Part-Time Student ☐

CITY   STATE

ZIP CODE   TELEPHONE (Include Area Code) ( )

ZIP CODE   TELEPHONE (INCLUDE AREA CODE) ( )

9. OTHER INSURED'S NAME (Last Name, First Name, Middle Initial)

10. IS PATIENT'S CONDITION RELATED TO:

11. INSURED'S POLICY GROUP OR FECA NUMBER

a. OTHER INSURED'S POLICY OR GROUP NUMBER

a. EMPLOYMENT? (CURRENT OR PREVIOUS)
☐ YES   ☐ NO

a. INSURED'S DATE OF BIRTH
MM DD YY   SEX   M☐   F☐

b. OTHER INSURED'S DATE OF BIRTH
MM DD YY   SEX   M☐   F☐

b. AUTO ACCIDENT?   PLACE (State)
☐ YES   ☐ NO

b. EMPLOYER'S NAME OR SCHOOL NAME

c. EMPLOYER'S NAME OR SCHOOL NAME

c. OTHER ACCIDENT?
☐ YES   ☐ NO

c. INSURANCE PLAN NAME OR PROGRAM NAME

d. INSURANCE PLAN NAME OR PROGRAM NAME

10d. RESERVED FOR LOCAL USE

d. IS THERE ANOTHER HEALTH BENEFIT PLAN?
☐ YES   ☐ NO   If yes, return to and complete item 9 a – d.

READ BACK OF FORM BEFORE COMPLETING & SIGNING THIS FORM.
12. PATIENT'S OR AUTHORIZED PERSON'S SIGNATURE I authorize the release of any medical or other information necessary to process this claim. I also request payment of government benefits either to myself or to the party who accepts assignment below.

SIGNED _____   DATE _____

13. INSURED'S OR AUTHORIZED PERSON'S SIGNATURE I authorize payment of medical benefits to the undersigned physician or supplier for services described below.

SIGNED _____

PATIENT AND INSURED INFORMATION

14. DATE OF CURRENT: ILLNESS (First symptom) OR
MM DD YY   INJURY (Accident) OR
PREGNANCY (LMP)

15. IF PATIENT HAS HAD SAME OR SIMILAR ILLNESS, GIVE FIRST DATE MM DD YY

16. DATES PATIENT UNABLE TO WORK IN CURRENT OCCUPATION
MM DD YY   MM DD YY
FROM   TO

17. NAME OF REFERRING PHYSICIAN OR OTHER SOURCE

17a. I.D. NUMBER OF REFERRING PHYSICIAN

18. HOSPITALIZATION DATES RELATED TO CURRENT SERVICES
MM DD YY   MM DD YY
FROM   TO

19. RESERVED FOR LOCAL USE

20. OUTSIDE LAB? $ CHARGES
☐ YES   ☐ NO

21. DIAGNOSIS OR NATURE OF ILLNESS OR INJURY. (RELATE ITEMS 1, 2, 3, OR 4 TO ITEM 24E BY LINE)
1. ⌊____.____   3. ⌊____.____
2. ⌊____.____   4. ⌊____.____

22. MEDICAID RESUBMISSION CODE   ORIGINAL REF. NO.

23. PRIOR AUTHORIZATION NUMBER

24.
A DATE(S) OF SERVICE						B Place of Service	C Type of Service	D PROCEDURES, SERVICES, OR SUPPLIES (Explain Unusual Circumstances)		E DIAGNOSIS CODE	F $ CHARGES	G DAYS OR UNITS	H EPSDT Family Plan	I EMG	J COB	K RESERVED FOR LOCAL USE
From			To					CPT/HCPCS	MODIFIER							
MM	DD	YY	MM	DD	YY											
1																
2																
3																
4																
5																
6																

25. FEDERAL TAX I.D. NUMBER   SSN ☐ EIN ☐

26. PATIENT'S ACCOUNT NO.

27. ACCEPT ASSIGNMENT? (For govt. claims, see back)
☐ YES   ☐ NO

28. TOTAL CHARGE $

29. AMOUNT PAID $

30. BALANCE DUE $

31. SIGNATURE OF PHYSICIAN OR SUPPLIER INCLUDING DEGREES OR CREDENTIALS (I certify that the statements on the reverse apply to this bill and are made a part thereof.)

SIGNED _____   DATE _____

32. NAME AND ADDRESS OF FACILITY WHERE SERVICES WERE RENDERED (If other than home or office)

33. PHYSICIAN'S SUPPLIER'S BILLING NAME, ADDRESS, ZIP CODE & PHONE #

PIN# _____   GRP# _____

PHYSICIAN OR SUPPLIER INFORMATION

(APPROVED BY AMA COUNCIL ON MEDICAL SERVICE 8/88)

PLEASE PRINT OR TYPE

FORM HCFA-1500 (12-90)
FORM OWCP-1500   FORM RRB-1500
FORM AMA OP050192

FORM 33A

Part Five   Numbered Forms and Worksheets

CHUMPVA

APPROVED OMB-0938-0008

Champus
BC/BS of RI
P.O.B 35
Providence RI 02901

☐☐ PICA

HEALTH INSURANCE CLAIM FORM

PICA ☐☐

1. MEDICARE	MEDICAID	CHAMPUS	CHAMPVA	GROUP HEALTH PLAN	FECA BLK LUNG	OTHER
☐ (Medicare #)	☐ (Medicaid #)	☐ (Sponsor's SSN)	☒ (VA File #)	☐ (SSN or ID)	☐ (SSN)	☐ (ID)

1a. INSURED'S I.D. NUMBER (FOR PROGRAM IN ITEM 1)
132-60-8001

2. PATIENT'S NAME (Last Name, First Name, Middle Initial)

3. PATIENT'S BIRTH DATE MM DD YY   SEX M ☐ F ☐

4. INSURED'S NAME (Last Name, First Name, Middle Initial)
Elbner Donald

5. PATIENT'S ADDRESS (No. Street)
6018 Orchard Lane

6. PATIENT RELATIONSHIP TO INSURED
Self ☒ Spouse ☐ Child ☐ Other ☐

7. INSURED'S ADDRESS (No. Street)
Sunset Lane

CITY   blgtn   STATE IN

8. PATIENT STATUS
Single ☐ Married ☐ Other ☐
Employed ☐ Full-Time Student ☐ Part-Time Student ☐

CITY   blgtn   STATE IN

ZIP CODE 47437-1237   TELEPHONE (Include Area Code) ( )

ZIP CODE 47437-1237   TELEPHONE (INCLUDE AREA CODE) ( )

9. OTHER INSURED'S NAME (Last Name, First Name, Middle Initial)

10. IS PATIENT'S CONDITION RELATED TO:

11. INSURED'S POLICY GROUP OR FECA NUMBER

a. OTHER INSURED'S POLICY OR GROUP NUMBER

a. EMPLOYMENT? (CURRENT OR PREVIOUS) ☐ YES ☐ NO

a. INSURED'S DATE OF BIRTH MM DD YY   SEX M ☐ F ☐

b. OTHER INSURED'S DATE OF BIRTH MM DD YY   SEX M ☐ F ☐

b. AUTO ACCIDENT?   PLACE (State) ☐ YES ☐ NO

b. EMPLOYER'S NAME OR SCHOOL NAME

c. EMPLOYER'S NAME OR SCHOOL NAME

c. OTHER ACCIDENT? ☐ YES ☐ NO

c. INSURANCE PLAN NAME OR PROGRAM NAME

d. INSURANCE PLAN NAME OR PROGRAM NAME

10d. RESERVED FOR LOCAL USE

d. IS THERE ANOTHER HEALTH BENEFIT PLAN? ☐ YES ☐ NO   If yes, return to and complete item 9 a – d.

READ BACK OF FORM BEFORE COMPLETING & SIGNING THIS FORM.
12. PATIENT'S OR AUTHORIZED PERSON'S SIGNATURE I authorize the release of any medical or other information necessary to process this claim. I also request payment of government benefits either to myself or to the party who accepts assignment below.

SIGNED   Signature on File   DATE   Today

13. INSURED'S OR AUTHORIZED PERSON'S SIGNATURE I authorize payment of medical benefits to the undersigned physician or supplier for services described below.

SIGNED   Signature on File

14. DATE OF CURRENT: MM DD YY   ILLNESS (First symptom) OR INJURY (Accident) OR PREGNANCY (LMP)

15. IF PATIENT HAS HAD SAME OR SIMILAR ILLNESS, GIVE FIRST DATE MM DD YY

16. DATES PATIENT UNABLE TO WORK IN CURRENT OCCUPATION FROM MM DD YY   TO MM DD YY

17. NAME OF REFERRING PHYSICIAN OR OTHER SOURCE

17a. I.D. NUMBER OF REFERRING PHYSICIAN
99-9999999

18. HOSPITALIZATION DATES RELATED TO CURRENT SERVICES FROM 5 11 YY   TO MM DD YY

19. RESERVED FOR LOCAL USE

20. OUTSIDE LAB? ☐ YES ☐ NO $ CHARGES

21. DIAGNOSIS OR NATURE OF ILLNESS OR INJURY. (RELATE ITEMS 1, 2, 3, OR 4 TO ITEM 24E BY LINE)
1. 200.00
2. 1800.00
3. ___.___
4. ___.___

22. MEDICAID RESUBMISSION CODE   ORIGINAL REF. NO.

23. PRIOR AUTHORIZATION NUMBER

24. A DATE(S) OF SERVICE From MM DD YY	To MM DD YY	B Place of Service	C Type of Service	D PROCEDURES, SERVICES, OR SUPPLIES (Explain Unusual Circumstances) CPT/HCPCS	MODIFIER	E DIAGNOSIS CODE	F $ CHARGES	G DAYS OR UNITS	H EPSDT Family Plan	I EMG	J COB	K RESERVED FOR LOCAL USE
3 11		11	4			8200	200 00	1				
3 18		22	1			52601	1800 00	1				

25. FEDERAL TAX I.D. NUMBER   SSN ☐ EIN ☒
99-9999999

26. PATIENT'S ACCOUNT NO.

27. ACCEPT ASSIGNMENT? (For govt. claims, see back) ☒ YES ☐ NO

28. TOTAL CHARGE $

29. AMOUNT PAID $

30. BALANCE DUE $

31. SIGNATURE OF PHYSICIAN OR SUPPLIER INCLUDING DEGREES OR CREDENTIALS (I certify that the statements on the reverse apply to this bill and are made a part thereof.)

SIGNED   DATE

32. NAME AND ADDRESS OF FACILITY WHERE SERVICES WERE RENDERED (If other than home or office)

33. PHYSICIAN'S SUPPLIER'S BILLING NAME, ADDRESS, ZIP CODE & PHONE #

PIN# LISW (GR9) Ret   GRP#

(APPROVED BY AMA COUNCIL ON MEDICAL SERVICE 8/88)

PLEASE PRINT OR TYPE

FORM HCFA-1500 (12-90)
FORM OWCP-1500   FORM RRB-1500
FORM AMA OP050192

FORM 34

Attending Dentist's Statement

Check one:

☐ Dentist's pre-treatment estimate

☑ Dentist's statement of actual services

Carrier name and address Minnesota Dental Ass.
873 2nd St
minn, mn 55014

PATIENT SECTION

1. Patient name first m.i. last	2. Relationship to employee	3. Sex m f	4. Patient birthdate MM DD YYYY	5. If full-time student school city
NANCY J. Hawkins	☐ self ☐ child ☑ spouse ☐ other	X	08 09	

6. Employee/subscriber name and mailing address	7. Employee/subscriber soc. sec. number	8. Employee/subscriber birthdate MM DD YYYY	9. Employee (company) name and address	10. Group number
Greg Hawkins 2301 Bushe Indpls, IN 46298	431-67-7980	11 10	Intemp Service 4130 N. Main Pkwy Indpls IN 4628	37/45

11. Is patient covered by another plan of benefits? Dental _____ Medical _____	12-a. Name and address of carrier(s)	12-b. Group no. (s)	13. Name and address of employer

14-a. Employee/subscriber name (if different than patient's)	14-b. Employee/subscriber soc. sec. number	14-c. Employee/subscriber birthdate MM DD YYYY	15. Relationship to patient ☐ self ☐ child ☐ spouse ☐ other _____

I have reviewed the following treatment plan. I authorize release of any information relating to this claim. I understand that I am responsible for all costs of dental treatment.

► Signature on file

Signed (Patient, or parent if minor) ___ Date ___

I hereby authorize payment directly to the below named dentist of the group insurance benefits otherwise payable to me.

► Signature on file

Signed (Insured person) ___ Date ___

DENTIST SECTION

16. Dentist name	24. Is treatment result of occupational illness or injury?	No	Yes	If yes, enter brief description and dates.
Dr Lane		X		

17. Mailing address	25. Is treatment result of auto accident?	X		
Medical & Dental Ass	26. Other accident?	X		

City, State, Zip	27. Are any services covered by another plan?			
3733 Professional Dr #300 Indpls IN 46260				

18. Dentist Soc. Sec. or T.I.N.	19. Dental licence no.	20. Dentist phone no.	28. If prosthesis, is this initial replacement?	(If no, reason for replacement)	29. Date of prior placement
99-9999999		317-123-4567			

21. First visit date current series	22. Place of treatment Office Hosp ECF Other	23. Radiographs or models enclosed?	No	Yes	How many?	30. Is treatment for orthodontics?	If services already commenced enter:	Date appliances placed	Mos. treatment remaining
01.21	X			X	1				

Identify missing teeth with "X"

FACIAL ... LINGUAL ... RIGHT UPPER PRIMARY LEFT PERMANENT LOWER ... LINGUAL ... FACIAL

32. Remarks for unusual services

31. Examination and treatment plan - List in order from tooth no. 1 through tooth no. 32 - Use charting system shown.							For administrative use only
Tooth # or letter	Surface	Description of service (including x-rays, prophylaxis, materials used, etc.) Line No.	Date service performed Mo. Day Year	Procedure number	Fee		
		1					
		2					
		3					
		4					
		5					
		6					
		7					
		8					
		9					
		10					
		11					
		12					
		13					
		14					
		15					

I hereby certify that the procedures as indicated by date have been completed and that the fees submitted are the actual fees I have charged and intend to collect for those procedures.

► _____ Date _____

Signed (Dentist)

Total Fee Charged	
Max. Allowable	
Deductible	
Carrier %	
Carrier pays	

FORM 35

Attending Dentist's Statement

Check one:

☐ **Dentist's pre-treatment estimate**

☐ **Dentist's statement of actual services**

Carrier name and address

P A T I E N T   S E C T I O N

| 1. Patient name
first   m.i.   last | 2. Relationship to employee
☐ self ☐ child
☐ spouse ☐ other | 3. Sex
m f | 4. Patient birthdate
MM DD YYYY | 5. If full-time student
school city |

| 6. Employee/subscriber name and mailing address | 7. Employee/subscriber
soc. sec. number | 8. Employee/subscriber
birthdate
MM DD YYYY | 9. Employee (company)
name and address | 10. Group number |

| 11. Is patient covered by another plan of benefits?
Dental _____
Medical _____ | 12-a. Name and address of carrier(s) | 12-b. Group no.(s) | 13. Name and address of employer |

| 14-a. Employee/subscriber name
(if different than patient's) | 14-b. Employee/subscriber
soc. sec. number | 14-c. Employee/subscriber birthdate
MM DD YYYY | 15. Relationship to patient
☐ self ☐ child
☐ spouse ☐ other |

I have reviewed the following treatment plan. I authorize release of any information relating to this claim. I understand that I am responsible for all costs of dental treatment.

► _____ Date _____

Signed (Patient, or parent if minor)

I hereby authorize payment directly to the below named dentist of the group insurance benefits otherwise payable to me.

► _____ Date _____

Signed (Insured person)

D E N T I S T   S E C T I O N

| 16. Dentist name | 24. Is treatment result of occupational illness or injury? | No | Yes | If yes, enter brief description and dates. |

| 17. Mailing address | 25. Is treatment result of auto accident?
26. Other accident? | | | |

| City, State, Zip | 27. Are any services covered by another plan? | | | |

| 18. Dentist Soc. Sec. or T.I.N. 19. Dental licence no. 20. Dentist phone no. | 28. If prosthesis, is this initial replacement? | | (If no, reason for replacement) 29. Date of prior placement |

| 21. First visit date current series 22. Place of treatment Office Hosp ECF Other 23. Radiographs or models enclosed? No Yes How many? | 30. Is treatment for orthodontics? | | If services already commenced enter: Date appliances placed Mos. treatment remaining |

Identify missing teeth with "X"

FACIAL
LINGUAL
RIGHT LINGUAL LEFT
UPPER LOWER PRIMARY PERMANENT
FACIAL

32. Remarks for unusual services

31. Examination and treatment plan - List in order from tooth no. 1 through tooth no. 32 - Use charting system shown.

Tooth # or letter	Surface	Description of service (including x-rays, prophylaxis, materials used, etc.) Line No.	Date service performed Mo. Day Year	Procedure number	Fee	For administrative use only
		1				
		2				
		3				
		4				
		5				
		6				
		7				
		8				
		9				
		10				
		11				
		12				
		13				
		14				
		15				

I hereby certify that the procedures as indicated by date have been completed and that the fees submitted are the actual fees I have charged and intend to collect for those procedures.

► _____ Date _____

Signed (Dentist)

Total Fee Charged	
Max. Allowable	
Deductible	
Carrier %	
Carrier pays	

FORM 36

Attending Dentist's Statement

Check one:

☐ Dentist's pre-treatment estimate

☑ Dentist's statement of actual services

Carrier name and address

Prudential Dental Plan
P.O. Box 210
Westbrook IL 61630

PATIENT SECTION

1. Patient name			2. Relationship to employee	3. Sex	4. Patient birthdate			5. If full-time student
first m.i. last			☑ self ☐ child	m f	MM DD YYYY			school city
Stacy J Bogan			☐ spouse ☐ other	X	12 01			

6. Employee/subscriber name and mailing address	7. Employee/subscriber soc. sec. number	8. Employee/subscriber birthdate			9. Employee (company) name and address	10. Group number
2130 Kristly Ln Indpls IN 46203	311-48-6120	MM 12	DD 01	YYYY	Bogan Studios 2900 cliff St Indpls IN 46330	

11. Is patient covered by another plan of benefits?	12-a. Name and address of carrier(s)	12-b. Group no.(s)	13. Name and address of employer
Dental _____ Medical _____			

14-a. Employee/subscriber name (if different than patient's)	14-b. Employee/subscriber soc. sec. number	14-c. Employee/subscriber birthdate MM DD YYYY	15. Relationship to patient ☐ self ☐ child ☐ spouse ☐ other ___

I have reviewed the following treatment plan. I authorize release of any information relating to this claim. I understand that I am responsible for all costs of dental treatment.

► Signature on file   Today

Signed (Patient, or parent if minor)   Date

I hereby authorize payment directly to the below named dentist of the group insurance benefits otherwise payable to me.

► Signature on file   Today

Signed (Insured person)   Date

DENTIST SECTION

16. Dentist name		24. Is treatment result of occupational illness or injury?	No	Yes	If yes, enter brief description and dates.
Patrick Zunkel DDS			X		
17. Mailing address		25. Is treatment result of auto accident?	X		
Medical & Dental Assi PC		26. Other accident?	X		
City, State, Zip		27. Are any services covered by another plan?	X		
Indpls, IN. 46260					

18. Dentist Soc. Sec. or T.I.N.	19. Dental licence no.	20. Dentist phone no.	28. If prosthesis, is this initial replacement?	(If no, reason for replacement)	29. Date of prior placement
99-9999999		317-123-4567			

21. First visit date current series	22. Place of treatment Office Hosp ECF Other	23. Radiographs or models enclosed? No Yes How many?	30. Is treatment for orthodontics?	If services already commenced enter.	Date appliances placed	Mos. treatment remaining
04·03	X	X	X			

Identify missing teeth with "X"

FACIAL / LINGUAL / PERMANENT / PRIMARY / RIGHT UPPER LOWER LEFT / LINGUAL / FACIAL

31. Examination and treatment plan - List in order from tooth no. 1 through tooth no. 32 - Use charting system shown.

Tooth # or letter	Surface	Description of service (including x-rays, prophylaxis, materials used, etc.) Line No.	Date service performed Mo. Day Year	Procedure number	Fee	For administrative use only
		1 Periodic Exam	04 03	00120	20 00	
		2 Bitewing - 2 films	04 03	00 272	12 00	
		3 Adult Prophylaxis	04 03	01110	37 00	
		4				
		5				
		6				
		7				
		8				
		9				
		10				
		11				
		12				
		13				
		14				
		15				

32. Remarks for unusual services

I hereby certify that the procedures as indicated by date have been completed and that the fees submitted are the actual fees I have charged and intend to collect for those procedures.

► Patrick Zunkel DDS   Date 04·03

Signed (Dentist)

Total Fee Charged	69	00
Max. Allowable		
Deductible		
Carrier %		
Carrier pays		

FORM 37

Attending Dentist's Statement

Check one:

☐ **Dentist's pre-treatment estimate**

☐ **Dentist's statement of actual services**

Carrier name and address

PATIENT SECTION

1. Patient name first m.i. last	2. Relationship to employee ☐ self ☐ child ☐ spouse ☐ other	3. Sex m f	4. Patient birthdate MM DD YYYY	5. If full-time student school city

6. Employee/subscriber name and mailing address	7. Employee/subscriber soc. sec. number	8. Employee/subscriber birthdate MM DD YYYY	9. Employee (company) name and address	10. Group number

11. Is patient covered by another plan of benefits? Dental _____ Medical _____	12-a. Name and address of carrier(s)	12-b. Group no.(s)	13. Name and address of employer

14-a. Employee/subscriber name (if different than patient's)	14-b. Employee/subscriber soc. sec. number	14-c. Employee/subscriber birthdate MM DD YYYY	15. Relationship to patient ☐ self ☐ child ☐ spouse ☐ other _____

I have reviewed the following treatment plan. I authorize release of any information relating to this claim. I understand that I am responsible for all costs of dental treatment.

► _____
Signed (Patient, or parent if minor)   Date

I hereby authorize payment directly to the below named dentist of the group insurance benefits otherwise payable to me.

► _____
Signed (Insured person)   Date

DENTIST SECTION

16. Dentist name	24. Is treatment result of occupational illness or injury?	No	Yes	If yes, enter brief description and dates.
17. Mailing address	25. Is treatment result of auto accident? 26. Other accident?			
City, State, Zip	27. Are any services covered by another plan?			
18. Dentist Soc. Sec. or T.I.N. 19. Dental licence no. 20. Dentist phone no.	28. If prosthesis, is this initial replacement?		(If no, reason for replacement) 29. Date of prior placement	
21. First visit date current series 22. Place of treatment Office Hosp ECF Other 23. Radiographs or models enclosed? No Yes How many?	30. Is treatment for orthodontics?		If services already commenced enter: Date appliances placed Mos. treatment remaining	

Identify missing teeth with "X"

FACIAL
LINGUAL
RIGHT UPPER LOWER   LEFT   PRIMARY   PERMANENT
LINGUAL
FACIAL

32. Remarks for unusual services

Tooth # or letter	Surface	31. Examination and treatment plan - List in order from tooth no. 1 through tooth no. 32 - Use charting system shown. Description of service (including x-rays, prophylaxis, materials used, etc.) Line No.	Date service performed Mo. Day Year	Procedure number	Fee	For administrative use only
		1				
		2				
		3				
		4				
		5				
		6				
		7				
		8				
		9				
		10				
		11				
		12				
		13				
		14				
		15				

I hereby certify that the procedures as indicated by date have been completed and that the fees submitted are the actual fees I have charged and intend to collect for those procedures.

► _____
Signed (Dentist)   Date _____

Total Fee Charged	
Max. Allowable	
Deductible	
Carrier %	
Carrier pays	

FORM 38

APPROVED OMB-0938-0008

CARRIER

□ PICA

HEALTH INSURANCE CLAIM FORM

PICA □□□

1. MEDICARE MEDICAID CHAMPUS CHAMPVA GROUP FECA OTHER	1a. INSURED'S I.D. NUMBER (FOR PROGRAM IN ITEM 1)

1. MEDICARE □ (Medicare #)   MEDICAID □ (Medicaid #)   CHAMPUS □ (Sponsor's SSN)   CHAMPVA □ (VA File #)   GROUP HEALTH PLAN □ (SSN or ID)   FECA BLK LUNG □ (SSN)   OTHER □ (ID)

1a. INSURED'S I.D. NUMBER   (FOR PROGRAM IN ITEM 1)

2. PATIENT'S NAME (Last Name, First Name, Middle Initial)

3. PATIENT'S BIRTH DATE   MM DD YY   SEX   M □ F □

4. INSURED'S NAME (Last Name, First Name, Middle Initial)

5. PATIENT'S ADDRESS (No. Street)

6. PATIENT RELATIONSHIP TO INSURED   Self □ Spouse □ Child □ Other □

7. INSURED'S ADDRESS (No. Street)

CITY   STATE

8. PATIENT STATUS   Single □   Married □   Other □
Employed □   Full-Time Student □   Part-Time Student □

CITY   STATE

ZIP CODE   TELEPHONE (Include Area Code)   (   )

ZIP CODE   TELEPHONE (INCLUDE AREA CODE)   (   )

9. OTHER INSURED'S NAME (Last Name, First Name, Middle Initial)

10. IS PATIENT'S CONDITION RELATED TO:

11. INSURED'S POLICY GROUP OR FECA NUMBER

a. OTHER INSURED'S POLICY OR GROUP NUMBER

a. EMPLOYMENT? (CURRENT OR PREVIOUS)   □ YES   □ NO

a. INSURED'S DATE OF BIRTH   MM DD YY   SEX   M □ F □

b. OTHER INSURED'S DATE OF BIRTH   MM DD YY   SEX   M □ F □

b. AUTO ACCIDENT?   PLACE (State)   □ YES   □ NO

b. EMPLOYER'S NAME OR SCHOOL NAME

c. EMPLOYER'S NAME OR SCHOOL NAME

c. OTHER ACCIDENT?   □ YES   □ NO

c. INSURANCE PLAN NAME OR PROGRAM NAME

d. INSURANCE PLAN NAME OR PROGRAM NAME

10d. RESERVED FOR LOCAL USE

d. IS THERE ANOTHER HEALTH BENEFIT PLAN?   □ YES   □ NO   If yes, return to and complete item 9 a – d.

READ BACK OF FORM BEFORE COMPLETING & SIGNING THIS FORM.
12. PATIENT'S OR AUTHORIZED PERSON'S SIGNATURE I authorize the release of any medical or other information necessary to process this claim. I also request payment of government benefits either to myself or to the party who accepts assignment below.

SIGNED _____   DATE _____

13. INSURED'S OR AUTHORIZED PERSON'S SIGNATURE I authorize payment of medical benefits to the undersigned physician or supplier for services described below.

SIGNED _____

14. DATE OF CURRENT: MM DD YY   ILLNESS (First symptom) OR INJURY (Accident) OR PREGNANCY (LMP)

15. IF PATIENT HAS HAD SAME OR SIMILAR ILLNESS, GIVE FIRST DATE   MM DD YY

16. DATES PATIENT UNABLE TO WORK IN CURRENT OCCUPATION   MM DD YY FROM   TO   MM DD YY

17. NAME OF REFERRING PHYSICIAN OR OTHER SOURCE

17a. I.D. NUMBER OF REFERRING PHYSICIAN

18. HOSPITALIZATION DATES RELATED TO CURRENT SERVICES   MM DD YY FROM   TO   MM DD YY

19. RESERVED FOR LOCAL USE

20. OUTSIDE LAB?   □ YES   □ NO $ CHARGES

21. DIAGNOSIS OR NATURE OF ILLNESS OR INJURY. (RELATE ITEMS 1, 2, 3, OR 4 TO ITEM 24E BY LINE)
1. _____   3. _____
2. _____   4. _____

22. MEDICAID RESUBMISSION CODE   ORIGINAL REF. NO.

23. PRIOR AUTHORIZATION NUMBER

24. A DATE(S) OF SERVICE		B Place of Service	C Type of Service	D PROCEDURES, SERVICES, OR SUPPLIES (Explain Unusual Circumstances)		E DIAGNOSIS CODE	F $ CHARGES	G DAYS OR UNITS	H EPSDT Family Plan	I EMG	J COB	K RESERVED FOR LOCAL USE
From MM DD YY	To MM DD YY			CPT/HCPCS	MODIFIER							
1												
2												
3												
4												
5												
6												

25. FEDERAL TAX I.D. NUMBER   SSN □ EIN □

26. PATIENT'S ACCOUNT NO.

27. ACCEPT ASSIGNMENT? (For govt. claims, see back)   □ YES   □ NO

28. TOTAL CHARGE $

29. AMOUNT PAID $

30. BALANCE DUE $

31. SIGNATURE OF PHYSICIAN OR SUPPLIER INCLUDING DEGREES OR CREDENTIALS (I certify that the statements on the reverse apply to this bill and are made a part thereof.)

SIGNED _____   DATE _____

32. NAME AND ADDRESS OF FACILITY WHERE SERVICES WERE RENDERED (If other than home or office)

33. PHYSICIAN'S SUPPLIER'S BILLING NAME, ADDRESS, ZIP CODE & PHONE #

PIN#   GRP#

(APPROVED BY AMA COUNCIL ON MEDICAL SERVICE 8/88)

PLEASE PRINT OR TYPE

FORM HCFA-1500 (12-90)
FORM OWCP-1500   FORM RRB-1500
FORM AMA OP050192

PATIENT AND INSURED INFORMATION

PHYSICIAN OR SUPPLIER INFORMATION

FORM 39

Attending Dentist's Statement

Check one:

☐ **Dentist's pre-treatment estimate**

☐ **Dentist's statement of actual services**

Carrier name and address

PATIENT SECTION

1. Patient name first m.i. last	2. Relationship to employee ☐ self ☐ child ☐ spouse ☐ other	3. Sex m	f	4. Patient birthdate MM DD YYYY	5. If full-time student school city

6. Employee/subscriber name and mailing address	7. Employee/subscriber soc. sec. number	8. Employee/subscriber birthdate MM DD YYYY	9. Employee (company) name and address	10. Group number

11. Is patient covered by another plan of benefits? Dental _____ Medical _____	12-a. Name and address of carrier(s)	12-b. Group no.(s)	13. Name and address of employer

14-a. Employee/subscriber name (if different than patient's)	14-b. Employee/subscriber soc. sec. number	14-c. Employee/subscriber birthdate MM DD YYYY	15. Relationship to patient ☐ self ☐ child ☐ spouse ☐ other

I have reviewed the following treatment plan. I authorize release of any information relating to this claim. I understand that I am responsible for all costs of dental treatment.

► _____

Signed (Patient, or parent if minor)   Date

I hereby authorize payment directly to the below named dentist of the group insurance benefits otherwise payable to me.

► _____

Signed (Insured person)   Date

DENTIST SECTION

16. Dentist name	24. Is treatment result of occupational illness or injury?	No	Yes	If yes, enter brief description and dates.
17. Mailing address	25. Is treatment result of auto accident? 26. Other accident?			
City, State, Zip	27. Are any services covered by another plan?			
18. Dentist Soc. Sec. or T.I.N. 19. Dental licence no. 20. Dentist phone no.	28. If prosthesis, is this initial replacement?		(If no, reason for replacement) 29. Date of prior placement	
21. First visit date current series 22. Place of treatment Office, Hosp, ECF, Other 23. Radiographs or models enclosed? No Yes How many?	30. Is treatment for orthodontics?		If services already commenced enter: Date appliances placed Mos. treatment remaining	

Identify missing teeth with "X"

FACIAL

(tooth chart: 1–16 / A–J top arch, LINGUAL, RIGHT UPPER LEFT, PRIMARY PERMANENT, LOWER, LINGUAL, 32–17 / T–K bottom arch, FACIAL)

32. Remarks for unusual services

31. Examination and treatment plan - List in order from tooth no. 1 through tooth no. 32 - Use charting system shown.

Tooth # or letter	Surface	Description of service (including x-rays, prophylaxis, materials used, etc.) Line No.	Date service performed Mo. Day Year	Procedure number	Fee	For administrative use only
		1				
		2				
		3				
		4				
		5				
		6				
		7				
		8				
		9				
		10				
		11				
		12				
		13				
		14				
		15				

I hereby certify that the procedures as indicated by date have been completed and that the fees submitted are the actual fees I have charged and intend to collect for those procedures.

► _____   Date _____

Signed (Dentist)

Total Fee Charged	
Max. Allowable	
Deductible	
Carrier %	
Carrier pays	

FORM 40

Attending Dentist's Statement

Carrier name and address

Check one:

☐ **Dentist's pre-treatment estimate**

☐ **Dentist's statement of actual services**

<table>
<tr><td rowspan="3">P A T I E N T</td><td colspan="2">1. Patient name
first   m.i.   last</td><td colspan="2">2. Relationship to employee
☐ self   ☐ child
☐ spouse ☐ other ____</td><td>3. Sex
m f</td><td>4. Patient birthdate
MM DD YYYY</td><td colspan="2">5. If full-time student
school   city</td></tr>
</table>

| 6. Employee/subscriber name and mailing address | 7. Employee/subscriber soc. sec. number | 8. Employee/subscriber birthdate MM DD YYYY | 9. Employee (company) name and address | 10. Group number |

| 11. Is patient covered by another plan of benefits? Dental _____ Medical _____ | 12-a. Name and address of carrier(s) | 12-b. Group no.(s) | 13. Name and address of employer |

| 14-a. Employee/subscriber name (if different than patient's) | 14-b. Employee/subscriber soc. sec. number | 14-c. Employee/subscriber birthdate MM DD YYYY | 15. Relationship to patient ☐ self ☐ child ☐ spouse ☐ other ____ |

I have reviewed the following treatment plan. I authorize release of any information relating to this claim. I understand that I am responsible for all costs of dental treatment.

▶ _____ Date _____
Signed (Patient, or parent if minor)

I hereby authorize payment directly to the below named dentist of the group insurance benefits otherwise payable to me.

▶ _____ Date _____
Signed (Insured person)

DENTIST SECTION

16. Dentist name	24. Is treatment result of occupational illness or injury?	No	Yes	If yes, enter brief description and dates.
17. Mailing address	25. Is treatment result of auto accident?			
	26. Other accident?			
City, State, Zip	27. Are any services covered by another plan?			
18. Dentist Soc. Sec. or T.I.N. 19. Dental licence no. 20. Dentist phone no.	28. If prosthesis, is this initial replacement?		(If no, reason for replacement)	29. Date of prior placement
21. First visit date current series 22. Place of treatment Office Hosp ECF Other 23. Radiographs or models enclosed? No Yes How many?	30. Is treatment for orthodontics?	If services already commenced enter.	Date appliances placed	Mos. treatment remaining

Identify missing teeth with "X"

31. Examination and treatment plan - List in order from tooth no. 1 through tooth no. 32 - Use charting system shown.

For administrative use only

Tooth # or letter	Surface	Description of service (including x-rays, prophylaxis, materials used, etc.) Line No.	Date service performed Mo. Day Year	Procedure number	Fee	
		1				
		2				
		3				
		4				
		5				
		6				
		7				
		8				
		9				
		10				
		11				
		12				
		13				
		14				
		15				

32. Remarks for unusual services

I hereby certify that the procedures as indicated by date have been completed and that the fees submitted are the actual fees I have charged and intend to collect for those procedures.

▶ _____ Date _____
Signed (Dentist)

Total Fee Charged	
Max. Allowable	
Deductible	
Carrier %	
Carrier pays	

FORM 41

INDEX

A

Accounts receivable (A/R), 89, 165
ADA dental claim forms, 95, 97
Adenocarcinoma, 50
Adjudication, 79, 165
Admitting privileges, 3, 165
Advanced life support (ALS) ambulance service, 79, 165
Adverse effect, 53, 165
Aging report, 155, 165
Aid to Families with Dependent Children (AFDC), 133, 165
AIDS testing
  patient request for, 136
  release of patient information regarding, 12
Alphanumerical codes, 79, 80, 165
American Dental Association (ADA)
  codes published by, 81. *See also* CDT-2 dental codes
  coding revisions by, 90
  function of, 89, 165
American Medical Association, 66
Appeal letter, 3, 166
Attending Dentist's Statement (ADA) dental form
  completion of, 148, 150-151
  description of, 148
  sample of, 149
Automobile insurance coverage, 144-145

B

Basic Life Support (BLS) Ambulance Service, 79, 166
Benefits, 3, 166

Benign hypertension, 62
Bilateral, 33, 166
Birthday rule, 111, 118, 119, 166
Blank forms/worksheets, 249-291
Bundle, 65, 166
Burns, scarring following, 58

C

Cancer
  coding for, 48
  description of, 46
Capitation, 155, 156, 166
Carcinoma in situ, 46. *See also* Cancer
Carcinomatosis, 51
CDT-1 dental codes, 90
CDT-2 dental codes
  Attending Dentist's Statement (ADA) dental form and, 148, 151
  dental claims for Medicare patients and, 152
  description of, 90
  manual layout for, 90-91
  selection of, 95
CHAMPUS (Civilian Health and Medical Program of the Uniformed Services)
  completing HCFA-1500 for, 141
  description of, 139-140, 166
  special cases involving, 140-141
CHAMPVA (Civilian Health and Medical Program of the Veterans Administration)
  completing HCFA-1500 for, 141
  description of, 139-140, 166
  special cases involving, 140-141
Chart, 3

Chief complaint (CC), 101, 166
Chronic hepatitis, 39
Clostridium botulinum, 58
Computerization, 157-158
Confidential Patient Information Record (CPIR)
  for dental patients, 95
  description of, 6
  emergency room care claims using information from, 27, 28
  release of information section of, 11, 12
  sample of, 8-11
Confidentiality, 12
Consultations
  description of, 3, 166
  gathering information about, 20
Contiguous malignancy, 51
Contingency, 143, 167
Coordination of benefits (COB), 111, 118, 167
Co-payment, 3, 167
Council on Dental Benefit Programs, 89, 90, 167
CPIN (clinical physician identification number), 125, 127, 128, 167
CPT codes
  description of, 66
  determining main term and, 71
  for immunizations, 84
  index use for, 71
  list of, 69
  location of correct, 66
  Medicare coding and, 80
  modifiers for, 76-77, 84

subterm indentations with, 73-74
use of, 66-68
Current Dental Terminology, Second Edition (CDT-2), 81, 89, 167. *See also* CDT-2 dental codes

D

Dental codes
  CDT-1, 90
  CDT-2, 90-91, 95, 148, 151, 152
  HCPCS, 81
Dental insurance coverage
  Medicare and, 152
  payment of claims and, 148
  predetermination of, 95
Dental Routing Slip, 95
Dental Treatment Record, 95, 96
Diagnosis
  description of, 33, 34, 167
  procedures for reaching, 34-35
Diagnostic codes. *See also specific types of codes*
  diagnosis and, 34-35
  E-Codes, 53, 54, 56-57
  hypertension, 62-63
  ICD-9-CM Codes for, 34
  ICD-9-CM Manual use for, 35, 38-42. *See also* ICD-9-CM Manual
  introduction to, 33
  late effect, 58
  for neoplasms, 46, 48, 50-51
  V-Codes, 53, 60
Digestive system, 38
Disability income insurance
  description of, 143, 144, 167
  Social Security, 144
Divorced parents, 120
Drug reactions, 56
Durable medical equipment regional carriers (DMERCS), 79, 167

E

E-codes
  description of, 53, 54, 167
  use of, 56-57
Emergency Room Patient Information Record, 24, 26
Emergency rooms, 24-27, 29
Endodontics, 4, 167
Entitlement programs, 143, 167
Eponyms, 65
ESRD (end-stage renal disease), 125, 168

Established patient, 4, 168
Explanation of benefits (EOB)
  description of, 4, 111, 113, 168
  sample forms of, 260, 264, 267
  sample letter for, 114
  to secondary carriers, 118

F

Family practice/practitioner, 4, 168
Fax machines, 12
Federal Register, 79, 81, 168
Fee-for-service
  completing insurance forms for, 102-108
  description of, 101, 168
First Report of Injury Form, 136, 137
Fiscal intermediary (FI), 79, 168

G

Gastritis, 56, 58
Gatekeeper, 4, 168
General surgeon, 4, 168
Generic name, 79, 168
Global package, 65, 168
Glossary, 165-173
Gynecology, 4, 168

H

HCFA-1500, 34
  birthday rule and, 118, 119
  for CHAMPUS/CHAMPVA, 141
  coordination of benefits on, 118
  dental claims for Medicare patients on, 152
  description of, 33, 168
  divorced parents on, 120
  fee for service or indemnity companies, 102-108
  for Medicaid patients, 134
  for patients with Medicare as secondary insurer, 129
  sample of, 102, 105, 107, 108
  spousal coverage on, 112-113
  when patient is not the insured, 109
  for Workers' Compensation claims, 136, 138
HCPCS codes
  Appendix C and, 84
  application of, 80-81
  code levels for, 80
  dental, 81
  dental claims for Medicare patients and, 152

description of, 80, 169
  immunization codes for, 84
  manual format for, 81, 82
  modifiers for, 84
  revision lists for, 84
Health Care Financing Administration Common Procedure Coding System, 80, 81, 169. *See also* HCPCS codes
Health Care Financing Administration (HCFA)
  annual codes of, 81
  description of, 33, 168
  insurance form of, 80-81
  Medicare and, 126, 129
Health care reform, 156
Health insurance. *See also* Dental insurance
  description of, 4, 168
  for preexisting conditions, 156
  primary and secondary, 5, 111. *See also* Primary insurance; Secondary insurance
Hemorrhoids, 41-42
Hernia, 38
HIV results, 12
Hospitals. *See also* Emergency rooms
  conditions for attending to patients in, 20, 24
  gathering information from records in, 20, 24
Hypertension, 62
Hypertension tables, 53, 62-63, 169

I

ICD-9-CM codes
  description of, 33-35, 169
examples of, 36
  rules for assignment of, 38-39
  using Index of Diseases, 41-42
ICD-9-CM Manual
  description of, 35
  E-codes in, 53, 54, 56-57
  how to use, 38-39
  Index of Diseases in, 41-42
  Table of Drugs and Chemicals, 56-57
  V-codes in, 53, 60
Identification cards, insurance company, 13
Immunization codes, 84
In situ, 46

Indemnity insurance
  completing insurance forms for, 102-108
  description of, 101, 169
Injury. See also Workers' Compensation Insurance Coverage
  automobile, 144-145
  reporting date of, 145
Inpatient care, 20
Insurance billing specialists
  impact of computerization on, 157-158
  impact of managed care on, 156-157
  job description for, 1, 6
Insurance companies
  documentation of treatment plans for, 20
  identification cards from, 13
  release of patient information to, 12
Insurer, 4, 169
Internal medicine, 4, 169
International Classification of Diseases, 9th Revision, Clinical Modification, 34. See also ICD-9-CM
Irritable bowel syndrome, 42

K

Kassebaum-Kennedy bill (1996), 156

L

Late effect codes, 53, 58, 169
Ledger card
  for dental patients, 95
  description of, 4, 169
  function of, 15, 20
  reporting emergency room care, 24, 27, 29
  sample of, 18, 23, 29, 116
Liability insurance, 101, 169
Litigation
  automobile, 145
  description of, 143, 169
Local Level III codes, 80, 81

M

Malignancy, contiguous, 51
Malignant hypertension, 62
Malignant neoplasms
  coding for, 48, 50-51
  description of, 46
Managed care
  description of, 4, 156, 169

impact on insurance billing specialists of, 156-157
Medicaid
  CHAMPUS/CHAMPVA and, 140
  for dental claims, 152, 153
  description of, 4, 134-135, 170
  eligibility for, 134
  Medicare coverage with, 132
  nonemergency vs. emergency visits and, 135
Medicaid Dental Claim Form 152, 153
Medicaid (MCD) identification number, 132
Medical necessity, 33, 170
Medical Records Department
  description of, 4, 170
  information on emergency room visits from, 24
Medical treatment records
  function of, 20
  sample of, 22
Medicare
  CHAMPUS/CHAMPVA and, 140
  coding for. See HCPCS codes
  for dental services, 152
  description of, 33, 126, 134, 170
  eligibility for, 126
  fee calculations used by, 130
  form to notify patient of lack of coverage under, 130, 131
  as insurance industry standard-bearer, 34
  Medicaid coverage in addition to, 132
  Medigap coverage and, 130-132
  as secondary coverage, 129
  as sole coverage, 126-128
Medicare Catastrophic Coverage Act of 1988, 34
Medicare group number, 125, 170
Medigap, 125, 130, 132, 170
Medi-Medi, 132
Melanoma, 50-51
Metastasize, 46, 48
Microfiche, 101, 170
Modifiers, 65, 170
Morphology, 34, 170
Multispecialty, 4, 170

N

National Correct Coding Primer, 80

National Level I codes, 80, 81. See also CPT codes
National Level II codes, 80, 81, 84. See also HCPCS codes
NEC (not elsewhere classifiable) code, 41
Neonate, 80, 169
Neoplasms
  coding rules for, 46, 48, 50-51
  description of, 46
  malignant, 46, 48, 50-51
New patient. See also Patient information
  Confidential Patient Information Record for, 8-11
  description of, 5, 170
  in emergency rooms, 24
  gathering information for, 6

O

Obstetrics, 5, 170
Office fee schedule, 5, 170
Office manager, 5, 170
On-call visits, emergency room, 24
Operative Report
  description of, 5, 170
  for emergency room procedures, 24
  sample of, 25
Oral surgeon, 5, 171
Orthodontics, 147, 171
Outpatient care, 20, 24

P

Parents, divorced, 120
Participating provider agreement (PAR), 130
Patient chart, 24
Patient information
  cautions regarding release of, 12
  elements of gathering, 6
  emergency room, 24-27, 29
  from hospital records, 20, 24, 25
  sample forms for, 8-11
  telephone requests for, 12
  written requests for, 12
Patient information forms
  for Rose Ann Altobelli, 176-179
  for Julie S. Justin, 180-183
  for Tom R. Willisse, 184-185
  for Terry P. Hammpton, 186-187
  for Richard O. Roberts, Jr., 188-189
  for Nicole M. Petroff, 190-191
  for Maria Blumquist, 192-193

for Robert R. Tillis, 194-195
for Ai Vang, 196-198
for James X. Moyer, Jr., 199
for Aleeshaa Mobutuu, 200-201
for Timothy Small, 202-203
for Richard Bacon, 204-206
for Barbara O'Leary, 207-208
for Willa F. Johnson, 209-211
for Mary Dawson, 212-213
for Gerald Steinbert, 214-215
for Hoyt Styvesant, 216-218
for Diana Higson, 218-219
for Everett B. White, 220-221
for Phillip P. Woods, 222-223
for Daniel O'Shea, 224-228
for Donald Ebner, 229-231
for Nancy J. Hawkins, 232-235
for Stacy J. Bogan, 236-237
for Stephanie McCullough, 238-239
for Keith Konklin, 240-242
for Aaron Marshall, 243-244
for Terrence James, 245-246
for Ben Williams, 247-248
Patient visits, 13-16
Pediatrician, 5, 171
Penicillin overdose, 56
Physicians' Current Procedural Terminology (CPT), 65, 171. *See also* CPT codes
Poisonings codes, 56-57
Post, 5, 171
Postpartum, 5, 171
Predetermination, 89, 171
Predetermination ADA dental claim form, 95, 97
Preexisting condition, 155, 156, 171
Pregnant patients, 12, 24
Primary care physician (PCP), 5, 171
Primary diagnosis, 101, 171
Primary insurance
  birthday rule and, 118
  description of, 5, 111, 171
  divorced parents and, 120
  filing claims for, 112, 113

Professional corporation (P.C.), 5, 171
Prophylaxis, 80, 171
Prosthesis, 147, 171

R

Receptionist, 5, 171
Reimbursement, 5, 171
Release of Information, 11, 12
Renal cell, 50
Residual effects coding, 58
Resource Based Relative Value Scale (RBRVS), 130
Route of administration, 80, 171
Routing slip
  CPT codes on, 66-68
  diagnosis on, 35
  function of, 13, 15
  path taken by, 15, 16
  researching information missing from, 20, 21
  samples of, 14, 17

S

Scarring, following burns, 58
Secondary diagnosis, 101, 172
Secondary insurance
  benefits description for, 118
  birthday rule and, 118, 119
  CHAMPUS/CHAMPVA as, 140
  description of, 5, 111, 113, 115, 172
  divorced parents and, 120
  filing claims for, 112, 113
  Medicare as, 129
  Medigap as, 130, 132
Sexual orientation, 12
Sexually transmitted diseases, 12
Social Security Disability Insurance (SSDI), 143, 144, 172
Sponsor, 139, 172
Spousal coverage, 112-113
Statement of Account, 29

Statement of Personal Injury – Possible Third Party Liability Statement DD Form 2527, 140
Subrogation, 139, 172
Subscriber, 5, 172
Supplemental Security Income (SSI), 133, 144, 172
Surgery, 20
Surgical package, 65, 172
Systemic, 80, 172

T

Table of Drugs and Chemicals (ICD-9-CM Manual), 56-57
Telephone, release of patient information by, 12
Third-party payer, 5, 172
Transurethral resection of prostate gland (TURP), 24
Treatment plans, 20, 22

U

Unbundle, 65, 172
Unilateral, 34, 172
UPIN (unique physician identification number), 125, 172
U.S. Public Health Service, 34

V

V-codes, 53, 60, 172
Veterans Administration, 34
Veterans Administration benefits, Medicare and, 128

W

Waiting periods, 156
Workers' Compensation Insurance Coverage
  description of, 5, 136, 138, 173
  First Report of Injury Form and, 136, 137
  Medicare and, 128
World Health Organization (WHO), 34, 173
Written requests for patient information, 12